VETERINARY SURGICAL SPECI
E. 21 MISSION AVE.
SPOKANE, WA. 99202
(509) 324-0055   Fax (509) 326-7213

Advances In
The Canine Cranial Cruciate Ligament

Advances In
The Canine Cranial Cruciate Ligament

Edited by

Peter Muir, BVSc, MVetClinStud, PhD, Diplomate ACVS, ECVS

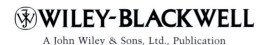

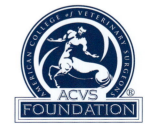

Edition first published 2010
© 2010 ACVS Foundation
This Work is a co-publication between the American College of Veterinary Surgeons Foundation and Wiley-Blackwell.

Blackwell Publishing was acquired by John Wiley & Sons in February 2007. Blackwell's publishing program has been merged with Wiley's global Scientific, Technical, and Medical business to form Wiley-Blackwell.

Editorial Office
2121 State Avenue, Ames, Iowa 50014-8300, USA

For details of our global editorial offices, for customer services, and for information about how to apply for permission to reuse the copyright material in this book, please see our Website at www.wiley.com/wiley-blackwell.

Authorization to photocopy items for internal or personal use, or the internal or personal use of specific clients, is granted by Blackwell Publishing, provided that the base fee is paid directly to the Copyright Clearance Center, 222 Rosewood Drive, Danvers, MA 01923. For those organizations that have been granted a photocopy license by CCC, a separate system of payments has been arranged. The fee code for users of the Transactional Reporting Service is ISBN-13: 978-0-8138-1852-8/2010.

Designations used by companies to distinguish their products are often claimed as trademarks. All brand names and product names used in this book are trade names, service marks, trademarks or registered trademarks of their respective owners. The publisher is not associated with any product or vendor mentioned in this book. This publication is designed to provide accurate and authoritative information in regard to the subject matter covered. It is sold on the understanding that the publisher is not engaged in rendering professional services. If professional advice or other expert assistance is required, the services of a competent professional should be sought.

Library of Congress Cataloging-in-Publication Data

Advances in the canine cranial cruciate ligament / editor, Peter Muir.
    p. ; cm. – (Advances in veterinary surgery)
    Includes bibliographical references and index.
    ISBN 978-0-8138-1852-8 (hardback : alk. paper) 1. Dogs–Surgery. 2. Cruciate ligaments–Surgery. I. Muir, Peter, BVSc.
II. American College of Veterinary Surgeons. III. Series: Advances in veterinary surgery.
    [DNLM: 1. Dog Diseases–surgery. 2. Ligaments, Articular. 3. Dogs–injuries. 4. Orthopedic Procedures–veterinary. 5. Rupture–veterinary. 6. Rupture, Spontaneous–veterinary. SF 991 A244 2010]
    SF992.M86A38 2010
    636.7'0897582059–dc22

2010013918

A catalog record for this book is available from the U.S. Library of Congress.

Set in 9.5 on 11.5 pt Palatino by Toppan Best-set Premedia Limited
Printed in Singapore by Markono Print Media Pte Ltd

1 2010

Dedication

This book is dedicated to Susannah Sample, to my family, and to all of my colleagues who have contributed effort to furthering understanding of the canine cruciate rupture arthropathy and the treatment of affected dogs.

Contents

About the Editor   xi

Contributors   xiii

Foreword   xvii
Kenneth A. Johnson

Foreword   xix
Mark D. Markel, American College of Veterinary Surgeons Foundation

Preface   xxi
Peter Muir

Acknowledgment   xxiii

1   Structure and Function   3

Introduction   3
Peter Muir

1 Morphology and Function of the Cruciate Ligaments   5
Hilde de Rooster, Tanya de Bruin, and Henri van Bree

2 Biomechanics of the Cruciate Ligaments   13
Susannah J. Sample, Ray Vanderby, Jr., and Peter Muir

3 Cruciate Ligament Remodeling and Repair   21
Connie S. Chamberlain and Ray Vanderby, Jr.

4 Meniscal Structure and Function   29
Antonio Pozzi and James L. Cook

5 Biomechanics of the Normal and Cranial Cruciate Ligament-Deficient Stifle   37
Antonio Pozzi and Stanley E. Kim

2   Etiopathogenesis of Cruciate Ligament Rupture   43

Introduction   43
Peter Muir

6 Histology of Cranial Cruciate Ligament Rupture   45
Kei Hayashi and Peter Muir

7 Genetics of Cranial Cruciate Ligament Rupture   53
Vicki Wilke

8 Cruciate Ligament Matrix Metabolism and Development of Laxity   59
Eithne Comerford

9 Stifle Morphology   65
Eithne Comerford

10 Role of Nitric Oxide Production and Matrix Protease Activity in Cruciate Ligament Degeneration   71
David E. Spreng

viii Contents

11 Role of Antibodies to Type I and II Collagen 77
Hilde de Rooster, Tanya de Bruin, and Eric Cox

12 Synovitis or Stifle Instability, Which Comes First? 81
Jason A. Bleedorn and Peter Muir

13 Role of Synovial Immune Responses in Stifle Synovitis 87
Peter Muir

3 Clinical Features 93

Introduction 93
Peter Muir

14 Epidemiology of Cranial Cruciate Ligament Rupture 95
James L. Cook

15 History and Clinical Signs of Cruciate Ligament Rupture 101
Peter Muir

16 Partial versus Complete Rupture of the Cranial Cruciate Ligament 105
Peter Muir

17 Caudal Cruciate Ligament Rupture 109
Peter Muir

18 Stress Radiography of the Stifle 113
Henri van Bree, Hilde de Rooster, and Ingrid Gielen

19 Stifle Ultrasonography 117
Cristi R. Cook

20 Computed Tomography of the Stifle 123
Ingrid Gielen, Jimmy Saunders, Bernadette Van Ryssen, and Henri van Bree

21 Magnetic Resonance Imaging of the Stifle 135
Peter V. Scrivani

4 Surgical Treatment 143

Introduction 143
Peter Muir

22 Arthroscopy versus Arthrotomy for Surgical Treatment 145
Brian S. Beale and Don A. Hulse

23 Joint Lavage 159
Peter Muir

24 Extracapsular Stabilization 163
James L. Cook

25 Tibial Plateau Leveling Osteotomy 169
Milan Milovancev and Susan L. Schaefer

26 Tibial Tuberosity Advancement 177
Randy J. Boudrieau

27 Intra-articular Stabilization 189
Paul A. Manley

28 Biomechanics of the Cranial Cruciate Ligament-Deficient Stifle Treated by Tibial Osteotomies 195
Antonio Pozzi and Stanley E. Kim

29 Arthroscopic Follow-Up after Surgical Stabilization of the Stifle 201
Brian S. Beale and Don A. Hulse

30 Cranial Cruciate Ligament Debridement 213
David E. Spreng

31 Surgical Treatment of Concurrent Meniscal Injury 217
James L. Cook and Antonio Pozzi

32 Meniscal Release 223
Antonio Pozzi and James L. Cook

33 Progression of Arthritis after Stifle Stabilization 229
John F. Innes

Contents   ix

34 Residual Lameness after Stifle
Stabilization Surgery   233
*Michael G. Conzemius and
Richard B. Evans*

5   Medical Management of Cruciate Rupture   239

Introduction   239
Peter Muir

35 Medical Therapy for Stifle Arthritis   241
Gayle H. Jaeger and Steven C. Budsberg

36 Rehabilitation for Dogs with Cranial
Cruciate Ligament Rupture   249
Courtney J. Arnoldy

6   Future Directions   255

Introduction   255
Peter Muir

37 Client-Specific Outcome Measures   257
John F. Innes

38 Total Knee Replacement
in the Dog   263
*Matthew J. Allen, William D. Liska,
and Katy L. Townsend*

39 Regenerative Medicine and Cranial
Cruciate Ligament Repair   271
Martha M. Murray and Patrick Vavken

40 Disease-Modifying Medical Therapy   277
Sara A. Colopy

Index   283

About the Editor

Peter Muir, BVSc, MVetClinStud, PhD, Diplomate ACVS, ECVS, obtained his veterinary degree in 1985 from Bristol University in the United Kingdom. After working in private practice in the UK, he returned to Bristol and obtained a PhD in veterinary science in 1990. He then moved to The University of Sydney to undertake training in small animal surgery, obtaining a Master's degree in 1992. He completed his surgery training at the University of Wisconsin-Madison and became a Diplomate of the American College of Veterinary Surgeons in 1995. After periods on faculty at the University of California, Davis, and the Royal Veterinary College, University of London, he returned to Madison as a faculty member, where he is a Professor of Small Animal Orthopaedic Surgery. He has authored many peer-reviewed publications on stifle arthritis and cranial cruciate ligament rupture and speaks regularly at international meetings on his work.

Contributors

Matthew J. Allen, Vet MB, PhD
Associate Professor
The Ohio State University
College of Veterinary Medicine
Department of Veterinary Clinical Sciences
601 Vernon L. Tharp Street
Columbus, OH 43210

Courtney J. Arnoldy, PT, DPT, CCRP
Physical Therapist
Certified Canine Rehabilitation Practitioner
University of Wisconsin-Madison
School of Veterinary Medicine
Department of Surgical Sciences
2015 Linden Drive
Madison, WI 53706

Brian S. Beale, DVM, Diplomate ACVS
Gulf Coast Veterinary Specialists
1111 West Loop South #160
Houston, TX 77027

Steven C. Budsberg, DVM, MS, Diplomate
ACVS
Professor
University of Georgia
College of Veterinary Medicine
Department of Small Animal Medicine and
Surgery
Athens, GA 30602

Jason A. Bleedorn, DVM
Clinical Instructor
University of Wisconsin-Madison
School of Veterinary Medicine
Department of Surgical Sciences
2015 Linden Drive
Madison, WI 53706

Randy J. Boudrieau, DVM, Diplomate ACVS,
ECVS
Professor
Tufts University
Cummings School of Veterinary Medicine
Department of Clinical Sciences
200 Westoboro Road
North Grafton, MA 01536

Connie S. Chamberlain, PhD
Research Associate
University of Wisconsin-Madison
School of Medicine and Public Health
Department of Orthopedics and Rehabilitation
1111 Highland Avenue
Madison, WI 53705

Sara A. Colopy, DVM, Diplomate ACVS
Clinical Instructor
University of Wisconsin-Madison
School of Veterinary Medicine
Department of Surgical Sciences
2015 Linden Drive
Madison, WI 53706

Eithne Comerford, MVB, PhD, CertVR, CertSAS,
PGCertHE, Diplomate ECVS, MRCVS
Senior Lecturer
University of Liverpool
School of Veterinary Science
Leahurst Campus
Chester High Road
Neston, CH64 7TE
United Kingdom

Michael G. Conzemius, DVM, PhD, Diplomate
ACVS
Endowed Professor
University of Minnesota
College of Veterinary Medicine
Department of Veterinary Clinical Sciences
1352 Boyd Avenue
St Paul, MN 55108

Cristi R. Cook, DVM, MS, Diplomate ACVR
Clinical Assistant Professor
University of Missouri
College of Veterinary Medicine
Department of Veterinary Medicine and Surgery
900 East Campus Drive
Columbia, MO 65211

James L. Cook, DVM, PhD, Diplomate ACVS
William & Kathryn Allen Distinguished
Professor of Orthopaedic Surgery
University of Missouri
College of Veterinary Medicine
Comparative Orthopaedic Laboratory
900 East Campus Drive
Columbia, MO 65211

Eric Cox, DVM, PhD, Diplomate ECPHM
Professor
Ghent University
Faculty of Veterinary Medicine
Department of Virology, Parasitology,
Immunology
Laboratory of Immunology
Salisburylaan 133
B-9820 Merelbeke
Belgium

Tanya de Bruin, DVM, PhD
De Graafschap dierenartsen
Schimmeldijk 1
Nl-7251 MX Vorden
The Netherlands

Hilde de Rooster, DVM, MVM, PhD, Diplomate
ECVS
Professor of Soft Tissue Surgery
Ghent University
Faculty of Veterinary Medicine
Department of Medicine and Clinical Biology of
Small Animals
Salisburylaan 133
B-9820 Merelbeke
Belgium

Richard B. Evans, PhD
Associate Professor
University of Illinois, Urbana-Champaign
1008 W Hazelwood
Urbana, IL 61802

Ingrid Gielen, DVM, PhD, MSC
Clinical Professor CT/MRI
Ghent University
Faculty of Veterinary Medicine
Department of Medical Imaging & Small Animal
Orthopaedics
Salisburylaan 133
9230 Merelbeke
Belgium

Kei Hayashi, DVM, PhD, Diplomate ACVS
Assistant Professor
University of California, Davis
Department of Surgical & Radiological Sciences
School of Veterinary Medicine
One Shields Avenue
Davis, CA 95616

Don A. Hulse, DVM, Diplomate ACVS
Professor
Texas A&M University
College of Veterinary Medicine
Department of Small Animal Clinical Sciences
College Station, TX 77843

John F. Innes, BVSc, PhD, CertVR, DSAS(orth),
MRCVS
Professor
University of Liverpool
School of Veterinary Science
Leahurst Campus
Chester High Road
Neston, CH64 7TE
United Kingdom

Gayle H. Jaeger, DVM, MSpVM, Diplomate
ACVS
VCA Newark Veterinary Specialty Group
1360 Marrows Rd
Newark, DE 19711

Kenneth A. Johnson, MVSc, PhD, FACVSc,
Diplomate ACVS, ECVS
Professor
The University of Sydney
Faculty of Veterinary Science
Sydney, NSW 2006
Australia

Stanley E. Kim, BVSc
Clinical Lecturer
University of Florida
College of Veterinary Medicine
Department of Small Animal Clinical Sciences
2015 SW 16th Ave
Gainesville, FL 32610

William D. Liska, DVM, Diplomate ACVS
Gulf Coast Veterinary Specialists
1111 West Loop South #160
Houston, TX 77027

Paul A. Manley, DVM, MSc, Diplomate ACVS
Professor
University of Wisconsin-Madison
School of Veterinary Medicine
Department of Surgical Sciences
2015 Linden Drive
Madison, WI 53706

Mark D. Markel DVM, PhD, Diplomate ACVS
Professor
University of Wisconsin-Madison
School of Veterinary Medicine
Department of Medical Sciences
2015 Linden Drive
Madison, Wisconsin 53706

Milan Milovancev, DVM, Diplomate ACVS
Wisconsin Veterinary Referral Center
360 Bluemound Road
Waukesha, WI 53188

Peter Muir, BVSc, MVetClinStud, PhD,
Diplomate ACVS, ECVS, MRCVS
Professor
University of Wisconsin-Madison
School of Veterinary Medicine
Department of Surgical Sciences
2015 Linden Drive
Madison, Wisconsin 53706

Martha Meaney Murray, MD
Assistant Professor
Harvard Medical School
Children's Hospital, Boston
Department of Orthopaedic Surgery
300 Longwood Ave
Boston, MA 02115

Antonio Pozzi, DMV, MS, Diplomate ACVS
Assistant Professor
University of Florida
College of Veterinary Medicine
Department of Small Animal Clinical Sciences
2015 SW 16th Ave
Gainesville, FL 32610

Susannah J. Sample, BS, MS, DVM
Research Assistant
University of Wisconsin-Madison
Comparative Orthopaedic Research Laboratory
School of Veterinary Medicine
2015 Linden Drive
Madison, WI 53706

Jimmy Saunders, DVM, PhD, Diplomate ECVDI
Professor of Diagnostic Imaging
Ghent University
Faculty of Veterinary Medicine
Department of Veterinary Medical Imaging and
Small Animal Orthopaedics
Salisburylaan 133
9230 Merelbeke
Belgium

Susan L. Schaefer, DVM, MS, Diplomate ACVS
Clinical Associate Professor
University of Wisconsin-Madison
School of Veterinary Medicine
Department of Surgical Sciences
2015 Linden Drive
Madison, WI 53706

Peter V. Scrivani, DVM, Diplomate ACVR
Assistant Professor
Cornell University
College of Veterinary Medicine
Department of Clinical Sciences
Ithaca, NY 14853

David E. Spreng, Dr.med.vet., Diplomate ECVS,
ACVECC
Associate Professor
University of Bern
Vetsuisse Faculty
Department of Clinical Veterinary Medicine
Laengassstr. 128
CH-3012 Bern
Switzerland

Katy L. Townsend, BVSc
Resident in Small Animal Surgery
The Ohio State University
College of Veterinary Medicine
Department of Veterinary Clinical Sciences
601 Vernon L. Tharp Street
Columbus, OH 43210

Henri van Bree, DVM, PhD, Diplomate ECVDI,
ECVS
Professor and Chair
Ghent University
Faculty of Veterinary Medicine
Department of Veterinary Medical Imaging and
Small Animal Orthopaedics
Salisburylaan 133
9230 Merelbeke
Belgium

Bernadette Van Ryssen, DVM, PhD
Professor of Small Animal Orthopaedic Surgery
Ghent University
Faculty of Veterinary Medicine
Department of Veterinary Medical Imaging and
Small Animal Orthopaedics
Salisburylaan 133
9230 Merelbeke
Belgium

Ray Vanderby, Jr., PhD
Professor
University of Wisconsin-Madison
School of Medicine & Public Health
Department of Orthopedics & Rehabilitation
1111 Highland Ave
Madison, WI 53705

Patrick Vavken, MD, MSc
Instructor
Harvard Medical School
Children's Hospital, Boston
Department of Orthopaedic Surgery
300 Longwood Ave
Boston, MA 02115

Vicki Wilke, DVM, PhD, Diplomate ACVS
Assistant Clinical Specialist
University of Minnesota
College of Veterinary Medicine
Department of Veterinary Clinical Sciences
St Paul, MN 55108

Contact information, including email addresses,
for contributors who are ACVS and ECVS
Diplomates is available from www.acvs.org and
www.ecvs.org, respectively.

Foreword

The creation of a comprehensive multi-author textbook that is exclusively devoted to just a single musculoskeletal structure—the canine cranial cruciate ligament—is unprecedented in the field of veterinary orthopaedics. However, this high degree of specificity in subject material is truly justified given the magnitude of the problem of cruciate ligament disease as a cause of severe, debilitating lameness in dogs. Looking back though the innumerable volumes of publications in the veterinary orthopaedic literature on the canine cruciate ligament, one publication remains a landmark. In 1952, Finnish veterinarian Saki Paatsama presented his doctoral thesis, entitled "Ligament Injuries in the Canine Stifle Joint: A Clinical and Experimental Study." Not only did Paatsama describe the characteristic cranial drawer sign, articular cartilage degeneration, and meniscal injury associated with cranial cruciate ligament rupture, he also reported one of the first of many surgical techniques intended to correct this problem.

During the ensuing six decades, this problem of canine cranial cruciate ligament disease continues to perplex; we still have no idea how to prevent it and very little understanding of the etiology in non-traumatic ligament rupture. Since the days of Patsaama, most of our effort has gone into developing better surgical techniques to stabilize the cranial cruciate ligament deficient stifle joint. Fortunately, however, we now appreciate that cruciate ligament rupture is rarely traumatic in dogs. This has led to more vigorous study of the exceedingly complex pathophysiology of this ligament disease, and the associated cascade of joint disease. Thus, it is most pleasing to see that a considerable section of this textbook has been devoted to a review of current knowledge of this aspect of the problem.

I commend Peter Muir on having assembled this fine anthology of contributions from authors worldwide. However, I do suspect that in another few years a second edition will be required, as I expect that we will see a rapid advance in our understanding of canine cruciate ligament disease.

Kenneth A. Johnson
Sydney, Australia

Foreword

The American College of Veterinary Surgeons (ACVS) Foundation is excited to present *The Canine Cranial Cruciate Ligament* as the inaugural book in a new book series entitled *Advances in Veterinary Surgery*. The ACVS Foundation is an independently chartered philanthropic organization devoted to advancing the charitable, educational, and scientific goals of the American College of Veterinary Surgeons. Founded in 1965, the ACVS sets the standards for the specialty of veterinary surgery. The ACVS, which is approved by the American Veterinary Medical Association, administers the board certification process for Diplomates in veterinary surgery and advances veterinary surgery and education. One of the principal goals of the ACVS Foundation is to foster the advancement of the art and science of veterinary surgery. The Foundation achieves these goals by: supporting investigations in the diagnosis and treatment of surgical diseases; increasing educational opportunities for surgeons, surgical residents, and veterinary practitioners; improving surgical training of residents and veterinary students; and bettering animal patients' care, treatment, and welfare. This collaboration with Wiley-Blackwell will benefit all who are interested in veterinary surgery by presenting the latest evidence-based information on a particular surgical topic.

This inaugural book is an outstanding example of the promise of this new series. *The Canine Cranial Cruciate Ligament* is edited by Dr. Peter Muir, a Diplomate of the American College of Veterinary Surgeons and a prominent scientist in orthopaedic research. He has assembled the leaders in the field of cranial cruciate ligament rupture and its treatment, presenting a cross-disciplinary and evidence-based approach to the literature in this important field. As you read through this book, you will find the latest information on the structure and function of the canine cranial cruciate ligament, the etiopathogenesis of cruciate rupture, the clinical features of dogs affected with this important condition, current surgical and medical treatments for affected dogs, and new directions that are beginning to appear in this important field of veterinary surgery. The ACVS Foundation is proud to partner with Wiley-Blackwell on this important new series and is proud to present this inaugural book in the series.

Mark D. Markel
Chair, Board of Trustees
ACVS Foundation

Preface

Although rupture of the cranial cruciate ligament has been recognized clinically in dogs for more than 50 years, research into this condition has largely focused on development of methods for surgical treatment of the unstable stifle, and not the disease mechanism. Rupture of the cranial cruciate ligament is one of the most common reasons dogs are presented to veterinarians for treatment of lameness. It has been a long-held clinical belief that the mechanism for cranial cruciate ligament rupture in dogs is similar to anterior cruciate ligament rupture in human beings. Historically, the dog has been a common animal model for research into the surgical treatment of anterior cruciate ligament rupture. Transection of the cranial cruciate ligament in experimental dogs has also been a common animal model for biomedical research studies of arthritis.

In the last 10 years, a growing body of work investigating the disease mechanism for cranial cruciate ligament rupture has been published. Although the etiopathogenesis is still not fully understood, collectively, this research has begun to challenge established views about what causes rupture of the cranial cruciate ligament and how canine patients with stifle arthritis should be managed. My goal for this writing project was to produce a book that summarizes state-of-the-art knowledge about the cruciate rupture arthropathy, provides a useful reference for a broad audience, and lays a foundation for development of future studies in this field.

Peter Muir

Acknowledgment

I would like to acknowledge the consistent support of Antonia Seymour and Erica Judisch of Wiley-Blackwell, and Dr. Mark Markel, Chair of the ACVS Foundation's Board of Trustees, for the *Advances in Veterinary Surgery* book series, as well as for this specific writing project. I am also extremely grateful to all of the organizations and foundations that have provided financial support for clinical research into the canine cruciate rupture arthopathy. Without these gifts, my work and the work of many others that is summarized in this book would not have been possible. Lastly, I would like to thank dog owners, dog breeders, and the American Kennel Club Canine Health Foundation for their interest in, and enthusiasm for, new knowledge regarding this important canine condition.

Peter Muir

Advances In
The Canine Cranial Cruciate Ligament

Section I

Structure and Function

Introduction

The anatomy of canine stifle is complex. Our understanding of the anatomy of the cranial and caudal cruciate ligaments has gradually evolved over time, particularly with regard to the microvascular anatomy of the ligaments. Recent work suggesting the existence of a blood-cruciate ligament barrier, analogous to the blood-brain barrier, is a particularly interesting finding, which may help in understanding the mechanisms that lead to gradual and progressive weakening and eventual rupture of the cranial cruciate ligament over time. In addition to their biomechanical role as joint stabilizers, the cranial and caudal cruciate ligaments likely have key functions in joint proprioception. In the future, it will be important to understand the physiological importance of such feedback loops, as current surgical treatments for the unstable stifle do not attempt to repair the ruptured cranial cruciate ligament.

This section provides a detailed discussion of stifle anatomy, including gross and microscopic anatomy of the cruciate ligaments.

1 Morphology and Function of the Cruciate Ligaments

Hilde de Rooster, Tanya de Bruin, and Henri van Bree

Introduction

In contrast to the plethora of veterinary publications on cruciate surgery in dogs, only a few papers deal with the microanatomy and the neurovascularity of the canine cruciate ligaments. However, understanding of the complex anatomy and function is imperative to elucidate the pathophysiology of cruciate disease and improve surgical intervention.

Morphology

Macroanatomy

The cranial cruciate ligament (CrCL) originates on the axial aspect of the lateral femoral condyle, very close to the articular margin (Figure 1.1). It extends diagonally across the joint space and attaches to the cranial intercondyloid area of the tibial plateau (Singleton 1957; Zahm 1965; Arnoczky & Marshall 1977). The tibial attachment site is bordered cranially by the cranial meniscotibial ligament of the medial meniscus and caudally by the cranial

Advances in the Canine Cranial Cruciate Ligament,
Edited by Peter Muir, © 2010 ACVS Foundation, This Work is a co-publication between the American College of Veterinary Surgeons Foundation and Wiley-Blackwell.

meniscotibial ligament of the lateral meniscus (Rudy 1974; Heffron & Campbell 1978; Figure 1.2). The CrCL is narrowest in its mid-region and fans out proximally and distally (Heffron & Campbell 1978). The length of the CrCL is positively correlated with body weight; taking the average length of the CrCL cranial and caudal borders, researchers have reported a mean length of 13.5–18.77 mm (Vasseur et al. 1985; Wingfield et al. 2000). The CrCL runs cranially, medially, and distally in an outward spiral as it passes from the femur to the tibia (Zahm 1965; Haut & Little 1969). Two demonstrably separate bundles are apparent (Figure 1.1; Arnoczky & Marshall 1977; Heffron & Campbell 1978). These components are termed craniomedial and caudolateral, based on their relative attachment sites onto the tibial plateau. The craniomedial subdivision is the most spiral and the longest, yet smaller component, and arises more proximally from the femur and inserts more cranially on the tibial attachment area, compared with the caudolateral subdivision. The fibers of the caudolateral component originate from the most lateral and distal part of the attachment area of the lateral femoral condyle, have a straighter path, and insert on the most caudal region of the tibial attachment area (Arnoczky & Marshall 1977; Heffron & Campbell 1978).

The caudal cruciate ligament (CaCL) is slightly longer and broader than the CrCL (Rudy 1974;

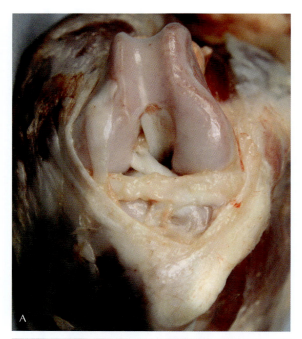

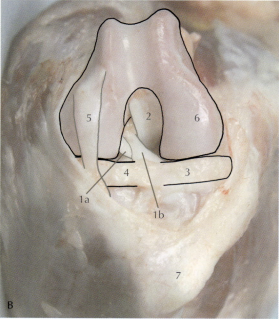

Figure 1.1 (A) Photograph and (B) line drawing of a flexed right stifle joint of a dog. Cranial view after removal of the infrapatellar fat pad. 1a: caudolateral bundle of the cranial cruciate ligament; 1b: craniomedial bundle of the cranial cruciate ligament; 2: caudal cruciate ligament; 3: medial meniscus; 4: lateral meniscus; 5: tendon of the long digital extensor; 6: medial humeral condyle; 7: tibial tuberosity.

Arnoczky & Marshall 1977; Harari 1993). Even its collagen fibrils are thicker than its cranial counterpart (Brunnberg 1989). The total midsection diameter is smallest as it fans out from the center, making the femoral and, to a lesser extent, the tibial attachments larger (Rudy 1974). In the dog, the CaCL also has two components, although they are less distinct and often inseparable (Heffron & Campbell 1978; Harari 1993).

Microanatomy

The cruciate ligaments are multifascicular structures, the base unit of which is collagen, and contain many wavy fascicular subunits (Figure 1.3A). Fascicles may be composed of 1–10 subfascicles, containing bundles of collagen fibers (Heffron & Campbell 1978; Yahia & Drouin 1989). At the osseous attachment sites of the CrCL, the collagen fibers are not arranged entirely parallel to the longitudinal axis of the ligament, and, especially in younger specimens, columns of chondroid cells do penetrate into the ligament (Figure 1.3B; Zahm 1965; Alm & Strömberg 1974). Where both cruciates are in contact, the collagen fibers are more densely packed and oriented tangential to the surface instead of parallel to the long axis (Vasseur et al. 1985). Fibers are formed by fibrils that are composed by organization of repeated collagen subunits (Alm & Strömberg 1974; Heffron & Campbell 1978; Vasseur et al. 1985). Their architecture is a combination of helical or planar, parallel, or twisted networks. The centrally located fibrils are nearly straight, whereas those at the periphery are arranged in a helical wave pattern (Zahm 1965; Alm & Strömberg 1974; Yahia & Drouin 1989).

Synovial envelope

Both the CrCL and the CaCL are covered by a fairly uniform fold of synovial membrane, which incompletely divides the stifle joint in the sagittal plane (Arnoczky et al. 1979). These enveloping epiligamentous membranes consist mainly of dense connective tissue, small fibroblasts, and some adipocytes; an intima and a thin subintimal layer can be distinguished (Heffron & Campbell

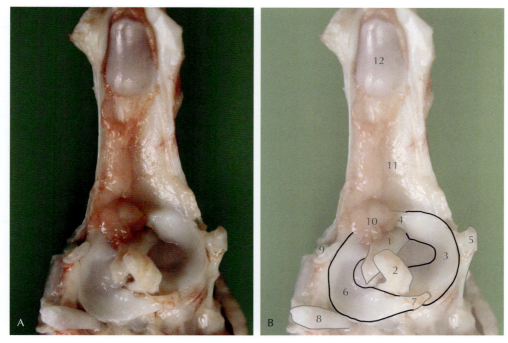

Figure 1.2 (A) Photograph and (B) line drawing of the left pelvic limb of a dog. Dorsal view on the tibial plateau after removal of the femur. 1: cranial cruciate ligament; 2: caudal cruciate ligament; 3: medial meniscus; 4: intermeniscal ligament; 5: medial collateral ligament; 6: lateral meniscus; 7: meniscofemoral ligament; 8: popliteal tendon; 9: tendon of the long digital extensor; 10: infrapatellar fat pad; 11: patellar tendon; 12: patella.

1978). The intima is a single layer of synoviocytes, and the subintimal layer is areolar tissue containing small vascular structures (Vasseur et al. 1985). Compared with the cruciate ligaments, the enveloping synovial membrane is relatively cellular (Heffron & Campbell 1978). Synovial lining does not occur on the surfaces of the cruciate ligaments that are in direct contact with each other (Vasseur et al. 1985). Under scanning electron microscopy, many small holes have been detected in the synovial membrane covering the cruciate ligaments, suggesting that the cruciate ligaments are also supplied with nutrients via the synovial fluid (Kobayashi et al. 2006).

Vascular supply

The major vascular contribution to the center of the stifle joint occurs from branches of the middle genicular artery, which arises from the popliteal artery, penetrates the caudal joint capsule, and passes craniodistally to the fossa intercondylaris, running cranially between the cruciate ligaments (Figures 1.4 and 1.5; Tirgari 1978). The vascular structures to the proximal part of the CrCL are more numerous and have larger diameters than those on the tibial side (Zahm 1965; Alm & Strömberg 1974).

The blood supply to both cruciate ligaments is predominantly of soft tissue origin; the contribution from the osseous attachments is negligible (Arnoczky et al. 1979; Kobayashi et al. 2006). The infrapatellar fat pad and the well-vascularized synovial membranes that form an envelope around the cruciate ligaments are the most important sources of vessels (Alm & Strömberg 1974; Tirgari 1978; Arnoczky et al. 1979; Kobayashi et al. 2006). The synovial vessels arborize into a finely meshed network of epiligamentous vessels, which ensheath the cruciate ligaments throughout their entire length (Figures 1.6 and 1.7; Arnoczky et al. 1979, Kobayashi et al. 2006). In general, the vascular arrangement and structural characteristics of

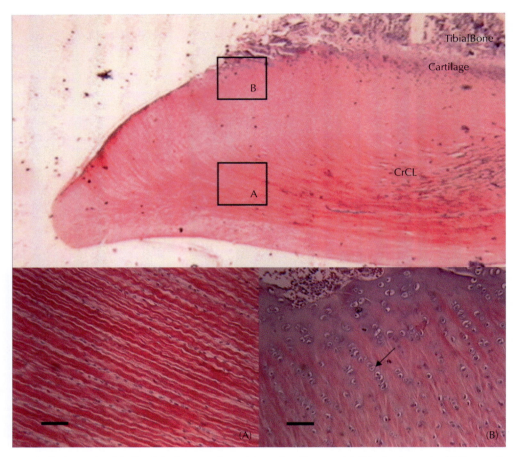

Figure 1.3 Histologic section (H&E stain) of a normal cranial cruciate ligament (CrCL) of a 4-month-old Riezenschnauzer. (A) Along the CrCL, dense collagen is aligned parallel to the long axis of the ligament. The collagen fibers have a regular accordion-like pattern. (B) At the attachment site of the CrCL, the collagen is not arranged entirely parallel to the long axis of the ligament. Columns of chondroid cells (arrow) do penetrate into the CrCL (bar = 100 μm). Reproduced from de Rooster et al. (2006), with permission from Wiley-Blackwell.

the vasculature inside the caudal and the CrCL are similar (Alm & Strömberg 1974; Arnoczky et al. 1979; Kobayashi et al. 2006). In the inner part of the cruciate ligaments, around and along the bundles of collagen fibers, an endoligamentous vascular network courses in the supporting connective tissue (Alm & Strömberg 1974; Arnoczky et al. 1979). The larger vessels, usually one artery accompanied by two veins, mainly course in a longitudinal direction both proximally and distally and lie parallel to the collagen fascicles (Alm & Strömberg 1974). Some of them have a tortuous path in the interfascicular areolar tissue. Only small capillaries branching from the longitudinal endoligamentous vessels running in a transverse direction encircle the collagen bundles. The core of the mid-portion of the CrCL is less well vascularized than the remainder of the ligament (Zahm 1965; Tirgari 1978; Arnoczky et al. 1979; Vasseur et al. 1985).

Anastomoses exist between extra- and intraligamentous blood networks (Alm & Strömberg 1974; Arnoczky et al. 1979; Kobayashi et al. 2006). Epiligamentous vessels penetrate transversely into the cruciate ligaments (Figure 1.7). Their branches ramify and anastomose with the endoligamentous vessels. There are numerous endosteal vessels at the ligamentous–osseous junctions; however,

Morphology and Function of the Cruciate Ligaments 9

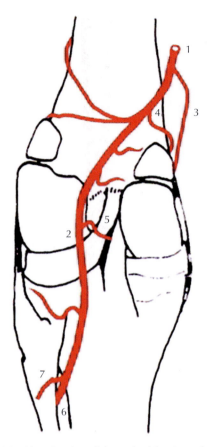

Figure 1.4 Line drawing of the major blood supply to the canine stifle joint. Caudal view. 1: femoral artery, 2: popliteal artery; 3: descending genicular artery, 4: proximal medial genicular artery, 5: middle genicular artery; 6: cranial tibial artery; 7: caudal tibial artery. Reproduced from de Rooster et al. (2006), with permission from Wiley-Blackwell.

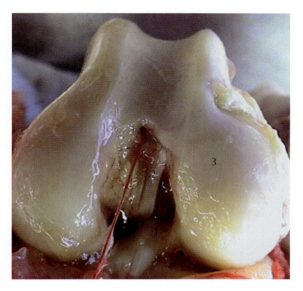

Figure 1.5 Photograph of the superficial vascularization of normal cruciate ligaments after injection of latex in a cadaver specimen of an adult dog. The infrapatellar fat pad and the synovial envelope are the most important sources of vessels. 1: cranial cruciate ligament; 2: caudal cruciate ligament; 3: lateral femoral condyle; 4: tibial plateau. Reproduced from de Rooster et al. (2006), with permission from Wiley-Blackwell.

communications with intrinsic endoligamentous vessels are quite poor, especially at the tibial attachment, where most of the endosteal vessels seem to terminate in subchondral loops instead of crossing the ligamentous–osseous junction (Alm & Strömberg 1974; Arnoczky et al. 1979; Kobayashi et al. 2006).

Innervation

Three major articular nerves arise from the saphenous nerve, tibial nerve, and common peroneal nerve to innervate the periarticular tissues of the canine stifle joint (Figure 1.8; O'Connor & Woodbury 1982). The main trunk of nerve bundles is found at the femoral end of the cruciate ligaments. Other nerves may contribute afferent fibers to a variable extent to the cruciate ligaments.

In dogs, the medial articular nerve, which branches from the saphenous nerve in the mid-thigh region, is the largest supply to the stifle joint (O'Connor & Woodbury 1982). Some of its branches course through the infrapatellar fat pad to terminate within the proximal or distal attachments of the cruciate ligaments or within the meniscal horns. Other branches of the medial articular nerve pass cranially through the joint capsule to extensively innervate the femoral attachment of the CaCL. The caudal articular nerve is variably present in dogs (O'Connor & Woodbury 1982). Its branches arise either directly from the tibial nerve or from a muscular branch of the tibial nerve. The caudal articular nerve runs to the caudal aspect of the joint capsule, where it

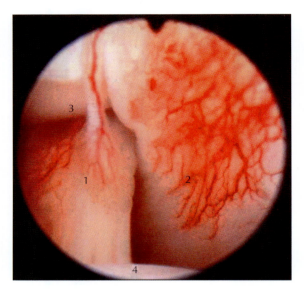

Figure 1.6 Arthroscopic view of the superficial vascularization of normal cruciate ligaments of an adult dog. The synovial vessels arborize to form a web-like network of periligamentous vessels that ensheath the cruciate ligaments. 1: cranial cruciate ligament; 2: caudal cruciate ligament; 3: lateral femoral condyle; 4: tibial plateau. Reproduced from de Rooster et al. (2006), with permission from Wiley-Blackwell.

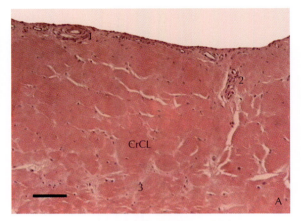

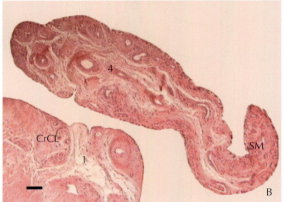

Figure 1.7 Histologic section (H&E stain) of a normal cranial cruciate ligament (CrCL) of an adult dog. (A) The CrCL is ensheathed by epiligamentous vessels (bar = 100 μm). (B) The well-vascularized synovial membrane (SM) forms an envelope over the CrCL (bar = 100 μm). 1: epiligamentous vessels; 2: anastomosis between epiligamentous and endoligamentous vessels; 3: hypovascular zone; 4: synovial vessels. Reproduced from de Rooster et al. (2006), with permission from Wiley-Blackwell.

may communicate with branches of the medial articular nerve. The lateral articular nerve branches from the common peroneal nerve at the level of the fibular head, deep to the biceps femoris muscle, and supplies the lateral aspect of the stifle joint (O'Connor & Woodbury 1982).

Nerves of differing sizes are located in the richly vascularized synovial tissue covering the cruciate ligaments (Yahia et al. 1992). From this peripheral synovium, axons radiate toward the center of the ligaments (Yahia et al. 1992). Within the cruciate ligaments, most nerves course along the epiligamentous and endoligamentous blood vessels in the interfascicular areolar spaces.

Neurohistologic studies identified various types of sensory nerve endings (receptors and free nerve endings) in the middle of the cruciate ligaments, well beneath the synovial sheath (Yahia et al. 1992). The highest number of mechanoreceptors was found in the proximal third of the CrCL, and the lowest, in the distal third (Arcand et al. 2000).

Functional anatomy

The cruciate ligaments resist forces that would cause the tibia to translate cranially relative to the femur and, to a lesser degree, resist forces that would cause tibial rotation (Arnoczky & Marshall 1977). The two components of the CrCL are not isometric, the main difference being the elongation of the craniomedial and the shortening of the

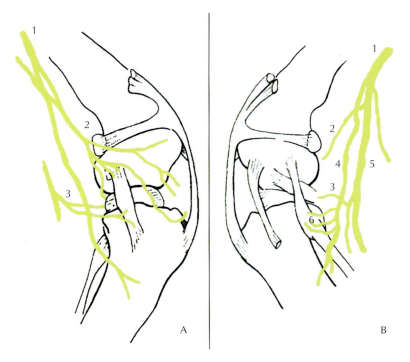

Figure 1.8 Line drawing of the major nerve supply to the canine stifle joint. (A) Medial view. (B) Lateral view. 1: saphenous nerve; 2: medial articular nerve; 3: posterior articular nerve; 4: common peroneal nerve; 5: tibial nerve; 6: lateral articular nerve. Reproduced from de Rooster et al. (2006), with permission from Wiley-Blackwell.

caudolateral component during flexion (Arnoczky & Marshall 1977; Heffron & Campbell 1978). The former is the major contributor to craniocaudal stability in stifle flexion. The latter only contributes when the craniomedial band is damaged or severely stretched (Wingfield et al. 2000). With the stifle in extension, both components are taut and limit cranial translation of the tibia relative to the femur (Arnoczky & Marshall 1977; Heffron & Campbell 1978).

As the stifle flexes, the cruciate ligaments are not only wrapped upon each other but also spiral on themselves (Singleton 1957; Arnoczky & Marshall 1977). The higher strain in the ligaments also limits the amount of normal internal rotation of the tibia on the femur (Zahm 1965; Arnoczky & Marshall 1977; Harari 1993). In extension, the medial and lateral collateral ligaments become the primary restraints of rotation, and the cruciate ligaments provide only a secondary check from the tension in both ligaments (Singleton 1957; Zahm 1965; Vasseur et al. 1985).

Together both cruciate ligaments are important secondary restraints against varus and valgus angulation. The cruciate ligaments become primary restraints if there is loss of collateral ligament support (Vasseur & Arnoczky 1981).

Overextension is prevented by tension in the cruciate ligaments, where the CrCL acts as the primary restraint (Arnoczky & Marshall 1977; Heffron & Campbell 1978). The caudolateral component of the CrCL is the primary contributor to restraining hyperextension (Heffron & Campbell 1978). The slightly longer caudal component of the CaCL can only be considered a secondary restraint (Singleton 1957; Arnoczky & Marshall 1977).

References

Alm A, Strömberg B. Vascular anatomy of the patellar and cruciate ligaments. A microangiographic and histologic investigation in the dog. Acta Chir Scand Suppl 1974;445:25–35.

Arcand MA, Rhalmi S, Rivard, C-H. Quantification of mechanoreceptors in the canine anterior cruciate ligament. Int Orthop 2000;24:272–275.

Arnoczky SP, Marshall JL. The cruciate ligaments of the canine stifle: An anatomical and functional analysis. Am J Vet Res 1977;38:1807–1814.

Arnoczky SP, Rubin RM, Marshall JL. Microvasculature of the cruciate ligaments and its response to injury. An experimental study in dogs. J Bone Joint Surg Am 1979;61:1221–1229.

Brunnberg L. Klinische Untersuchungen zu Ätiologie und Pathogenese der Ruptur des Ligamentum cruciatum craniale beim Hund. 2. Mitteilung: Zur Ätiologie und Diagnose der Ruptur des Ligamentum cruciatum craniale beim Hund. Kleintierprax 1989;34: 445–449.

de Rooster H, de Bruin T, van Bree H. Morphologic and functional features of the canine cruciate ligaments. Vet Surg 2006;35:769–780.

Harari J. Caudal cruciate ligament injury. Vet Clin North Am Small Anim Pract 1993;23:821–829.

Haut RC, Little RW. Rheological properties of canine anterior cruciate ligaments. J Biomech 1969;2:289–298.

Heffron LE, Campbell JR. Morphology, histology and functional anatomy of the canine cranial cruciate ligament. Vet Rec 1978;102:280–283.

Kobayashi S, Baba H, Uchida K, et al. Microvascular system of anterior cruciate ligament in dogs. J Orthop Res 2006;24:1509–1520.

O'Connor BL, Woodbury P. The primary articular nerves to the dogs knee. J Anat 1982;134:563–572.

Rudy RL. Stifle joint. In: *Canine Surgery*, Archibald J (ed). Santa Barbara, CA: American Veterinary Publications, 1974, pp. 1104–1115.

Singleton WB. The diagnosis and surgical treatment of some abnormal stifle conditions in the dog. Vet Rec 1957;69:1387–1394.

Tirgari M. The surgical significance of the blood supply of the canine stifle joint. J Small Anim Pract 1978; 19:451–462.

Vasseur PB, Arnoczky SP. Collateral ligaments of the canine stifle joint: Anatomic and functional analysis. Am J Vet Res 1981;42:1133–1137.

Vasseur PB, Pool RR, Arnoczky SP, et al. Correlative biomechanical and histologic study of the cranial cruciate ligament in dogs. Am J Vet Res 1985;46: 1842–1854.

Wingfield C, Amis AA, Stead AC, et al. Cranial cruciate stability in the Rottweiler and racing Greyhound: An *in vitro* study. J Small Anim Pract 2000;41:193–197.

Yahia LH, Drouin G. Microscopical investigation of canine anterior cruciate ligament and patellar tendon: Collagen fascicle morphology and architecture. J Orthop Res 1989;7:243–251.

Yahia LH. Newman NM, St Georges M. Innervation of the canine cruciate ligaments. A neurohistological study. Anat Histol Embryol 1992; 21:1–8.

Zahm H. Die Ligamenta decussata in gesunden und arthrotischen Kniegelenk des Hundes. Kleintierprax 1965;10:38–47.

2 Biomechanics of the Cruciate Ligaments

Susannah J. Sample, Ray Vanderby, Jr., and Peter Muir

Introduction

The canine cranial cruciate ligament (CrCL) is the most widely studied ligament in veterinary medicine. Over the past 40 years, studies of the CrCL have focused primarily on either surgical methods to replace its function after rupture or furthering understanding of histologic and mechanical age-related degradation. Unlike in humans, little is known about the specific biomechanical properties of the CrCL in dogs. More detailed biomechanical descriptions of the CrCL are needed as technologies for ligament replacement procedures in dogs evolve.

Biomechanical properties refer to the relationship between the length and tension of a given biologic material. This chapter will give a short overview of the biomechanical properties of ligaments and summarize what is known about the biomechanics of the canine CrCL. Biologic factors and disease conditions that are known to influence the biomechanical properties of ligaments will also be discussed, as will the biomechanics of graft

---

Advances in the Canine Cranial Cruciate Ligament, Edited by Peter Muir, © 2010 ACVS Foundation, This Work is a co-publication between the American College of Veterinary Surgeons Foundation and Wiley-Blackwell.

materials that have been considered for possible cruciate repair.

Ligament composition

Ligaments have a hierarchical architecture (Figure 2.1) and consist of a combination of water and longitudinally running collagen fibers, which are mostly type I collagen (70%–80% of tissue dry weight and >90% of collagen), with a small amount of type III collagen (3%–10%). Minimal amounts of types V, X, XII, and XIV, elastin, and proteoglycans are also components.

The hierarchical architecture of a ligament influences its mechanical properties. A ligament is made up of multiple smaller structures called fiber bundles (Figures 2.1 and 2.2). Each fiber bundle, in turn, is composed of the basic fibers of the ligament and includes fibroblasts; fibroblasts are the primary cells that make up both ligament and tendon. Ligament fibers have varying amounts of crimp (Figure 2.2). Crimp is a sort of wave within collagen fibers (Figures 2.1 and 2.2) and is the primary driving force behind the nonlinear stress–strain relationship that exists initially when the ligament undergoes tensile loading. Crimp facilitates progressive recruitment of fibers to resist load. Crimped fibers also help to provide resistance at extremes of joint motion.

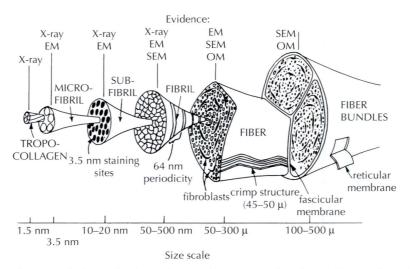

Figure 2.1 Diagram illustrating the hierarchical organization of ligaments and tendons. A ligament has a hierarchical structure, starting at the level of individual fibroblasts. These cells are arranged to create a series of fibril structures, which eventually results in the formation of fibers. Fiber bundles or fascicles then combine to create the ligament itself. It should be noted that tendons also possess this basic hierarchical architecture. EM: electron microscopy; SEM: scanning electron microscopy; OM: optical microscopy. Reproduced from SEB Symposia XXXIV 1980, The mechanical properties of biological tissues, with permission from the Society of Experimental Biology.

The strength of ligaments and tendons relates to the diameter of its composite fibrils; thicker fibrils have a greater effect on tensile strength and are considered the determinants thereof (Ottani et al. 2001). In horses, the effect of exercise on collagen fibril diameter has been of great interest, particularly with regard to superficial and deep digital flexor tendon injury. Studies have shown that exercise initially increases fibril diameter, but exercise-induced microdamage results in a decrease in fibril diameter (Cherdchutham et al. 2001).

The CrCL is unique in architecture and function. It is a continuum of fibers from a distal cranial medial orientation on the lateral femoral condyle to the cranial central interspinous area of the tibial plateau. These fibers are recruited differentially throughout stifle flexion so that the fibers are often defined by functional bundles. Most commonly, two bundles are described, the cranial medial bundle (CM) and the caudal lateral bundle (CL). In extension, both fiber bundles are tight and parallel. In flexion, the structure twists when the femoral attachment of the CrCL rolls back. When this occurs, the CL bundle becomes slack, while the CM bundle remains load-bearing. The reduced number of CrCL fibers that are load-bearing during flexion consequently makes them more vulnerable to overstretch damage.

Biomechanical properties

Because ligaments are designed to transfer load from bone to bone in a longitudinal direction, uniaxial tensile tests are used to characterize the structural and material properties of ligaments using force–deformation and stress–strain curves, respectively. Typically, all CrCL testing is carried out with the stifle extended to recruit fibers from both fiber bundles. This provides a best case scenario for strength and stiffness and comparable biomechanical properties. Stifle loadings in any off-axis direction and/or with some stifle flexion would result in different stiffness and strength.

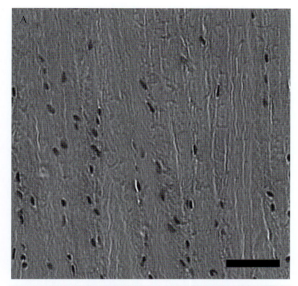

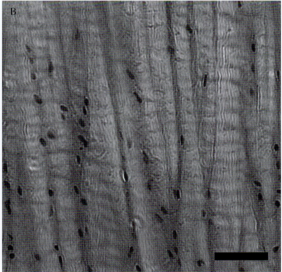

Figure 2.2 Longitudinal section of intact cranial cruciate ligament (CrCL) from a 1.5-year-old female beagle viewed using bright light (A) and circularly polarized light (B). Intact CrCL from young dogs has a hierarchically organized structure. Birefringence of the extracellular matrix collagen and the crimped structure are clearly visible in polarized light as bright and dark repeating bands within the ligament fibers. Crimp is a wave-like feature of ligaments that exists at the level of the fiber and is the primary reason for a ligament's nonlinear elasticity. Bar = 50 µm.

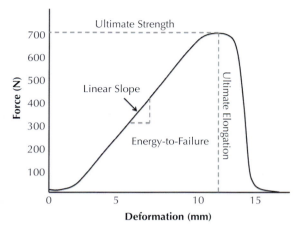

Figure 2.3 Typical force–deformation curve for ligament during uniaxial tensile testing. The force–deformation curve of ligament can be divided into three regions. The toe region is the initial nonlinear part of the curve, which is primarily due to the existence of crimp at the level of the fiber. In this region, small forces result in a large degree of lengthening because of the crimped nature of the collagen fibers. The second is the linear region, which occurs after crimp has been maximally stretched. The linear slope of this region is reflective of the material's stiffness. The final region is the point at which a ligament begins to rupture; the peak of this part of the curve gives the material's ultimate strength and ultimate elongation values.

All ligaments are viscoelastic in their mechanical behavior. That is, their stretch will increase during sustained loads (creep) and the tensile load required to maintain a fixed position will decrease with time (relaxation). Although important, these biomechanical characteristics are often considered secondary. Thus, testing protocols "precondition" specimens with repeated loads and test at a constant rate of loading to minimize secondary effects, producing a standard force versus deformation curve that can be used for biomechanical comparison.

Force–deformation curve

Structural properties are described using a force–deformation curve, which can be divided into three regions (Figure 2.3). The first is the toe region, which is nonlinear and has a low initial stiffness; in this region, due to the crimped nature of the collagen fibers, small forces result in a relatively large degree of lengthening. The next region is the linear region, which displays a high degree of stiffness due to the collagen fibers being stretched. The last region is the point at which the ultimate strength has been reached, which is the point at which the ligament is no longer able to sustain a given force and consequently ruptures. Structural properties of a ligament can be derived from the force–deformation curve. The linear stiffness is the slope of the linear portion of the curve; stiffness is an extensive material property, meaning that it depends both on the material being measured and its size or boundary conditions. The ultimate strength and ultimate elongation of the material are then determined at the point of rupture, and the energy-to-failure is the area under the curve prior to failure.

Stress–strain curve

Stress is defined as load divided by cross-sectional area (MPa), and is calculated using known load data and a cross-sectional measurement of the ligament. Strain can be thought of as deformation, and is defined as the change in length divided by original length; during uniaxial tensile testing, strain can be directly determined. The stress–strain curve can be divided into three portions (Figure 2.4). The first is the toe region, at which point large changes in strain result in minimal stress being applied; it is in this region that the "un-crimping" of the collagen fibers occurs as they are being recruited to bear load. The next is the linear region, which occurs when the ligament fibers themselves are being stretched. The slope of this linear region defines Young's modulus (also known as elastic modulus or modulus); Young's modulus describes the properties of the composite material including all its solid and fluid constituents. The last region occurs when the ligament begins to rupture. As fibers begin to rupture, stiffness decreases. The point before this decrease in stiffness defines the ultimate stress and ultimate strain of the tissue. When sufficient fiber damage has occurred and the elongation continues, the remaining fibers rupture and the ligament breaks. The area under the curve before failure is called

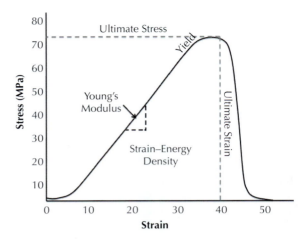

Figure 2.4 Typical stress–strain curve for ligament during uniaxial tensile testing. A stress–strain curve is determined by calculating the amount of strain (deformation) that occurs as a result of varying levels of tensile (or compressive) loading. The slope of the linear aspect of the stress–strain curve defines Young's Modulus. A material's yield point occurs once the material begins to deform plastically prior to rupture. The point or rupture is where the ultimate stress and ultimate strain are defined.

strain–energy density, or the energy stored in the elastic ligamentous material.

Viscoelasticity

A ligament, like all soft collagenous connective tissues, is considered a viscoelastic material, in that it exhibits both viscous and elastic properties when undergoing deformation, and therefore has time-dependent mechanical behavior. Two characteristic material properties that are exhibited by viscoelastic materials are creep and relaxation. Creep describes how a ligament continues to stretch under a sustained force. Relaxation describes how the tensile force required to keep a stretched ligament at a constant length diminishes over time. As a consequence of relaxation, the stiffness of a viscoelastic material depends upon the rate at which load is applied. For a fast rate of loading, the viscoelastic CrCL will be stiffer than if it is stretched slowly. Another vicoelastic property is hysteresis or energy dissipation; if a ligament is loaded and then unloaded, its stress–strain curve will not follow the same path because some energy is lost during loading. However, during repetitive loading and unloading, its stress–strain curve does synchronize, which underscores the importance for preconditioning before experimental ligament biomechanical testing.

Biologic factors

There are a number of non-disease-related factors that affect ligament biomechanical properties, including age, body weight, phenotype, whether animals are gonadectomized, and use/disuse (Laros et al. 1971; Vasseur et al. 1985; Duval et al. 1999).

In dogs, the effect of age on CrCL mechanical properties has been of particular interest. Skeletal maturity has been shown to increase strength, stiffness, and other mechanical properties of ligaments. However, significant weakening occurs in the CrCL with age. Decreases in modulus, ultimate stress, and strain–energy density have been reported, particularly in dogs weighing more than 15 kg (Vasseur et al. 1985).

It is well recognized that excessive body condition is a risk factor for cruciate rupture (see Chapter 14). Specific breeds of dog are also at increased risk, such as the Mastiff, Akita, and Rottweiler, while others, such as the greyhound, seem to be relatively protected from the condition (Duval et al. 1999; Whitehair et al. 1993). It is not clear why some breeds are predisposed to cruciate rupture, although differences in histologic, metabolic, anatomic, and immune cell population between the species have all been considered possible explanations (Wingfield et al. 2000; Comerford et al. 2005, 2006; Muir et al. 2007). Neutering of either gender also increases the prevalence of CrCL rupture, suggesting that sex hormones may affect CrCL mechanical properties (Slauterbeck et al. 2004).

As is seen with bone, immobilization results in significant decreases in ligament strength. A study using a 9-week rabbit stifle immobilization model showed that CrCL cross-sectional area was significantly decreased and ultimate strain was significantly increased with immobilization, although decreases in modulus were not significant, and no changes in ultimate stress were found (Newton et al. 1995). Pelvic limb disuse also results in impaired

ligament healing; the CrCL of male rats that underwent hindlimb suspension for 3 weeks had significantly decreased ultimate strength, ultimate stress, and elastic modulus versus controls (Provenzano et al. 2003). Relatively few studies have been performed on the biomechanical effects of remobilization on previously immobilized ligament, but over time material properties appear to be restored before structural properties (Woo et al. 1999).

Sites of ligament rupture

In human beings and dogs, most CrCL/anterior cruciate ligament tears occur through the body of the ligament, although the cause of rupture in human beings is most commonly considered to be trauma, whereas in dogs, most ruptures are not associated with obvious trauma. It has been shown that in animals with normal stifles, tensile tests of the femur–CrCL–tibia complex often result in avulsion fractures of the CrCL tibial insertion site, as opposed to tears through the CrCL body (Goldberg et al. 1982; Klein et al. 1982). This suggests that the mechanism resulting in CrCL rupture in the majority of dogs is due to a pathologic process that results in degradation of CrCL material properties. Much work has been focused on the specific histologic changes that occur in ligaments that have ruptured, such as the development of chondroid transformation of ligament fibroblasts, alterations to collagen structure, changes in collagen fiber crimp, and loss of ligament fibroblasts. However, the cause and timeline of these changes and how they relate to the progression of the cruciate rupture arthropathy and development of CrCL rupture remain unclear (Vasseur et al. 1985; Narama et al. 1996; Hayashi et al. 2003). It should be noted that avulsion fractures do occur clinically in dogs, although they appear to be most commonly associated with obvious trauma and present with an acute onset of severe lameness (Reinke 1982).

Synovitis and ligament biomechanics

Development of synovitis and joint degradation has been clearly associated with CrCL transection models that create joint instability (Lipowitz et al.

1985), but the relationship between synovitis and joint instability in the canine cruciate rupture arthropathy remains controversial. In one study examining the effect of synovitis on ligament biomechanics in a rabbit model, the presence of chronic synovitis significantly decreased ligament strength. Histologically, these ligaments showed a loss of normal fiber orientation, a disorganized cellular pattern, changes in the interstitial matrix, and some infiltration of inflammatory cells within the ligament body (Goldberg et al. 1982). Given the known effects of synovitis on ligament strength, the hypothesis that synovitis precedes cruciate rupture in affected dogs fits with the clinical observation that mid-body CrCL ruptures are typically found clinically.

Another study looked at Wistar rats, which are predisposed to spontaneous synovitis. In these animals, a correlation was found between stifle synovitis and chondroid metaplasia of the cruciate ligaments; these changes were not age related (Sasaki et al. 1998). Taken together, these data support the hypothesis that stifle synovitis is a key factor that promotes joint degradation and diminished ligament strength in dogs with the cruciate rupture arthropathy. Although this relationship between synovitis and ligament structural properties remains little studied, the possibility of osteoarthritis and cruciate failure being a consequence of synovitis merits further investigation.

Isometric points

With finite sized areas of CrCL insertion, it is not possible for all CrCL fibers to be isometric throughout flexion, so the CM and CL bundles have differing biomechanics. Surgical protocols, however, require the most isometric points to be used for joint stabilization or ligament reconstruction. Stabilization of the cruciate-deficient canine stifle occurs through either intra-capsular or extracapsular techniques. The extracapsular stabilization method is an established method that is still commonly employed today. The general concept of this method is to align a suture outside of the joint capsule in the direction of the previously existing CrCL. Biomechanically, the placement of such sutures should not be considered so simplistically. Ideally, sutures should be placed isometrically,

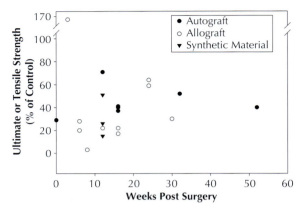

Figure 2.5 Strength of ligament replacements. Although allografts, autografts, and numerous synthetic materials have been tested as possible replacement materials for ruptured cranial cruciate ligaments (CrCL) in experimental dogs, none have proven to have the same mechanical properties as an intact CrCL. The lack of strength seen in these materials over time, compounded by the synovitis typically seen in clinical patients, remains a barrier to their successful use in the canine clinical patient.

meaning that during motion the suture attachment sites should remain a constant distance apart, thus preventing laxity of the suture material and consequent cranial translation of the joint. Numerous studies have looked at identification of isometric points (Guénégo et al. 2007; Roe et al. 2008), with the recently developed "tight-rope" procedure being one of the latest techniques designed to provide bone to bone fixation.

Biomechanics of grafts

The use of intra-articular grafts for restoration of joint stability has been well established in human orthopaedics. However, in dogs with the cruciate rupture arthropathy, the use of grafts in CrCL-deficient stifles has fallen out of favor in the clinical setting. Various allografts, autografts, and synthetic materials have been tested in experimental animals, but none have shown to be mechanically equivalent to an intact CrCL (Figure 2.5). One challenge of using grafts to replace CrCLs in dogs is that grafts lose strength over time (Cabaud et al. 1980; Shino et al. 1984; Curtis et al. 1985; Vasseur et al. 1985; McFarland et al. 1986;

Yoshiya et al. 1986; van Rens et al. 1986; Johnson et al. 1989; Thorson et al. 1989). Unlike experimental dogs used in these studies, client-owned dogs affected with the cruciate rupture arthropathy typically exhibit moderate to severe synovitis at the time of surgical treatment. Therefore, without a disease-modifying treatment, using grafts in these patients would be even less likely to provide long-term stifle stability compared with experimental dogs.

Conclusion

The biomechanical properties of the cruciate ligaments are essential for stifle joint stabilization. It is the degradation of these properties that ultimately leads to cruciate rupture and the loss of joint stability. Until materials that display the key properties of ligaments are developed, or a means to reconstruct or replace the CrCL is found, stabilization of stifles in dogs with CrCL rupture will continue to be a challenge. The lack of understanding regarding the mechanisms involved in the development of CrCL rupture in affected dogs, particularly with regard to synovitis, remains a barrier to the development of better surgical treatments.

References

Cabaud EH, Feagin JA, Rodkey WG. Acute anterior cruciate ligament injury and augmented repair. Am J Sports Med 1980;8:395–401.

Cherdchutham W, Becker CK, Spek ER, et al. Effects of exercise on the diameter of collagen fibrils in the central core and periphery of the superficial digital flexor tension in foals. Am J Vet Res 2001;62: 1563–1570.

Comerford EJ, Tarlton JF, Innes JF, et al. Metabolism and composition of the canine anterior cruciate ligament relate to differences in knee joint mechanics and predisposition to ligament rupture. J Orthop Res 2005; 23:61–66.

Comerford EJ, Tarlton JF, Wales A, et al. Ultrasound differences in cranial cruciate ligaments from dogs of two breds with a differing predisposition to ligament degeneration and rupture. J Comp Pathol 2006;134: 8–16.

Curtis RJ, Delee JC, Drez DJ. Reconstruction of the anterior cruciate ligament with freeze dried fascia lata allografts in dogs. Am J Sports Med 1985;13: 408–414.

Duval JM, Budsberg SC, Flo GL, Sammarco JL. Breed, sex and body weight as risk factors for rupture of the cranial cruciate ligament in young dogs. J Am Vet Med Assoc 1999;215:811–814.

Goldberg VM, Burstein A, Dawson M. The influence of an experimental immune synovitis on the failure mode and strength of the rabbit anterior cruciate ligament. J Bone Joint Surg Am 1982;64:900–906.

Guénégo L, Zahra A, Madelénat A, et al. Cranial cruciate ligament rupture in large and giant dogs. A retrospective evaluation of a modified lateral extracapuslar stabilization. Vet Comp Orthop Traumatol 2007; 20:43–50.

Hayashi K, Frank JD, Dubinsky C, et al. Histologic changes in ruptured canine cranial cruciate ligament. Vet Surg 2003;32:269–277.

Johnson SG, Hulse DA, Hogan HA, et al. System behavior of commonly used cranial cruciate ligament reconstruction autographs. Vet Surg 1989;18:459–465.

Klein L, Player JS, Heiple KG, et al. Isotopic evidence for resorption of soft tissues and bone in immobilized dogs. J Bone Joint Surg Am 1982;64:225–230.

Laros GS, Tipton CM, Cooper RR. Influence of physical activity on the ligament insertions in the knees of dogs. J Bone Joint Surg Am 1971;53:275–285.

Lipowitz AJ, Wong PL, Stevens JB. Synovial membrane changes after experimental transection of the cranial cruciate ligament in dogs. Am J Vet Res 1985;46: 1166–1170.

McFarland EG, Morrey BF, An KN, et al. The relationship of vascularity and water content to tensile strength in a patellar tendon replacement of the anterior cruciate in dogs. Am J Sports Med 1986;14:436–448.

Muir P, Schaefer LS, Manley PA, et al. Expression of immune response genes in the stifle joint of dogs with oligoarthritis and degenerative cranial cruciate ligament rupture. Vet Immunol Immunopathol 2007;119: 214–221.

Narama I, Masuoka-Nishiyama M, Matsuura T, et al. Morphogenesis of degenerative changes predisposing dogs to rupture of the cranial cruciate ligament. J Vet Med Sci 1996;58:1091–1097.

Newton PO, Woo SL, MacKenna DA, et al. Immobilization of the knee joint alters the mechanical and ultrastructural properties of the rabbit anterior cruciate ligament. J Orthop Res 1995;13:191–200.

Ottani V, Raspanti M, Ruggeri A. Collagen structure and functional implications. Micron 2001;32:251–260.

Provenzano PP, Martinez DA, Grindeland RE, et al. Hindlimb unloading alters ligament healing. J Appl Physiol 2003;94:314–324.

Reinke JD. Cruciate ligament avulsion injury in the dog. J Am Anim Hosp Assoc 1982;18:257–264.

Roe SC, Kue J, Gemma J. Isometry of potential suture attachment sites for the cranial cruciate ligament deficient canine stifle. Vet Comp Orthop Traumatol 2008;21:215–220.

Sasaki S, Nagai H, Mori I, et al. Spontaneous synovitis in Wistar rats. Toxicol Pathol 1998;26:687–690.

Shino K, Kawasaki T, Hirose H, et al. Replacement of the anterior cruciate ligament by an allogeneic tendon graft. J Bone Joint Surg Br 1984;66:672–681.

Slauterbeck JR, Pankratz K, Xu KT, et al. Canine ovariohysterectomy and orchiectomy increases the prevalence of ACL injury. Clin Orthop Relat Res 2004;429:301–305.

Thorson E, Rodrigo JJ, Vasseur P, et al. Replacement of the anterior cruciate ligament. A comparison of autografts and allografts in dogs. Acta Orthop Scand 1989;60:555–560.

van Rens TJG, van den Berg AF, Huiskes R, et al. Substitution of the anterior cruciate ligament: A long term histologic and biomechanical study with autogenous pedicled grafts of the iliotibial band in dogs. Arthroscopy 1986;2:139–154.

Vasseur PB, Pool RR, Arnoczky SP, Lau RE. Correlative biomechanical and histologic study of the cranial cruciate ligament in dogs. Am J Vet Res 1985;46:1842–1854.

Whitehair JG, Vasseur PB, Willits NH. Epidemiology of cranial cruciate ligament rupture in dogs. J Am Vet Med Assoc 1993;203:1016–1019.

Wingfield C, Amis AA, Stead AC, Law HT. Comparison of the biomechanical properties of Rottweiler and racing greyhound cranial cruciate ligaments. J Small Anim Pract 2000;41:303–307.

Woo SL, Debski RE, Withrow JD, et al. Biomechanics of knee ligaments. Am J Sports Med 1999;27:533–543.

Yoshiya S, Andrish JT, Manley MT, et al. Augmentation of anterior cruciate ligament reconstruction in dogs with prostheses of different stiffnesses. J Ortho Res 1986;4:475–485.

3 Cruciate Ligament Remodeling and Repair

Connie S. Chamberlain and Ray Vanderby, Jr.

Introduction

Multiple factors adversely affect the healing capacity of the cranial cruciate ligament (CrCL), including complex ligament anatomy, biomechanical forces, nutritional delivery, and the biologic milieu. These factors prevent a ruptured CrCL from regenerating its native tissue or recapitulating mechanical function. With little intrinsic healing potential, ruptures of the CrCL are often reconstructed. The repair process may extend from months to years and the injured ligament or replacement graft never fully recovers the original mechanical properties (Levenson et al. 1965; Lin et al. 2004). CrCL grafts usually lengthen (Feagin & Curl 1976; Sherman & Bonamo 1988; Kaplan et al. 1990) and their initial tissue strength can drop by ~50% after remodeling. Reconstructed stifles are often less stable and fail to restore normal joint kinematics. These deficiencies contribute to premature joint degeneration, osteoarthritis, and compromised function. This chapter will briefly discuss the biologic processes for natural CrCL healing as well as the biologic steps

occurring during healing of a reconstructed CrCL graft.

Healing potential of the extracapsular ligament

For comparison, consider healing of an extracapsular ligament (e.g., a medial collateral ligament [MCL]; Figure 3.1). A robust healing cascade occurs consisting of hemostasis and inflammation, proliferation, and remodeling (Frank et al. 1983; Clark 1985, 1993; Chamberlain et al. 2009). Hemostasis and inflammation immediately follow injury and are characterized by the formation of a hematoma organized into a fibrinogen mesh, and the accumulation of neutrophils, monocytes/macrophages, and T lymphocytes (Chamberlain et al. 2009). These inflammatory cells rid injured tissue of debris and secrete cytokines and growth factors that modulate inflammation, attract fibroblasts to the injury, and stimulate subsequent activities in the healing cascade. The proliferative phase follows the inflammatory stage and consists of increased fibroblasts, myofibroblasts, additional macrophages, and endothelial cells (Chamberlain et al. 2009). These cells and their products form granulation tissue within the injured region. Remodeling is the final phase of healing and follows proliferation. The earlier infiltration of

---

Advances in the Canine Cranial Cruciate Ligament,
Edited by Peter Muir, © 2010 ACVS Foundation, This Work is a co-publication between the American College of Veterinary Surgeons Foundation and Wiley-Blackwell.

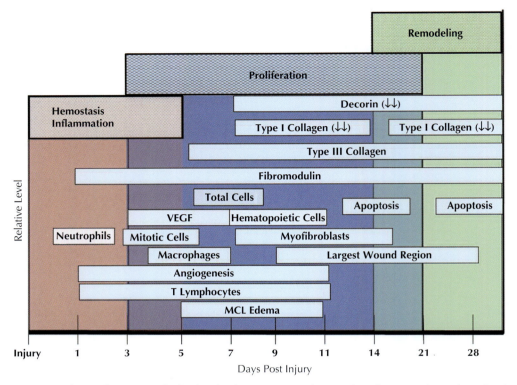

Figure 3.1 Process of normal, extracapsular healing by the rat MCL. Healing involves three complex and overlapping processes, including hemostasis and inflammation, proliferation, and remodeling. Hemostasis and inflammation involves clot formation and the infiltration of inflammatory cells, such as neutrophils, macrophages, and T lymphocytes, immediately after injury. Proliferation is characterized by the formation of granulation tissue, including fibroblast proliferation and angiogenesis. Remodeling is the final phase and involves cell number reduction and scar formation. For review, see Chamberlain et al. (2009).

fibroblasts, inflammatory cells, and endothelial cells diminish to basal levels during this stage (Chamberlain et al. 2009). This phase of healing lasts many months in ligaments, resulting in scar-like neo-ligamentous tissue that can still be found 2 years post injury (Frank et al. 1983). The cellular profile of the remodeling ligament is somewhat similar to uninjured tissue compared with the previous inflammatory or proliferative phases, but complete functional recovery may never occur. With or without surgical intervention, the injured MCL will heal, but it results in tissue that is more scar-like than the native tissue and mechanically inferior.

Healing potential of the completely ruptured CrCL

Unlike the extracapsular MCL, the intracapsular CrCL does not heal without early surgical intervention. A native CrCL is a highly organized, dense connective tissue composed of dense parallel collagen bundles, exhibiting birefringence and crimping under polarized light (Hayashi et al. 2003a). Small blood vessels and fusiform- and ovoid-shaped fibroblasts surround the collagen bundles. A synovial membrane surrounds the CrCL and consists of dense connective tissue,

Cruciate Ligament Remodeling and Repair 23

Table 3.1 Healing potential of the cranial cruciate ligament after complete or partial rupture, or surgical repair[a]

Time post injury	Complete rupture	Partial rupture	Surgical repair
Immediately	No hematoma	Possible hematoma	
1 week	Necrosis, inflammation	Necrosis, inflammation, provisional matrix, fibroblast proliferation throughout	Inflammation, provisional matrix
2 weeks	Edema, ligament retraction, fibroblast proliferation of ends	Necrosis, no granulation tissue formation, fibroblast proliferation throughout ligament	Proliferation, granulation tissue
4 weeks	Collagen formation, ligament resorption	No granulation tissue formation, fibroblast proliferation throughout ligament, collagen formation	Fibroblast proliferation, collagen formation
6 weeks	Collagen formation, ligament resorption	Fibroblast proliferation	Collagen formation
8 weeks	Collagen formation, ligament resorption	Fibroblast proliferation	Collagen formation
10 weeks	Collagen formation, ligament resorption		Collagen formation

[a]For review, see O'Donoghue et al. (1966).

small fibroblasts, and some adipocytes (Heffron & Campbell 1978; Hayashi et al. 2003a).

Healing phases are summarized in Table 3.1. Immediately after complete CrCL rupture, the synovial joint fluid bathes the ligament and prevents clot formation and union of the ligament ends (O'Donoghue et al. 1966). The lack of hematoma precludes formation of a provisional matrix and granulation tissue to start the healing process. One week after rupture, the CrCL undergoes necrosis and inflammatory cell infiltration; B and T lymphocytes, macrophages, dendritic cells, and IgG, IgM, and IgA plasma cells infiltrate the inflamed synovium (O'Donoghue et al. 1966; Lemburg et al. 2004). The extracellular matrix (ECM) collagenous structure is partially lost or disorganized, lacks birefringence, and exhibits little or no crimp (Hayashi et al. 2003a,b). At 2 weeks, the CrCL becomes edematous, the injured ends retract, and fibroblasts proliferate and accumulate near the ruptured ends and decrease within the inner ligament (O'Donoghue et al. 1966; Hayashi et al. 2003b). Atypical spheroid-shaped fibroblasts appear with the typical fusiform- and ovoid-shaped fibroblasts (Hayashi et al. 2003b).

Surviving centralized spheroid fibroblasts undergo chondroid transformation and become devitalized as a result of inadequate blood flow, tissue hypoxia, and oxidative stress (Hayashi et al. 2003a,b). A diminished blood supply to the ruptured ligament also results in the resorption of the ligament (O'Donoghue et al. 1966). Occasionally the ruptured CrCL will fuse to the caudal cruciate ligament and maintain vascularity. Similar to a partial CrCL rupture, contact to a blood supply limits necrosis. By 8 weeks, the remaining CrCL segment shortens, precluding the possibility of suturing the ends together (O'Donoghue et al. 1966). Similar to the rabbit, after 3–12 months, few remnants of ligament exist and stifles show signs of osteoarthritis, with cartilaginous damage localizing primarily at the femoral condyle (Hefti et al. 1991).

Healing potential of the partially ruptured CrCL

The partially torn CrCL initially exhibits a weak healing response (Table 3.1). Partial CrCL ruptures form a hematoma and produce an organized fibrin meshwork to promote an early inflammatory response (Hefti et al., 1991). At one week post injury the ligament remains intact, and a gelatinous provisional matrix fills the gap (O'Donoghue et al. 1966). Between 2 and 4 weeks, proliferating fibroblasts infiltrate the entire ligament, but formation of granulation tissue is delayed (O'Donoghue et al. 1966). Fibroblast proliferation continues throughout the ligament and the partially torn CrCL develops longitudinally oriented collagen fibers in the defect by 10 weeks (O'Donoghue et al. 1966). Although partial ruptures form a hematoma and provisional matrix (unlike complete ruptures), the partial defect remains incompletely filled and therefore functionally deficient.

Healing potential of the surgically repaired CrCL

Surgical repair of the CrCL via suturing the ligament ends together immediately after injury can provide some degree of healing (Table 3.1). Similar to the extracapsular MCL, the sutured CrCL undergoes inflammation, proliferation, and remodeling, albeit a slower process. Granulation tissue forms in the sutured region, the inflammatory response progressively subsides, and the region of scar formation stabilizes. At 1 and 2 weeks post surgery, the ligament forms a provisional matrix consisting of inflammatory cells (O'Donoghue et al. 1966). By week 4, fibroblast proliferation and collagen formation increases within the defect (O'Donoghue et al. 1966). Between 6 and 10 weeks, the newly formed collagen within the defect blends with the intact portion of the CrCL. However, tensile strength of the ligament remains substantially weaker than the uninjured CrCL (O'Donoghue et al. 1966). This promising healing outcome is described when a transected ligament was surgically repaired. A typical injury results in frayed ends, complicating successful closure of the ligament ends. Additionally, if repair is not completed immediately after rupture, the ligament ends undergo necrosis and resorb, inhibiting successful surgical intervention.

Healing potential of the reconstructed CrCL graft

Rupture of the CrCL may involve reconstruction with an autograft or allograft because of the poor functional outcomes with nonoperative treatment. In a process that is slower and less efficient than MCL healing, a CrCL graft undergoes a complex healing process that includes synovialization, avascular necrosis, revascularization, cellular proliferation, and remodeling. At the time of transplantation, the central core of the graft is avascular. After transplantation, a synovial layer forms around the graft, providing a blood supply to the transplanted tissue. The inner core remains avascular and acellular for up to 3 months post surgery, but the peripheral graft repopulates with fibroblasts. The lack of vascularity and cellularity within the ligament core results in central graft necrosis, leading to collagen destruction. Eventually, vascular buds originating from the infrapatella fat pad and synovial tissue forms within the graft. The vessels progress from the epiligament to the central portion of the graft and by 4–6 months, specimens typically revascularize. Vascularization helps to transport inflammatory cells and supply nutrients to the healing tissue. Infiltrating vessels also contribute to cellular repopulation of the graft. Avascular necrosis may be limited or prevented if vascularized autografts or grafts with preserved peritendinous connective tissue are used (Lambert 1983; van Rens et al. 1986; Butler et al. 1989a,b; Sckell et al. 1999).

Cell proliferation follows revascularization of the ligament graft. Limited proliferation of intrinsic graft tendon cells occurs, even without a peritendinous connective tissue or vascularized graft. Allografts, however, need further processing (e.g., deep freezing) to eradicate the intrinsic cells. Fresh allografts cause a severe inflammatory reaction and rejection response, implying some degree of intrinsic cellular influence after grafting. Proliferating cells, including fibroblasts, neutrophils, circulating M1, and resident M2 macrophages, initially appear within the bone–graft interface (Kawamura et al. 2005). Circulating M1 macrophages remain in the blood stream until the initiation of an immune response. After injury, cells travel to the compromised site and promote inflammation, resulting in phagocytosis and tissue

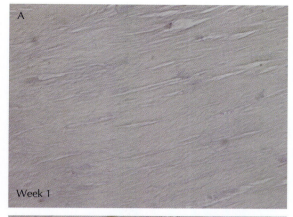
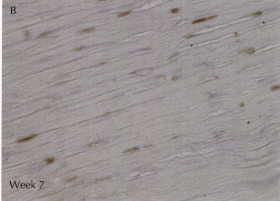

Figure 3.2 Macrophage localization within the reconstructed CrCL. Immunohistochemistry of the circulating M1 macrophages within a reconstructed rat CrCL at (A) 1 and (B) 7 weeks post transplantation. Similar to the canine-reconstructed CrCL, few macrophages localize to the graft at week 1 post injury. As time progresses, more cells infiltrate the ligament. (600×)

destruction. In contrast, the resident M2 macrophages are intrinsic cells that reduce inflammation and stimulate healing. With time, cell proliferation progresses from the interface to the outer and inner graft (Figure 3.2). Neutrophils and macrophages, derived from the bone marrow or synovial membrane, accumulate within the outer graft by day 4 (Kawamura et al. 2005). Proliferating cells, M1, and M2 macrophages continue to progress into the inner graft and are evident by 14 days post transplantation (Kawamura et al. 2005). Few to no neutrophils or T lymphocytes localize to the inner graft (Kawamura et al. 2005).

Evidence suggests that the macrophages differentiate into a fibroblast phenotype to synthesize collagen (Vaage & Lindblad 1990).

During remodeling, the graft undergoes restructuring of collagen fibers and proteoglycan content. The graft is very similar to the original CrCL in morphology, including crimp pattern and fibroblast morphology, but the size of the collagen fibrils, and the distribution of glycosaminoglycans remain significantly different from the original tissue. Additionally, the graft remains mechanically inferior to the uninjured tissue. When CrCL are reconstructed *in vitro* and placed in a testing machine, grafts pull out from the osseous tunnel. A study in sheep demonstrated that at 3 weeks after CrCL reconstruction, the load to failure of the graft averaged 5% of the normal ligament graft, 37.8 ± 17.8 N versus intact 759.2 ± 114.1 N. The graft failure now was typically in the intra-articular portion (Meller et al. 2008). Graft load to failure improved to 15% of the normal ligament after 6 weeks and exhibited a decline in grip-to-grip elongation (Meller et al. 2008). By 12 and 24 weeks, the strength of the graft improved to 41% and 69% of the normal ligament, respectively (Meller et al. 2008), but the graft strength remained far less than the normal CrCL even 52 weeks after transplantation. Thus, the remodeling process certainly does not regenerate the CrCL.

Healing potential of the reconstructed graft interface tissue

CrCL reconstruction requires healing of the tendon graft and bone tunnels in the femur and tibia. Repair of the CrCL proceeds via formation of a fibrovascular interface tissue between the graft and bone, bone ingrowth into the graft–bone interface, and progression of collagen fiber continuity between tendon and bone to result in a reestablished graft-osseous junction (Rodeo et al. 1993, 1999). After CrCL reconstruction, the graft and original cancellous bone fills with fibroblast-deposited fibrovascular tissue at the interface (Figure 3.3). Inflammatory cells and type III collagen initially accumulate in the interface granulation tissue. A few neutrophils and T lymphocytes are found within the granulation tissue in the first week after surgery (Kawamura et al. 2005). After

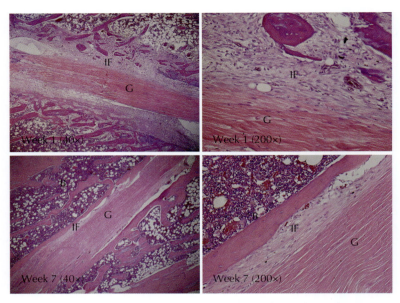

Figure 3.3 Hematoxylin and eosin staining of the rat-reconstructed CrCL graft 1 and 7 weeks post surgery. Similar to the dog, at 1 week post transplantation, the reconstructed graft contains a paucity of cells, and the interface tissue exhibits a cellularly active and inflamed region. Seven weeks post transplantation, cells continue to reside in the less inflamed interface but also infiltrate the reconstructed graft. Additionally, bone ingrowth into the tendon graft becomes more apparent. B: bone; IF: interface; G: graft.

neutrophil numbers decrease, M1 macrophages, followed by M2 macrophages, appear. While the inflammatory cells infiltrate the granulation tissue, new bone also permeates the interface. Chondroid cells then appear from the side of the bone tunnel and degrade the granulation tissue and deposit type II collagen. The granulation tissue is progressively replaced with maturing lamellar bone. As healing progresses, numerous cells consisting of osteoblasts and osteoclasts scatter throughout the tunnel. Graft incorporation initiates at the fixation sites and progresses toward the articular tunnel entrance, where graft motion may impair early graft incorporation. Approximately 3–4 weeks after surgery, an indirect graft insertion forms perpendicular collagen fibers resembling Sharpey's fibers (Gulotta et al. 2007). The type III collagen-positive fibers are present 1 year after surgery and the number and size are associated with the pull-out strength of the graft (Gulotta et al. 2007). It should be noted that there is healing at the interface, but the reconstruction tunnels do not fill with cancellous bone.

Summary

Without surgical repair, the CrCL cannot form a hematoma or subsequent granulation tissue, and the ligament eventually degenerates. Healing of repaired tissue in a synovial environment is incomplete and functionally undesirable. Surgical reconstruction of the CrCL can improve outcome but launches a healing and remodeling cascade that is slow and not functionally regenerative. Many factors modulate the ineffective healing response between tendon graft and bone, including the presence of inflammatory cells in the graft, limited bone ingrowth into the tendon graft, graft-tunnel motion, the paucity of undifferentiated progenitor cells, and lack of a coordinated signaling cascade toward regenerative healing (Gulotta et al. 2007). Reconstruction of a CrCL using graft tissue improves healing and functional outcome but does not regenerate native ligament tissue. The reconstructed CrCL undergoes synovialization, avascular necrosis, vascularization, cellular proliferation, and remodeling but still results in mechanically compromised tissue. The interface between graft and bone likewise undergoes a repair process involving the development of a fibrovascular interface, bone ingrowth, and collagen fiber continuity. Studies have quantified deficiencies in the healing and remodeling processes in repaired or reconstructed CrCLs. Recent advances show that the above CrCL healing cascades and graft healing processes can be modulated. Advances such as tissue engineering, targeted delivery of bioactive molecules, or healing augmented with platelet rich plasma provide optimism that treatments will become available to improve and accelerate the repair or reconstruction of a ruptured CrCL.

References

Butler DL, Grood ES, Noyes FR, et al. Mechanical properties of primate vascularized vs. nonvascularized patellar tendon grafts; changes over time. J Orthop Res 1989a;7:68–79.

Butler DL. Kappa Delta Award paper. Anterior cruciate ligament: Its normal response and replacement. J Orthop Res 1989b;7:910–921.

Chamberlain CS, Crowley E, Vanderby R. The spatiotemporal dynamics of ligament healing. Wound Repair Regen 2009;17:206–215.

Clark RA. Cutaneous tissue repair: Basic biologic considerations. J Am Acad Dermatol 1985;13:701–725.

Clark RA. Biology of dermal wound repair. Dermatol Clin 1993;11:647–666.

Feagin JA, Jr., Curl WW. Isolated tear of the anterior cruciate ligament: 5-year follow-up study. Am J Sports Med 1976;4:95–100.

Frank C, Schachar N, Dittrich D. Natural history of healing in the repaired medial collateral ligament. J Orthop Res 1983;1:179–188.

Gulotta LV, Rodeo SA. Biology of autograft and allograft healing in anterior cruciate ligament reconstruction. Clin J Sports Med 2007;26:509–524.

Hayashi K, Frank JD, Dubinsky C, et al. Histologic changes in ruptured canine cranial cruciate ligament. Vet Surg 2003a;32:269–277.

Hayashi K, Frank JD, Hao Z, et al. Evaluation of ligament fibroblast viability in ruptured cranial cruciate ligament of dogs. Am J Vet Res 2003b;64:1010–1016.

Heffron LE, Campbell JR. Morphology, histology and functional anatomy of the canine cranial cruciate ligament. Vet Rec 1978;102:280–283.

Hefti FL, Kress A, Fasel J, et al. Healing of the transected anterior cruciate ligament in the rabbit. J Bone Joint Surg Am 1991;73:373–383.

Kaplan N, Wickiewicz TL, Warren RF. Primary surgical treatment of anterior cruciate ligament ruptures: A long-term follow-up study. Am J Sports Med 1990;18: 354–358.

Kawamura S, Ying L, Kim HJ, et al. Macrophages accumulate in the early phase of tendon-bone healing. J Orthop Res 2005;23:1425–1432.

Lambert KL Vascularized patellar tendon graft with rigid internal fixation for anterior cruciate ligament insufficiency. Clin Orthop Relat Res 1983;172:85–89.

Lemburg AK, Meyer-Lindenberg A, Hewicker-Trautwein M. Immunohistochemical characterization of inflammatory cell populations and adhesion molecule expression in synovial membranes from dogs with spontaneous cranial cruciate ligament rupture. Vet Immunol Immunopathol 2004;97:231–240.

Levenson SM, Geever EF, Crowley LV, et al. The healing of rat skin wounds. Ann Surg 1965;161:293–308.

Lin TW, Cardenas L, Soslowsky, LJ. Biomechanics of tendon injury and repair. J Biomech 2004;37:865–877.

Meller R, Willbold E, Hesse E, et al. Histologic and biomechanical analysis of anterior cruciate ligament graft to bone healing in skeletally immature sheep. Arthroscopy 2008;24:1221–1231.

O'Donoghue DH, Rockwood CA, Jr., Frank GR, et al. Repair of the anterior cruciate ligament in dogs. J Bone Joint Surg Am 1966;48:503–519.

Rodeo SA, Arnoczky SP, Torzilli PA, et al. Tendon-healing in a bone tunnel. A biomechanical and histological study in the dog. J Bone Joint Surg Am 1993;75:1795–1803.

Rodeo SA, Suzuki K, Deng XH, et al. Use of recombinant human bone morphogenetic protein-2 to enhance tendon healing in a bone tunnel. Am J Sports Med 1999;27:476–488.

Sherman MF, Bonamo JR. Primary repair of the anterior cruciate ligament. Clin J Sports Med 1988;7:739–750.

Sckell A, Leunig M, Fraitzl CR, et al. The connective-tissue envelope in revascularisation of patellar tendon grafts. J Bone Joint Surg Br 1999;81:915–920.

Vaage J, Lindblad WJ. Production of collagen type I by mouse peritoneal macrophages. J Leukoc Biol 1990;48:274–280.

van Rens TJ, van den Berg AF, Huiskes R, et al. Substitution of the anterior cruciate ligament: A long-term histologic and biomechanical study with autogenous pedicled grafts of the iliotibial band in dogs. Arthroscopy 1986;2:139–154.

4 Meniscal Structure and Function

Antonio Pozzi and James L. Cook

Surgical anatomy

The menisci are crescent-shaped wedges of fibrocartilage that rest on the peripheral aspects of the articular surfaces of the proximal tibia. They function to effectively deepen the medial and lateral tibial fossae for articulation with the condyles of the femur (Figure 4.1). They are thickest abaxially and taper to thin, unattached edges axially. The superior femoral surfaces are slightly concave to accommodate the femoral condyles, thus providing greater articular contact area and improved stifle joint congruity. In dogs, the medial meniscus is larger than the lateral and more ovoid in shape. The lateral meniscus is smaller and more circular (Hulse & Shires 1983; Arnoczky 1993; Evans 1993; Carpenter & Cooper 2000).

Both medial and lateral menisci have attachments that influence their mobility and function (Figure 4.2). The medial meniscus is firmly attached to the tibia through cranial and caudal meniscotibial ligaments. Strong attachments are also present between the abaxial aspect of the medial meniscus and the medial collateral ligament. The abaxial periphery of the medial meniscus is also attached to the joint capsule via short ligaments that blend with the joint capsule (sometimes referred to as the coronal ligaments). A cranial meniscotibial ligament anchors the lateral meniscus to the tibial plateau caudolateral to the cranial cruciate ligament (CrCL). Small caudal meniscotibial ligaments may or may not be present in dogs and can be attached cranial or caudal to the caudal cruciate ligament (CaCL) insertion when present. However, the lateral meniscus differs from the medial meniscus in that the caudal pole of the lateral meniscus is attached firmly to the femur through the meniscofemoral ligament, which inserts onto the caudomedial aspect of the intercondylar notch, caudal to the CaCL. In addition, the abaxial border of the lateral meniscus lacks a firm attachment to the lateral collateral ligament or joint capsule, and instead forms a groove where the popliteal tendon slides between the meniscus and joint capsule during stifle motion. The resultant mobility of the lateral meniscus helps to explain the decreased incidence of severe lateral meniscal tears concurrent to CrCL insufficiency when compared to the medial meniscus in dogs (Ralphs & Whitney 2002). The intermeniscal or transverse ligament connects the cranial poles of the lateral and medial menisci and blends with fibers from the cranial meniscotibial ligaments. The intermeniscal ligament lies just cranial to the tibial attachment of the CrCL and is

---

Advances in the Canine Cranial Cruciate Ligament,
Edited by Peter Muir, © 2010 ACVS Foundation, This Work is a co-publication between the American College of Veterinary Surgeons Foundation and Wiley-Blackwell.

30 Structure and Function

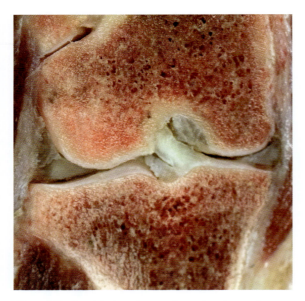

Figure 4.1 Frontal plane image of a cadaveric specimen showing the congruity provided by the menisci to the femoral and tibial articulation. The wedge-shaped menisci fill the space between the femoral and the tibial condyles.

covered by the infrapatellar fat pad. A comprehensive understanding of meniscal anatomy is integral to understanding disease mechanisms and for avoiding iatrogenic damage to these important structures during surgical treatment of stifle disorders.

Structure and composition

The menisci consist of highly differentiated cells of various phenotypes arranged in an intricately arranged extracellular matrix (ECM). Meniscal cells vary from fusiform, fibroblastic to rounded, chondrocytic phenotypes depending on location. The morphological similarities of these meniscal cells to those of other musculoskeletal tissues suggest specific functions in connective tissue synthesis and maintenance for each phenotype. For example, cells in the periphery of menisci are similar to those in ligaments and tendons, while cells in the central region are similar to hyaline cartilage (Helio Le Graverand et al. 2001). The ECM associated with the cells in these different regions also mimics the composition and function of the respective tissues.

The ECM of menisci is composed primarily of water, collagens, and proteoglycan aggregates (Adams & Ho 1987; Stephan et al. 1998; Cook et al. 1999; Noone et al. 2002). Although meniscal tissue contains several different molecular species of collagen, type I collagen accounts for about 90% of the total collagen present (Eyre & Wu 1983). Other types of collagen are also present and demonstrate regional differences. For example type I collagen is more abundant in the periphery, while type II is predominant in the axial third of the meniscus (Cheung 1987). This arrangement is most likely related to the specific biomechanical functions of each region (Bullough et al. 1970). On the meniscal surfaces, the collagen fibrils are randomly oriented and form a mesh. Just beneath this layer the collagen bundles show a more irregular orientation. Deep to these layers in the peripheral meniscus, the collagen fibers are organized in large bundles, which are circumferentially arranged from cranial to caudal attachments sites. Small radial fibers, also called "tie fibers," are arranged across the circumferential fibers and connect the abaxial region to the axial regions, where type II collagen fibers and proteoglycan predominate. The tie fibers provide structural rigidity by resisting the splitting force that arises from compressive loading to the axial region and helping to transfer it to a radial load, which the circumferential fibers can resist.

Several types of proteoglycan exist in the meniscus. In the adult dog, a relatively constant distribution of 60% chondroitin-6-sulfate, 25% chondroitin-4-sulfate, 10% chondroitin, and 5% dermatan sulfate is found (Adams & Muir 1981). The distribution of the proteoglycan depends on the region of the meniscus. The inner third is approximately 8% proteoglycan and the outer third is only 2% proteoglycan.

Neurovascular anatomy

The menisci are relatively avascular. Both menisci demonstrate a common pattern and distribution of blood vessels that arise from the medial and lateral genicular arteries (Arnoczky & Warren 1983). Within the synovial and capsular tissue of the stifle, an extensive perimeniscal capillary plexus supplies the peripheral border of the

Meniscal Structure and Function 31

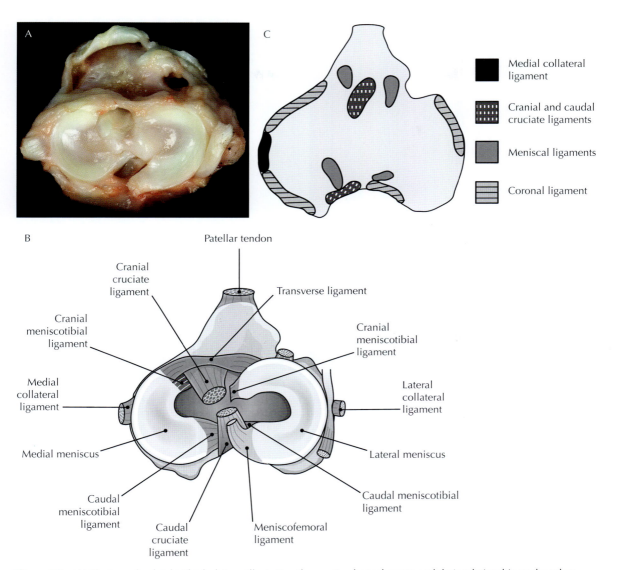

Figure 4.2 (A) Photograph of right tibial plateau illustrating the meniscal attachments and their relationship to the other intra-articular structures. (B) Drawing of the tibial plateau showing the meniscal ligaments. (C) Drawing of the tibial plateau after removal of the menisci and the other structures, showing the footprints of the meniscal and cruciate ligaments. Copyright © Samantha J. Elmhurst at www.livingart.org.uk.

meniscus throughout its attachment to the joint capsule. These vessels are limited to the peripheral 10% to 25% of the meniscus. Synovial vessels are also found in regions where there is no direct contact between meniscus and cartilage (Arnoczky & Warren 1983). Although the peripheral portion of the menisci is vascularized, most of the meniscus is avascular and must rely to a large degree on synovial sources of nutrition. Alternative mechanisms for nutrition are diffusion or mechanical pumping of synovial fluid from compression of the tissue during stifle motion (Arnoczky et al. 1980). These regional differences have profound implications for meniscal pathology and treatment considerations (Figure 4.3).

The innervation of the meniscus is not as well delineated as its blood supply. Nerve fibers originating from the perimeniscal tissue radiate into

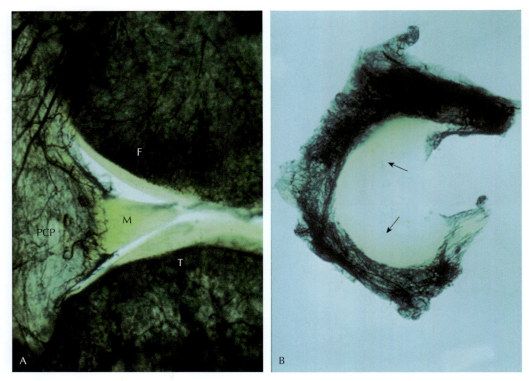

Figure 4.3 (A) Frontal plane section of the medial compartment of a dog's stifle prepared with Spalteholz technique showing the perimeniscal capillary plexus forming the red–red zone of the meniscus. Notice that the red–red or vascular zone is only about 25% of the radial width, which corresponds to about a 2-mm-wide region of peripheral tissue. PCP: perimeniscal capillary plexus; F: femur; M: avascular zone of the meniscus; T: tibia. (B) View of the entire medial meniscus. The avascular axial margin of the medial meniscus is indicated (arrows). Figure 4.3A was reproduced from Arnoczky and Warren (1983), with permission from SAGE Publications. Figure 4.3B was courtesy of Dr. Stephen Arnoczky.

the peripheral 30% of the meniscus and are most dense in the cranial and caudal horns. Nerve fibers in the menisci appear to predominately serve propioceptive and mechanoreceptive roles with little, if any, nociceptive function recognized. Meniscal-derived sensory signals during loading may contribute to protective neuromuscular reflex control of joint motion.

Biomechanical and material properties

The meniscus demonstrates a complex set of material properties that vary nonlinearly with location (inhomogeneous) and direction (anisotropic). These properties are important for the biomechanical functions of the meniscus, such as load transmission at the tibiofemoral articulation, shock absorption, and stability. These functions are vital for the normal homeostasis of the cartilage and the function of the stifle. The tensile properties of meniscal tissue are closely related to the collagen fiber architecture. Variations in tensile stiffness and strength of meniscal tissue correspond to local differences in collagen ultrastructure and fiber bundle orientation.

In compression, the meniscal tissue should be considered a biphasic composite material because of its composition of 75% in water and 25% in collagen and proteoglycan. During loading, most of the water is forced to flow through the matrix to redistribute within the tissue or exudate from the tissue. The high frictional drag forces associated with the water flow through the porous-permeable solid matrix give rise to time-dependent viscoelastic behaviors such as creep and stress relaxation. The significance of the viscoelastic behavior of the meniscus is that when the joint is loaded for long periods, the contact area increases, thereby reducing the stress per unit area of the tissue. The concentration of proteoglycans influences the viscoelastic behavior of the meniscus because their negative charges counteract fluid flow.

Material properties are also very important for meniscal behavior in tension. Variations in tensile stiffness and strength are found in different regions and relate to local differences in collagen fiber ultrastructure and fiber bundle orientation. Intact tie fibers are also very important as they restrain motion between circumferential fibers and improve the stiffness characteristics of the meniscus (Bullough et al. 1970). The importance of the integrity of the collagen network cannot be overemphasized because disruption of this precise collagen ultrastructure directly results in alterations in tissue biomechanics predisposing to tearing and clinically significant loss of meniscal function (Thieman et al. 2009).

Meniscal function

The material properties of the meniscus are closely related to its function. The combination of low compressive stiffness and low permeability suggests that the menisci are highly efficient shock absorbers in the stifle. This is crucial for the activities of dogs. When the menisci are subjected to loading during weight bearing activities, they act as "firm pillows" between the femoral and tibial condyles. Based on their viscoelastic properties, the wedge-shaped menisci also adapt to the incongruent articular surfaces until fluid flow ceases as equilibrium is reached. Repeated compressive loading and unloading of menisci create a circulation pathway that is important for tissue nutrition and joint lubrication (Arnoczky et al. 1980).

Another important concept for understanding the role of the meniscus as a shock absorber is the hoop tension theory. Shrive et al. (1978) proposed that the meniscus is able to absorb high loads across the joint by converting the compressive forces into radially directed forces. The theory has been confirmed in dogs by direct measurement of hoop strain and contact pressures of the medial meniscus (Pozzi et al. 2010b). As the meniscus is loaded, the cranial and the caudal attachments of the meniscus are tensioned along with the circumferential fibers to prevent the meniscus from extruding (Figure 4.4). The tension developed in the circumferential fibers from the cranial to the caudal attachments is called "hoop tension." The integrity of both collagen network and meniscal attachments is critical for the hoop tension to develop. A transection of the meniscus or its attachments disrupts completely the primary functions of the meniscus because it eliminates the hoop tension (Pozzi et al. 2008, 2010a).

The meniscus contributes to stifle stability and joint kinematics by enhancing congruity between the convex tibial plateau and the round femoral condyle. The increased congruity is important for static stability. In the normal stifle, the CrCL is considered a primary restraint, while the menisci act as secondary stabilizers. In the CrCL-deficient stifle, the menisci become primary stabilizers of the uncontrolled translation and rotation of the joint. The caudal pole of the medial meniscus is particularly important in providing this stability and, as such, is at highest risk of injury if excessive femorotibial motion is present, such as in the CrCL-deficient stifle (Pozzi et al. 2006).

The contributions of the menisci to joint congruity and stability in both intact and CrCL-deficient stifles suggest that a functionally intact meniscus should be preserved whenever possible. This approach may be especially important in the CrCL-deficient stifle that may significantly benefit from the stabilizing effects of the meniscus for improving already disrupted joint kinematics. If this approach is selected, protecting the menisci by stabilizing the joint with a technique that most optimally reestablishes normal kinematics becomes crucial. On the other hand, it could be argued that leaving intact menisci in a CrCL-deficient stifle puts them at an unacceptable risk for subsequent damage, driving the need for additional surgery. This latter argument has been used as the rationale for meniscal release or meniscectomy in tibial plateau leveling osteotomy (TPLO) and tibial tuberosity advancement (TTA) treated CrCL-deficient stifles for the last 15 years (see Chapters 25 & 26). Meniscal release eliminates

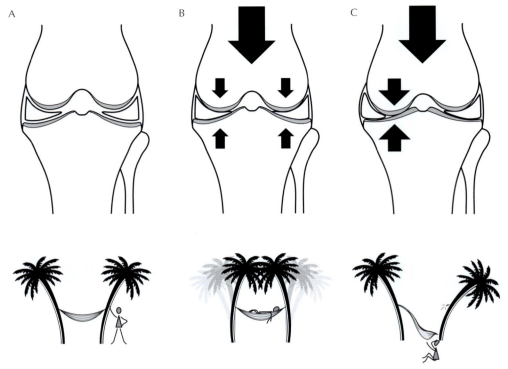

Figure 4.4 Schematic depiction of the hoop tension theory. (A,B) The intact meniscus acts as a hammock hanging under tension between the palms. The hammock holds a person only if it is firmly secured to the palms. Similarly, the meniscus acts as a load-bearing structure only if its ligaments are firmly anchored to the tibia. (C) If the anchorage of the hammock is cut, the person falls on the ground. The failure of the hammock is caused by its inability to develop the tension between the two palms. Similarly, a transected meniscus (meniscal release) cannot develop the hoop tension (tension between the palms) to function as a load-bearing structure. Copyright © Samantha J. Elmhurst at www.livingart.org.uk.

important functions in the stifle joint but may decrease the risk of subsequent meniscal tear. As such, the surgeon needs to make treatment decisions regarding the menisci carefully and with informed client consent (see Chapters 31 and 32).

References

Adams ME, Ho YA. Localization of glycosaminoglycans in human and canine menisci and their attachments. Connect Tissue Res 1987;16:269–279.

Adams ME, Muir H. The glycosaminoglycans of canine menisci. Biochem J 1981;197:385–389.

Arnoczky SP. Pathomechanics of cruciate ligaments and meniscal injuries. In: Disease Mechanisms in Small Animal Surgery, Bojrab MJ (ed.), second edition. Philadelphia: Lea & Febiger, 1993, pp. 764–776.

Arnoczky SP, Warren RF. The microvasculature of the meniscus and its response to injury: An experimental study in the dog. Am J Sports Med 1983;11:131–141.

Arnoczky SP, Marshall JL, Joseph A, et al. Meniscal diffusion: An experimental study in the dog. Trans Orthop Res Soc 1980;5:42.

Bullough PG, Munuera L, Murphy J, et al. The strength of the menisci of the knee as it relates to their fine structure. J Bone Joint Surg Br 1970;52:564–567.

Carpenter DH, Cooper RC. Mini review of canine stifle joint anatomy. Anat Histol Embryol 2000;29:321–329.

Cheung HS. Distribution of type I, II, III, V in the pepsin solubilized collagen in bovine menisci. Connect Tissue Res 1987;16:343–356.

Cook JL, Tomlinson JL, Kreeger JM, Cook CR. Induction of meniscal regeneration in dogs using a novel biomaterial. Am J Sports Med 1999;27:658–665.

Evans HE. The skeleton, arthrology, the muscular system. In: Miller's Anatomy of the Dog, Evans HE (ed.), third edition. Philadelphia: WB Saunders, 1993, pp. 122–384.

Eyre DR, Wu JJ. Collagen of fibrocartilage: A distinctive molecular phenotype in bovine meniscus. FEBS Lett 1983;158:265–270.

Helio Le Graverand MP, Ou Y, Schield-Yee T, et al. The cells of the rabbit meniscus: Their arrangement, interrelationship, morphological variations and cytoarchitecture. J Anat 2001;198:525–535.

Hulse DA, Shires PK. The meniscus: Anatomy, function and treatment. Comp Cont Ed Pract Vet 1983;5:765–774.

Noone TJ, Millis DL, Korvick DL, et al. Influence of canine recombinant somatotropin hormone on biomechanical and biochemiscal properties of the medial meniscus in stifles with altered stability. Am J Vet Res 2002;63:419–426.

Pozzi A, Kowaleski MP, Apelt D, et al. Effect of medial meniscal release on tibial translation following tibial plateau leveling osteotomy. Vet Surg 2006;35:486–494.

Pozzi A, Litsky AS, Field J, et al. Effect of medial meniscal release on load transmission following tibial plateau leveling osteotomy. Vet Comp Orthop Traumatol 2008;17:198–203.

Pozzi A, Kim SE, Lewis DD. Effect of transection of the caudal menisco-tibial ligament on medial femorotibial contact mechanics. Vet Surg 2010a, in press.

Pozzi A, Tonks CA, Ling H. Medial meniscus contact mechanics and strain following serial meniscectomies in a cadaveric dog study. Vet Surg 2010b, in press.

Ralphs SC, Whitney WO. Arthroscopic evaluation of menisci in dogs with cranial cruciate ligament injuries: 100 cases (1999–2000). J Am Vet Med Assoc 2002;221:1601–1604.

Stephan JS, McLaughlin RM, Griffith G. Water content and glycosaminoglycan disaccharide concentration of the canine meniscus. Am J Vet Res 1998;59:213–216.

Shrive NG, O'Connor JJ, Goodfellow JW, et al. Load-bearing in the knee joint. Clin Orthop 1978;131:279–287.

Thieman KM, Pozzi A, Ling HY, et al. Contact mechanics of simulated meniscal tears in cadaveric canine stifles. Vet Surg 2009;38:803–810.

5 Biomechanics of the Normal and Cranial Cruciate Ligament-Deficient Stifle

Antonio Pozzi and Stanley E. Kim

Normal stifle

The stifle is a complex, diarthrodial, synovial joint that allows motion in three planes (Figure 5.1). The round femoral condyles articulate with the flat tibial condyles with a range-of-motion about the medial–lateral axis of approximately 120°. Normal stifle angles range from 160° in full extension, to 40° in full flexion (Jaegger et al. 2002; Allen et al. 2009). The flexion–extension motion occurs through a combination of rolling and gliding of the femur on the tibia. With rolling alone, the femoral condyle would roll off the tibial plateau before maximum flexion is achieved, whereas with gliding alone, the femoral shaft would impinge on the tibia. Rollback is asymmetric: femorotibial contact translates more caudally on the lateral than on the medial plateau, resulting in internal tibial rotation during stifle flexion (Vasseur & Arnoczky 1981). This change in rotational constraint over a range-of-motion, which also occurs in the human knee, has been termed the "screw-home" mechanism.

Due to the slight tibial translation in the sagittal plane that is coupled with flexion and extension, it is clear that the stifle does not function as a pure hinge joint. Medial–lateral and proximal–distal translation is tightly constrained by the collateral ligaments but still allow for rotation about the medial–lateral and longitudinal axes. Although the rotational motion about the medial–lateral axis far exceeds the motion about the other two axes, approximately 20° of varus–valgus and internal–external rotation occurs over an entire walking-gait cycle in normal dogs (Korvick et al. 1994). Understanding stifle kinematics in three dimensions rather than simply attempting to address craniocaudal stability is important for the treatment of cranial cruciate ligament (CrCL) deficiency. Both lack of neutralization (e.g., tibial osteotomies) and absolute constraint (e.g., extracapsular stabilization) of internal–external rotation may lead to abnormal mechanical stresses on the articular surfaces and progression of osteoarthritis (Chailleux et al. 2007; Kim et al. 2008).

The patellofemoral joint is an important contributor to complex stifle biomechanics. The patella acts as a pulley mechanism to improve efficiency of stifle extension, as it increases the lever arm of the quadriceps mechanism by lengthening the distance between the quadriceps muscle force and the center of flexion–extension rotation

---

Advances in the Canine Cranial Cruciate Ligament,
Edited by Peter Muir, © 2010 ACVS Foundation, This Work is a co-publication between the American College of Veterinary Surgeons Foundation and Wiley-Blackwell.

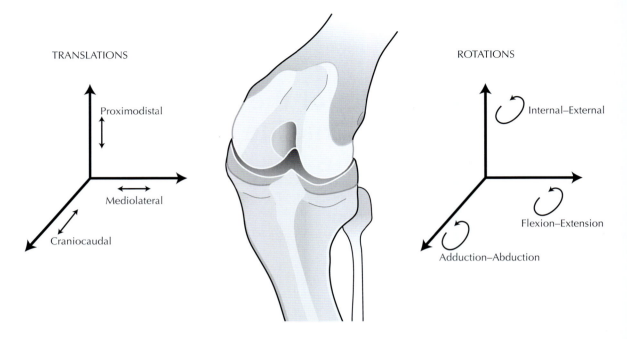

Figure 5.1 Drawing illustrating the six degrees of freedom of the femorotibial articulation. The femur and the tibia rotate and translate about the three axes shown in the drawing. Copyright © Samantha J. Elmhurst at www.livingart.org.uk.

of the stifle. In doing so, a significant force compressing the patella against the femoral condyle is generated as the muscle contracts. This retropatellar force is an important contributor to the stability of the patellofemoral joint and results in a force acting on the distal femur in the cranial–caudal direction. The balance of extensor and flexor moments acting at the stifle joint contributes to dynamic stability (Tepic et al. 2002).

Unlike most other diarthrodial joints in the dog, the bony congruency between the femoral condyle and the tibial plateau adds little to the stability of the stifle. Rather, primary and secondary soft tissue stabilizers provide stability to the stifle. The CrCL acts as a primary stabilizer for both cranial–caudal translation and internal–external rotation. The caudal cruciate ligament (CaCL) has a primary role in limiting caudal tibial translation and also helps to limit excessive internal–external rotation (Arnoczky & Marshall 1977). The menisci act as secondary stabilizers. The degree to which they contribute to joint stability is dependent on the condition of the primary stabilizers, in particular the CrCL. In a CrCL-deficient stifle, the medial meniscus plays a role in primary stabilization, acting as a wedge opposing femoral condyle translation and rotation (Pozzi et al. 2006). The increased mobility of the lateral meniscus does not allow it to act as a wedge between the femur and the tibia, and may protect it from impingement and tearing. Other passive stabilizers include the collateral ligaments and the joint capsule.

The dynamic stability of the stifle in various daily activities is provided by a delicate interplay between passive stabilizers and active musculature. The stifle is controlled mostly by two-joint muscles that cross either the hip and the stifle, or the stifle and the hock. Contraction of one of these muscles alone produces movement of all the joints that the muscle crosses. To isolate movement at a single joint, the two-joint muscles contract with other muscles, frequently with a one-joint synergist. Synergism between muscle–tendon units crossing the stifle is found between the quadriceps and the hamstrings, which simultaneously contract during activity (co-

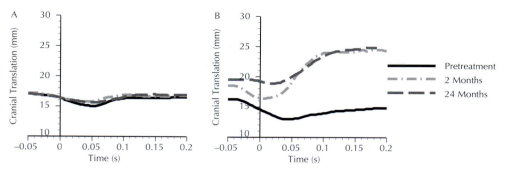

Figure 5.2 Craniocaudal translation of the tibia relative to the femur during the stance phase of gait in cranial cruciate ligament (CrCL) intact (A) and CrCL-deficient (B) dogs. Data represent baseline before CrCL transection or sham CrCL transection, 2 months after surgery, and 24 months after surgery. Note that there are clear changes in tibial translation after CrCL transection, whereas there is relatively little laxity in the intact CrCL during locomotion. Over time, cranial translation of the tibia becomes incrementally worse, suggesting that periarticular fibrosis does not provide much dynamic stability to the CrCL-deficient stifle. Reproduced from Tashman et al. (2004), with permission from Wiley-Blackwell.

contraction). Co-contraction is considered an important mechanism in functional adaptation in human patients with anterior cruciate ligament deficiency, but further research is needed to understand its role in dogs.

The clinician needs to understand all the motions in the stifle joint that are normally limited by the ligaments, to perform and interpret manual stress tests and correctly determine the abnormality. The term *instability* has been used to describe an abnormal motion that exists to the joint due to a ligament injury. The term *laxity* simply indicates increases in motion or looseness detected during palpation tests or stifle examination, without providing direct indication of whether abnormal motion occurs *in vivo*. The goal of a comprehensive stifle examination is to detect an increase in the amount of motion (translation or rotation) or an abnormal position (subluxation) to determine the specific anatomic defect that is present. The manual stress examinations are designed to test only one or two motions at a time. Therefore, the diagnosis cannot be based solely on the abnormal motion detected with a single manual stress. The diagnosis requires knowledge of stifle biomechanics and which ligaments limit each of the possible motions in the stifle. Ultimately, the clinical examination must be interpreted considering the stifle in a six degrees of freedom system, recognizing that six possible motions may occur three dimensions.

Cranial cruciate ligament-deficient stifle

The CrCL contributes to passive restraint of the stifle by limiting cranial translation of the tibia relative to the femur, excessive internal rotation of the tibia, and hyperextension of the stifle (Arnoczky & Marshall 1977). *In vivo* kinematic studies have demonstrated that most changes after CrCL transection are noted in the stance phase of the gait (Korvick et al. 1994; Tashman et al. 2004). Approximately 10 mm of cranial tibial translation is consistently observed and sustained throughout stance. Femorotibial alignment is restored during swing phase and is therefore largely unaffected by CrCL deficiency at a walk. The initial pattern of cranial translation progressively changes over time. Tashman et al. demonstrated that by 2 years after CrCL transection, the position of the tibia at the terminal swing is shifted cranially by approximately 5 mm (Figure 5.2). Thus, the decrease in dynamic instability was considered an indication of more persistent tibial subluxation throughout the gait cycle rather than a return toward normal stifle kinematics (Tashman et al. 2004). The *in vivo* investigations by Tashman et al. and Korvick et al. were performed in normal dogs with acute, experimental CrCL transection. It is likely that stifles affected by naturally occurring CrCL insufficiency in clinical dogs may not exhibit the same magnitude of subluxation, as

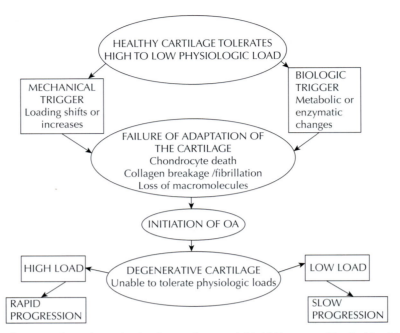

Figure 5.3 Diagram illustrating the pathomechanics theory of osteoarthritis (OA) proposed by Andriacchi et al. (2004). This theory suggests that the mechanical environment of the stifle influences the initiation and progression of osteoarthritis of the stifle. A healthy stifle can tolerate increased or decreased loads on the cartilage without developing osteoarthritis. In contrast, a joint with abnormal kinematics and contact pressure (i.e., shift of contact areas) responds to high or low loads with progression of osteoarthritis. Therefore, decreasing load on degenerated cartilage may decrease progression of osteoarthritis. Notice that biologic, as well as mechanical, factors can act as the trigger for osteoarthritis.

periarticular fibrosis often exists at the time of complete CrCL rupture (Hayashi et al. 2004).

The cranial tibial subluxation occurring during the stance phase of gait may be driven by the quadriceps contraction among other factors (Korvick et al. 1994; Tashman et al. 2004). In the dog, the moment across the joint is flexor from ground contact until mid-stance, and then extensor until the end of the stance phase (Colborne et al. 2005). Quadriceps contraction at extended joint angles produces CrCL strain, but in the CrCL-deficient stifle in flexion, quadriceps contraction cannot load the CrCL or cause tibial subluxation. Thus, during the swing phase, quadriceps activation on a flexed stifle does not cause subluxation, suggesting that the swing phase is CrCL independent in the dog (Korvick et al. 1994; Tashman et al. 2004).

The CrCL is a passive restraint to excessive internal tibial rotation, and *ex vivo* studies simulating weight-bearing demonstrated 14° internal tibial rotation after CrCL transection (Warzee et al. 2001; Kim et al. 2009). Articular surface geometry and lower tension in the lateral collateral ligament with the stifle in extension were thought to have induced this axial rotational malalignment (Warzee et al. 2001; Kim et al. 2009). Excessive peak internal rotation in CrCL-deficient stifles, however, has not been observed *in vivo* (Tashman et al. 2004). This suggests the muscular forces about the stifle, which have not been reproduced in bench-top studies, are the primary stabilizers against abnormal axial rotation, and the CrCL is a secondary rotational stabilizer at a walk or trot. High-demand activities, however, may generate higher axial torques that overcome muscular compensation, and elicit abnormal rotational stability in CrCL-deficient stifles. Such investigations have yet to be performed in the dog.

Joints and joint structures are complex systems whose components are interdependent on one another and are constantly altering their cellular and molecular mechanisms to maintain and restore tissue homeostasis. In the stifle, CrCL function is fundamentally important in maintaining tissue homeostasis of other structures such as the meniscus and cartilage. In an attempt to maintain stifle function and tissue homeostasis, these abnormal stresses on compensating joint structures can then result in their adaptation or their failure. This concept has led to the idea that there is an envelope of function or a range of loading that is compatible with overall homeostasis. Loads above or below this "zone of homeostasis" may lead to pathologic changes. *In vivo* three-dimensional kinematic studies have shown that the dog has little capability for eliminating craniocaudal instability via neuromuscular compensation to stay in the "zone of homeostasis" (Korvick et al. 1994; Tashman et al. 2004; Anderst & Tashman 2009). In addition, both cadaveric and *in vivo* studies have reported abnormal contact mechanics and increased tangential shear loading caused by femorotibial subluxation (Pozzi et al. 2006; Anderst & Tashman 2009). These alterations in stifle biomechanics are likely an important factor in osteoarthritis progression in the CrCL-deficient stifle. Cranial tibial subluxation results in a spatial shift of loading patterns to where articular cartilage is unable to accommodate these loads, inducing osteoarthritis (Andriacchi et al. 2004; Figure 5.3). Cartilage metabolism is dependent on the maintenance of the mechanical stimuli that the chondrocytes are adapted for (Carter et al. 2004). Therefore, reduced or increased loading of specific regions of the articular cartilage may trigger cartilage breakdown. To prevent osteoarthritis, surgical treatment of the CrCL-deficient stifle should aim at restoring normal joint function. For an optimal outcome, not only craniocaudal instability should be restored, but also normal three-dimensional kinematics and contact mechanics should be obtained after surgical stabilization of the joint. While aiming at normal joint biomechanics is crucial when selecting surgical techniques for stifle stabilization or CrCL repair, joint adaptation should be taken into account when selecting the treatment for the CrCL-deficient stifle. For example, a dog with a chronic CrCL-deficient stifle may be at a too advanced adaptation stage to allow significant improvement of its joint biomechanics. In this case, arthroscopy or arthrotomy

and meniscal treatment, followed by rehabilitation, may be selected over a stabilization technique (Tivers et al. 2009). Further work needs to be done to understand how differences in stage of CrCL rupture may play a role in treatment selection.

References

Allen MJ, Leone KA, Lamonte K, et al. Cemented total knee replacement in 24 dogs. Vet Surg 2009;38: 555–567.

Anderst WJ, Tashman S. The association between velocity of the center of closest proximity on subchondral bones and osteoarthritis progression. J Orthop Res 2009;27:71–77.

Andriacchi TP, Mündermann A, Smith RL, et al. A framework for the in vivo pathomechanics of osteoarthritis at the knee. Ann Biomed Eng 2004;32:447–457.

Arnoczky SP, Marshall JL. The cruciate ligaments of the canine stifle: An anatomical and functional analysis. Am J Vet Res 1977;38:1807–1814.

Carter DR, Beaupre GS, Wong M, et al. The mechanobiology of articular cartilage development and degeneration. Clin Orthop Relat Res 2004;427:S69–77.

Chailleux N, Lussier B, De Guise J, et al. In vitro 3-dimensional kinematic evaluation of 2 corrective operations for cranial cruciate ligament-deficient stifle. Can J Vet Res 2007;71:175–180.

Colborne GR, Innes JF, Comerford EJ, et al. Distribution of power across the hind limb joints in Labrador retrievers and greyhounds. Am J Vet Res 2005;66: 1563–1571.

Hayashi K, Manley PA, Muir P. Cranial cruciate ligament physiology in dogs with cruciate disease: A review. J Am Anim Hosp Assoc 2004;40:385–390.

Jaegger G, Marcellin-Little DJ, Levine D. Reliability of goniometry in Labrador retrievers. Am J Vet Res 2002;63:979–986.

Kim SE, Pozzi A, Kowaleski MP, et al. Tibial osteotomies for cranial cruciate ligament insufficiency in dogs. Vet Surg 2008;37:111–125.

Kim SE, Pozzi A, Banks SA, Conrad B, et al. Effect of tibial plateau leveling osteotomy on femorotibial contact mechanics and stifle kinematics. Vet Surg 2009;38:33–39.

Korvick DL, Pijanowski GJ, Schaeffer DJ. Three-dimensional kinematics of the intact and cranial cruciate ligament-deficient stifle of dogs. J Biomech 1994;27: 77–87.

Pozzi A, Kowaleski MP, Apelt D, et al. Effect of medial meniscal release on tibial translation after tibial plateau leveling osteotomy. Vet Surg 2006;35:486–494.

Tashman S, Anderst W, Kolowich P, et al. Kinematics of the ACL deficient canine knee during gait: Serial changes over two years. J Orthop Res 2004;22: 931–941.

Tivers MS, Commerford EJ, Owen MR. Does a fabella-tibial suture alter the outcome for dogs with cranial cruciate ligament insufficiency undergoing arthrotomy and caudal pole medial meniscectomy? Vet Comp Orthop Traumatol 2009;22:283–288.

Tepic S, Damur DM, Montavon PM. Biomechanics of the stifle joint. *Proceedings of the 1st World Orthopaedic Veterinary Congress.* Munich, Germany, 2002, pp. 189–190.

Vasseur PB, Arnoczky SP. Collateral ligaments of the canine stifle joint: Anatomic and functional analysis. Am J Vet Res 1981;42:1133–1137.

Warzee CC, Dejardin LM, Arnoczky SP, et al. Effect of tibial plateau leveling on cranial and caudal tibial thrusts in canine cranial cruciate-deficient stifles: An in vitro experimental study. Vet Surg 2001;30:278–286.

Section II

Etiopathogenesis of Cruciate Ligament Rupture

Introduction

Historically cranial cruciate ligament (CrCL) rupture in dogs has been considered a consequence of accidental injury, with subsequent development of stifle arthritis. However, particularly since the late 1980s, this paradigm has been challenged. It was established that a high risk of contralateral CrCL rupture existed in affected dogs and that the typical history and clinical signs of CrCL rupture could not easily be explained by traumatic injury. Recent work has clearly shown that stifle arthritis precedes the development of CrCL rupture and associated stifle instability in the majority of affected dogs. A logical extension of this paradigm shift in thinking is to ask the following question: What causes stifle arthritis to develop in affected dogs with clinically stable stifles? A comprehensive understanding of the answer to this question will likely drive new developments in the clinical management of canine patients affected with the cruciate rupture arthropathy.

6 Histology of Cranial Cruciate Ligament Rupture

Kei Hayashi and Peter Muir

Pathology of cranial cruciate ligament rupture

The exact etiopathogenesis of canine cranial cruciate ligament (CrCL) rupture is not defined. Although acute CrCL rupture does occur with trauma, a number of previous studies have suggested that the majority of CrCL ruptures are the result of chronic degenerative changes within the ligament (Vasseur et al. 1985; Hayashi et al. 2003a).

Development of progressive CrCL rupture appears to involve a gradual degeneration of CrCL itself, inflammatory disease in the stifle joint, partial CrCL rupture, and, eventually, complete rupture. After rupture, secondary changes such as progressive arthritis and meniscal injury often develop. Initially, slight weakening or stretching of the CrCL may not cause lameness but can produce mild joint instability and therefore promote arthritic joint degeneration. However, it is unclear whether this represents the initial phase of the arthropathy, or whether development of stifle synovitis is the initial event. Dogs with incip-

ient cruciate rupture often have a stable joint clinically, but are presented with lameness, effusion of the stifle joint, and synovitis. Complete CrCL rupture produces obvious instability of the stifle joint, resulting in more severe joint pain, lameness, and progressive degenerative changes within the joint. Clinical observations have demonstrated that these changes consist of periarticular osteophyte formation, capsular thickening, and meniscal damage. As these changes progress, the joints may become more stable, although a recent experimental study suggests that periarticular fibrosis does little to improve dynamic instability during locomotion (Tashman et al. 2004). Dogs with advanced or end-stage pathologic changes within the stifle may have little palpable passive instability because of extensive periarticular fibrosis. After a partial or complete CrCL rupture, some degree of tissue repair response arises in the epiligamentous region of the CrCL (Hayashi et al. 2003a). In human anterior cruciate ligament (ACL), distinct histologic phases of tissue repair, including an inflammatory phase, an epiligamentous repair phase, a proliferative phase, and a remodeling phase develop after rupture (Murray et al. 2000). Whether similar phases exist in dogs is not known. Expansion of the volume of the epiligamentous tissue does occur in the dog during a repair phase that lasts many weeks. However, a bridging scar does not form in the rupture site.

Advances in the Canine Cranial Cruciate Ligament,
Edited by Peter Muir, © 2010 ACVS Foundation, This Work is a co-publication between the American College of Veterinary Surgeons Foundation and Wiley-Blackwell.

Eventually, synovial tissue covers the ruptured ends of the CrCL.

Histologic features of cruciate ligament

The CrCL is a complex structure consisting of an extracellular matrix and a diverse population of cells. It has distinctive histologic features typical of dense collagenous connective tissues (ligaments and tendons). The extracellular matrix proteins in CrCL are primarily composed of type I collagen. Bundles of collagen fibers are longitudinally oriented, mostly running parallel to one another. Normal CrCL collagen fibers have a recurrent undulating wave or crimped structure (Figure 6.1; Hayashi et al. 2003a). The human ACL has been shown to also contain collagen types III, IV, V, and VI, and other extracellular matrix molecules including glycosaminoglycans, fibronectin, laminin, entactin, tenascin, and undulin (Neurath & Stofft 1992). The matrix of the CrCL represents a complicated regulatory network of proteins, glycoproteins, viscoelastic fibers, and glycosaminoglycans with multiple functional interactions.

The predominant cell type in the CrCL is the fibroblast. Ligament fibroblasts are arranged in long parallel rows between collagen fiber bundles. In human ACL, three different phenotypes of fibroblasts have been described: fusiform or spindle-shaped, ovoid, and spheroid (Murray & Spector 1999). The cytoplasm of fusiform fibroblasts is intimately attached to the extracellular collagen and follows the crimped waveform of the fibers. Ovoid and spheroid fibroblasts are situated in the loose connective tissue between collagen fibers. It is presently unclear whether these cells represent differing metabolic states of the same cells or whether they are distinctly different fibroblasts.

A histologic study of human ACL identified three histologically different zones along the anteromedial bundle as it coursed from the femoral to the tibial attachment (Murray & Spector 1999). Two of the zones, the fusiform and ovoid, were located in the proximal one quarter of the bundle. The third spheroid zone occupied the distal three quarters of the fiber bundles. The fusiform cell zone was characterized by a high number density of longitudinally oriented cells with fusiform-shaped nuclei, longitudinal blood vessels, and high crimp lengths. The cytoplasm of the cells in this zone appeared to be intimately attached to the extracellular collagen and followed the crimp waveform of the fibers. The ovoid cell zone was characterized by a high number density of cells with ovoid-shaped nuclei, longitudinal vessels, and high crimp lengths. In this zone as well, the cytoplasm of the cells appeared to follow the waveform of the adjacent collagen. The spheroid cell zone was characterized by a low density of spheroid cells, few blood vessels, and a short crimp length. Cells were noted within and among fascicles, as well as within lacunae. The role of the various fibroblast phenotypes in the maintenance of the human ACL is not known.

The histologic structure of the cruciate ligament is not homogeneous. In ACL, it has been reported that there is a zone where the tissue resembles fibrocartilage (Petersen & Tillmann 1999). The fibrocartilaginous zone is located 5–10 mm proximal of the tibial ligament insertion in the anterior portion of the ligament. Within this zone, the cells are arranged in columns and the cell shape is round to ovoid. Transmission electron microscopy reveals typical features of chondrocytes. These chondrocyte-like cells are surrounded by a felt-like pericellular matrix, a high content of cellular organelles, and short processes on the cell surface. The pericellular collagen is positive for type II collagen. An avascular zone is located within the fibrocartilage of the anterior part where the ligament faces the anterior rim of the intercondylar fossa. It has been proposed that the stimulus for the development of fibrocartilage within dense connective tissue is shearing and compressive stress (Milz et al. 2005). In the ACL, this biomechanical situation may occur when the ligament impinges on the anterior rim of the intercondylar fossa when the knee is fully extended (Quasnichka et al. 2005).

Histopathology of the canine cranial cruciate ligament

The canine CrCL undergoes a partial fibrocartilagenous transformation as described in human ACL, which may represent chronic and irreversible degeneration. This idiopathic degeneration is

Histology of Cranial Cruciate Ligament Rupture   47

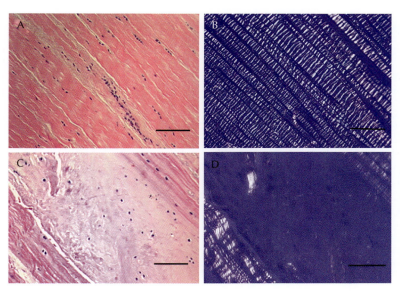

Figure 6.1 Longitudinal sections of intact (A,B) and ruptured CrCL (C,D) from a 2-year-old ovariohysterectomized beagle and a 7-year-old castrated male golden retriever, respectively, viewed using bright light (A,C) and circularly polarized light (B,D) microscopy. (A,B) Intact CrCL from young dogs has a hierarchically organized structure. Birefringence of the extracellular matrix collagen and the crimped structure of collagen fiber bundles are clearly visible in polarized light. (C,D) The disorganized regions of the extracellular matrix in ruptured CrCL exhibit loss of birefringence and crimp, as well as loss of ligament fibroblasts. Bars = 100 μm. Reproduced from Hayashi et al. (2003a), with permission from Wiley-Blackwell.

a common histologic finding of intact CrCL, despite its grossly normal appearance. A histologic study reported that the CrCL of dogs weighing more than 15 kg consistently had microscopic evidence of degenerative changes by 5 years of age (Vasseur et al. 1985). These changes are characterized by loss of ligamentocytes, metaplasia of surviving ligamentocytes to chondrocytes, and failure to maintain collagen fiber bundles, which progressed in severity with age. The CrCL in dogs weighing less than 15 kg generally had less severe alterations than those in heavier dogs, and the onset of the degenerative process was delayed by several years. The deep core region of the CrCL deteriorates earlier than the superficial epiligamentous region, and the mid-portion of the CrCL deteriorates earlier than regions close to bony attachments.

In ruptured CrCL, more severe changes such as hyalinization, mineralization, and cloning of chondrocyte-like cells can also occur. However, inflammatory or reparative responses are rarely observed (Hayashi et al. 2003a). Significant loss of fibroblasts from the core region of ruptured CrCL occurs. In contrast, cell number densities are similar in ruptured and intact CrCL in the epiligamentous region (Hayashi et al. 2003a,b). In ruptured CrCL, numbers of typical ligament fibroblasts (fusiform and ovoid cells) are decreased, and in the core region numbers of cells exhibiting chondroid transformation (spheroid cells) are increased (Figures 6.1–6.3). The structure of the extracellular matrix collagen in the core region is extensively disrupted in ruptured CrCL. Rupture of the CrCL is also associated with disruption of the hierarchical architecture of extracellular matrix collagen, with loss of the normal crimp and loss of birefringence (Figures 6.1, 6.2, and 6.4). A histologic study reported that crimp was no longer detectable in many ligament specimens from dogs with CrCL rupture (Figures 6.1, 6.4, and 6.5) (Hayashi et al. 2003a). Interestingly, in the ruptured CrCL specimens in which crimp was still detectable, crimp length was significantly increased, and crimp angle tended to be lower, compared with intact CrCL from young dogs (Figure 6.5; Hayashi et al. 2003a). These data suggest that the remaining organized collagen experiences mechanical over-

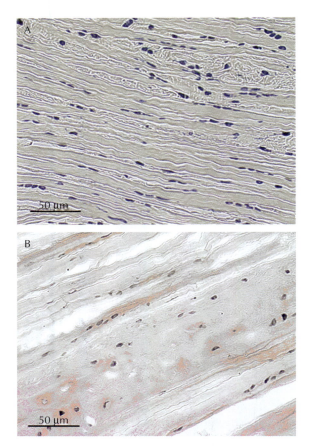

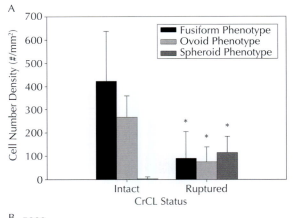

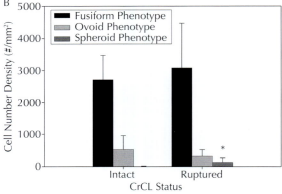

Figure 6.2 Photomicrographs of longitudinal frozen sections of intact cranial cruciate ligament (CrCL) from a 2-year-old ovariohysterectomized beagle (A) and an 8-year-old ovariohysterectomized Labrador retriever (B) obtained via bright light microscopy. Specimens were stained histochemically for lactate dehydrogenase (LDH), a marker of cell viability. (A) Central part of the core region of the intact CrCL from a young dog. Notice parallel rows of fusiform and ovoid LDH-stained ligament fibroblasts, with an organized extracellular matrix containing crimped collagen fibers. (B) Central part of the core region of the intact CrCL from an old dog. Notice the decreased number of ligament fibroblasts; many cells are devitalized (weak staining for LDH) with an ovoid phenotype. Collagen fibers within the extracellular matrix have also been disrupted. Bar = 50 μm.

Figure 6.3 Relationship of cell number densities to cranial cruciate ligament (CrCL) rupture status in the core (A) and epiligamentous (B) regions of interest. *Columns are significantly different from intact CrCL ($p < 0.05$). Reproduced from Hayashi et al. (2003a), with permission from Wiley-Blackwell.

load that elongates the crimp within the collagen fibers, as progressive CrCL rupture develops over time, thereby causing the collagen to have a longer crimp length and a smaller crimp angle. These findings also support the general hypothesis that microinjury to the ligament from mechanical overload may form an important part of the mechanically induced signaling events that orchestrate CrCL remodeling and may be a key factor in the mechanism that leads to gradual CrCL rupture over time.

Fibroblast viability and metabolism are different in young intact, aged intact, and ruptured CrCL (Hayashi et al. 2003b). Metabolically active viable fibroblasts detected by a metabolic marker, lactate dehydrogenase (LDH), were seen in all intact and ruptured CrCLs. However, the number of nonviable cells in the core region of ruptured CrCLs was greater than that in intact CrCLs of young and aged dogs (Figures 6.6 and 6.7).

Histology of Cranial Cruciate Ligament Rupture   49

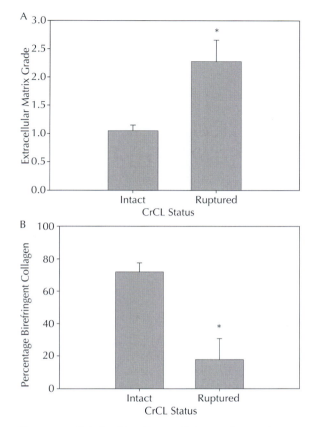

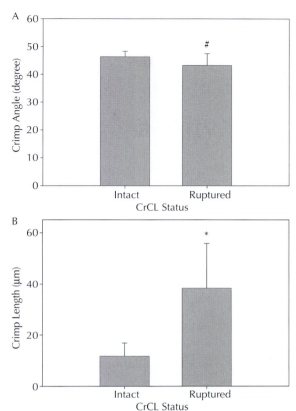

Figure 6.4 Relationship of extracellular matrix organization (A) and collagen birefringence (B) to cranial cruciate ligament (CrCL) rupture status in the core region of interest. CrCL were graded using a numerical rating scale (1: highly organized fibrous tissue structure with parallel alignment and dense packing of collagen fibers; 2: partially disrupted organized fibrous structure of collagen fibers; 3: total loss of organized fibrous structure of collagen with homogenous appearance of the extracellular matrix), and values represent the mean of five fields of view. *Columns are significantly different from intact CrCL ($p < 0.05$). Reproduced from Hayashi et al. (2003a), with permission from Wiley-Blackwell.

Figure 6.5 Relationship of crimp angle (A) and crimp length (B) to cranial cruciate ligament (CrCL) rupture. *Significantly different from intact CrCL ($p < 0.05$). #Lower crimp angle compared with intact CrCL ($p < 0.15$). Reproduced from Hayashi et al. (2003a), with permission from Wiley-Blackwell.

Cruciate ligament adaptation and repair

Ruptured CrCLs have significantly higher amounts of immature collagen cross-links, total and sulfated GAGs and water content (cartilage-like material), and concentration of pro-MMP-2 (gelatinase), compared with those of the intact ligament (Comerford et al. 2004). These findings suggest that the extracellular matrix of ruptured CrCL has increased matrix turnover. Cartilage-like tissue is more vulnerable to disruption under normal tensile loading. Therefore, CrCL degeneration with fibrocartilaginous transformation may predispose CrCL to pathological rupture.

However, areas of fibrocartilage are also observed in grossly normal CrCL in low-risk breeds (greyhounds), when intrinsic extracellular matrix changes in the CrCLs of labrador retriever (high-risk breed) are compared with those in greyhounds (Comerford et al. 2006). Transmission electron microscopy revealed that the collagen fibril diameters of greyhounds were larger than

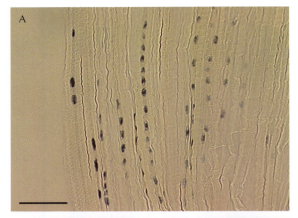

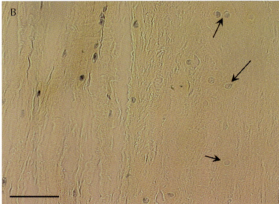

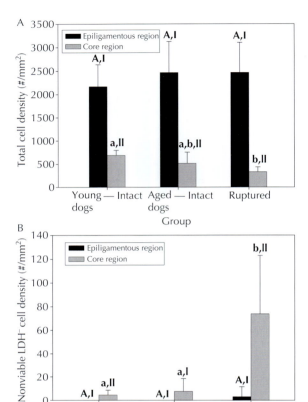

Figure 6.6 Photomicrographs of longitudinal frozen sections of ruptured cranial cruciate ligament (CrCL) from a 6-year-old ovariohysterectomized Labrador retriever obtained via bright light microscopy. Specimens were stained histochemically for lactate dehydrogenase (LDH), a marker of cell viability. (A) Periphery of the main axial tissue component (core) region of the ruptured CrCL. Notice parallel rows of fusiform and ovoid LDH-stained ligament fibroblasts, with an organized extracellular matrix containing crimped collagen fibers. (B) Central part of the core region of the ruptured CrCL. Notice the low number of ligament fibroblasts; many cells are devitalized (loss of LDH-positive staining) with a spheroid phenotype (black arrows). Most of the collagen fibrils within the extracellular matrix have been disrupted. Bar = 50 μm. Reproduced from Hayashi et al. (2003b), with permission from the American Veterinary Medical Association.

Figure 6.7 Relationship of total cell number densities to CrCL disease status in the epiligamentous and core regions of the CrCL (A), and relationship of nonviable lactate dehydrogenase (LDH) LDH⁻ cell densities to CrCL disease status in the epiligamentous and core regions of the CrCL (B). Columns within a region with differing upper or lower case letters are significantly different ($p < 0.05$). Columns within a CrCL status group with differing Roman numerals are significantly different. Reproduced from Hayashi et al. (2003b), with permission from the American Veterinary Medical Association.

those of Labrador retrievers, which may relate to tissue maturity and tissue's mechanical properties. Histology revealed that the fibrocartilagenous areas were found in both breeds. These observations suggest that the formation of fibrocartilage is clearly not a disadvantage to the healthy racing greyhounds and cannot be regarded as pathological degeneration in this breed. Fibrocartilage would appear to protect CrCLs in the greyhounds, but it may be indicative of a mild degenerative change in high-risk breeds that is a risk factor for rupture. It is currently unclear whether CrCL degeneration and transformation into fibrocartilage is a key pathologic change that is an important risk factor for eventual CrCL rupture in certain breeds of dog.

Conclusion

Taken together, current literature suggests that progressive rupture of the CrCL during the development of stifle instability is associated with histological changes to the matrix that include loss of ligament fibroblasts and chondroid transformation of surviving cells. Disruption of matrix collagen includes loss of crimp. Two central hypotheses have been proposed regarding the initial mechanism that leads to CrCL degeneration and then rupture:

1. A primary defect in the ligament tissue itself or in the metabolism of the CrCL that leads to partial rupture of the CrCL and development of microinstability of the stifle
2. Activation of synovial immune responses and development of a chronic synovitis that promotes CrCL degeneration, as ligament nutrition and metabolism are related to synovial fluid physiology.

These hypotheses are discussed further in other chapters in this section. Confirmation that one or both of these hypotheses is correct should be a focus of future work studying the mechanism for the CrCL rupture arthropathy in the dog.

References

Comerford EJ, Innes JF, Tarlton JF, Bailey AJ. Investigation of the composition, turnover, and thermal properties of rupture cranial cruciate ligaments of dogs. Am J Vet Res 2004;65:1136–1141.

Comerford EJ, Tarlton JF, Wales A, et al. Ultrastructural differences in cranial cruciate ligaments from dogs of two breeds with a differing predisposition to ligament degeneration and rupture. J Comp Pathol 2006;134: 8–16.

Hayashi K, Frank JD, Dubinsky C, et al. Histologic changes in ruptured canine cranial cruciate ligament. Vet Surg 2003a;32:269–277.

Hayashi K, Frank JD, Hao Z, et al. Evaluation of ligament fibroblast viability in ruptured cranial cruciate ligament of dogs. Am J Vet Res 2003b;64:1010–1016.

Milz S, Benjamin M, Putz R. Molecular parameters indicating adaptation to mechanical stress in fibrous connective tissue. Adv Anat Embryol Cell Biol 2005;178:1–71.

Murray MM, Spector M. Fibroblast distribution in the anteromedial bundle of the human anterior cruciate ligament: The presence of alpha-smooth muscle actin-positive cells. J Orthop Res 1999;17:18–27.

Murray MM, Martin SD, Martin TL, Spector M. Histological changes in the human anterior cruciate ligament after rupture. J Bone Joint Surg Am 2000; 82:1387–1397.

Neurath MF, Stofft E. Structure and function of matrix components in the cruciate ligaments. An immunohistochemical, electron-microscopic, and immunoelectron-microscopic study. Acta Anat 1992;145:387–394.

Petersen W, Tillmann B. Structure and vascularization of the cruciate ligaments of the human knee joint. Anat Embryol 1999;200:325–334.

Quasnichka HL, Anderson-MacKenzie JM, Tarlton JF, et al. Cruciate ligament laxity and femoral intercondylar notch narrowing in early-stage knee osteoarthritis. Arthritis Rheum 2005;52:3100–3109.

Tashman S, Anderst W, Kolowich P, et al. Kinematics of the ACL-deficient canine knee during gait: Serial changes over two years. J Orthop Res 2004;22: 931–941.

Vasseur PB, Pool RR, Arnoczky SP, Lau RE. Correlative biomechanical and histologic study of the cranial cruciate ligament in dogs. Am J Vet Res 1985;46: 1842–1854.

7 Genetics of Cranial Cruciate Ligament Rupture

Vicki Wilke

Introduction

Specific breeds of dogs appear to have an increased risk of cranial cruciate ligament (CrCL) rupture, while other breeds almost never experience the condition. This suggests a genetic predisposition. In addition, some breeds present with CrCL rupture at an early age, usually less than 2 years old, and often will have bilateral CrCL rupture. Again, the young age at presentation supports a heritable cause to the condition. The other typical presentation of this condition is a degenerative process that occurs when the animal is middle aged to older. It is unknown whether this difference in clinical presentation may represent variable expressivity of the disease, implying some dogs are more severely affected than others, or different etiopathogeneses. Environmental modifiers may also affect the expression of the trait; some potential modifiers include body condition score, sex, neuter status, and nutrition.

At present, CrCL rupture is considered a binary trait; dogs either are affected or are unaffected. The current gold standard of diagnosis is surgical confirmation of a ruptured CrCL, either completely or partially, which is typically paired with some other procedure. No phenotypic test has yet been evaluated to determine its correlation to CrCL rupture, although stifle radiographs are routinely performed as part of the diagnostic workup. Ideally, a genetic test would be utilized to identify dogs that are predisposed to the condition. This would allow identification of carriers of the trait and development of selective breeding strategies or counseling of clients on environmental modification to minimize the impact of the clinical course of the disease.

Screening

As previously mentioned, surgical confirmation is the gold standard for diagnosis of CrCL rupture. However, as clinicians, it is common to examine patients, particularly older patients, and detect the hallmarks of chronic CrCL rupture: a medial buttress, decreased range of motion, and crepitus within the stifle. Yet the patient is not before us for evaluation of lameness. These patients are considered to have chronic CrCL rupture and are nonetheless clinically not "affected" by the condition. In the more routine presentation, an animal is presented to the veterinarian for acute or chronic lameness, and either a partial or complete, unila-

Advances in the Canine Cranial Cruciate Ligament,
Edited by Peter Muir, © 2010 ACVS Foundation, This Work is a co-publication between the American College of Veterinary Surgeons Foundation and Wiley-Blackwell.

teral or bilateral CrCL rupture is diagnosed. In both of these clinical scenarios dogs are affected with CrCL rupture, yet most veterinarians are unlikely to perform surgery on an animal unless it is clinically affected with the condition. In the former scenario, the condition may not become a clinical problem until the patient is much older, if at all. If our goal is to reduce the incidence of the disease, what then is a reliable screening method to detect affected animals? Are two-view standard radiographs sensitive enough to detect early disease, without detectable instability and/or accompanying lameness? The ideal would be a combination of a genetic susceptibility test with concurrent supportive physical and radiographic examination findings.

Status ascertainment

CrCL rupture has a variable age of onset. This makes identification of an unaffected individual difficult, as they may be genetically predisposed but may not yet have developed the clinical course of the disease. In two separate studies, age of onset was evaluated for CrCL rupture. One study evaluated all Labrador retrievers presenting to a veterinary teaching hospital within a specified period of time, and another evaluated all breeds of dogs. For Labrador retrievers, only 6% were 8 years or older at the time of diagnosis of CrCL rupture, and when evaluating all breeds, only 11.3% were 11 years of age or older at time of CrCL rupture diagnosis (Rooney et al. 2002, Reif & Probst 2003). Therefore, one can reasonably assume that a dog over 8 years of age, and more conservatively over 11 years of age, is unlikely to develop CrCL rupture.

Population stratification

Rupture of the CrCL has been reported to be associated with different causes, including trauma, immune-mediated mechanisms (Niebauer et al. 1987; Galloway & Lester 1995; Lawrence et al. 1998), age-related degeneration of the CrCL (Vasseur et al. 1985), obesity (Whitehair et al. 1993), and conformational abnormalities such as a patella luxation (Aiken et al. 1995) and a narrowed

femoral intercondylar notch (Aiken et al. 1995; Shelbourne et al. 1998). This makes population stratification important for genetic analyses as not all affected individuals may be considered to have a genetic predisposition to the condition. Conversely, not stratifying the population based on the most likely cause of CrCL rupture will "dilute" the results and/or lead to false-positive associations between genetics and the trait. In summary, future genetic analyses should strive to properly ascertain the most likely cause of CrCL when selecting cases.

Segregation analysis

In initial studies, the Newfoundland breed of dog was selected for analyses based on a high incidence (22.4%) of the CrCL rupture trait (Wilke et al. 2006). Results of segregation analysis performed on a population of 411 Newfoundlands indicated that CrCL likely has an autosomal recessive mode of inheritance with 51% penetrance (Wilke et al. 2006). Penetrance is the proportion of individuals that have the mutation and express the phenotype; it is often confused with, but *is not*, equivalent to the level of expression of a trait. In this population, 92 Newfoundlands (53 female, 39 male) were CrCL rupture affected (22%) and 319 (182 female, 137 male) were CrCL rupture unaffected. The frequency of the recessive allele was 0.60. Heritability (narrow sense) was also estimated to be 0.27. This indicates an effect of environment on the expression of CrCL rupture. For comparison, a trait that is purely genetic has a heritability of 1.0.

Candidate gene analyses

The comparative candidate gene approach is dependent on the existence of a known mutation for a specific disorder in a particular species and the occurrence of the same disorder in the species of interest. No known comparative candidate gene exists that has been shown to cause the development of CrCL rupture.

The biological candidate gene approach relies on presumed knowledge of gene functions and their potential role in the disease etiology. In a study in a population of Newfoundland dogs, several genes were selected for analyses based on their known association with joint hypermobility in cattle or primary arthritis formation in humans. This included *Cartilage Oligomeric Matrix Protein* (*COMP*), *Collagen Type 9 alpha 1 and 2* (*COL9A1* and *COL9A2*), and *Fibrillin 1* (*FBN1*). Based on Chi-square analyses, there was no significant association between single nucleotide polymorphisms (SNPs) found within these genes and CrCL rupture status (affected and unaffected), although some suggestion of an association was found between *COL9A1* (located on chromosome 12 *Canis familiaris autosome* [CFA] 12) and CrCL rupture-affected status ($p = 0.10$; Wilke et al. 2005).

A more recent study evaluated microsatellite markers that are closely located to the genes *COL9A1*, *COL9A2*, and *COL9A3* in a population of boxers with a high incidence of CrCL rupture (Temwichitr et al 2007). Data from this study suggest that the genes studied are not related to CrCL rupture in the population studied. However, the microsatellites they identified could be possible candidates for other collagenopathies.

To further define the genetic basis of CrCL rupture, a genome-wide association study (GWAS), using microsatellites (MSATs), was performed in a population of Newfoundlands. A microsatellite is a variable repeating segment of DNA, usually found in a noncoding segment. A GWAS, or positional candidate gene approach, uses first the identification of a chromosomal region that is associated with a disorder, and then identification of all genes located in that region. The genes are then organized by function and selected according to possible involvement in development of CrCL rupture. A subset of the recruited Newfoundland dogs population ($n = 90$) were selected for the GWAS based on their degree of interrelationships within the pedigree and the statistical likelihood that they segregated into homozygous unaffected and homozygous affected animals (Macrossan et al. 2005). Age and other potential contributors to cause of CrCL rupture were not considered for population selection; cases were classified as either affected or unaffected with CrCL rupture.

A total of 495 of 532 MSATs were informative in the selected population with an average interval of 5.5 cM between markers. Comparisons of genotypes and allele frequencies were made between CrCL rupture affected and unaffected dogs. Eighty six markers were considered statistically significant based on the nominal $p < 0.05$, while four markers (located on four chromosomes) were significant when false discovery rate was controlled at the 0.05 level using the Storey and Tibshirani method (Storey et al. 2003, Wilke et al. 2009). The MSATs are CPH19 located on CFA 3, FH3702 located on CFA 5, REN147D07 located on CFA 13, and FH3750 located on CFA 24.

These markers were validated on the basis of genotyping additional closely located MSATs and genes. Validation of the significant markers is necessary to determine the biological importance of the identified markers and hence identification of which chromosomal regions to study further. Initial validation of the four markers confirmed significance of three chromosomes (CFA 3, 5, and 13, Table 7.1). Positional candidate genes located on CFA 3 have been sequenced for mutation identification: *Versican core protein precursor* (*VCAN*) and *Aggrecan core protein precursor* (*cartilage-specific protein core protein* [*CSPCP*]). Proteoglycans are major components of extracellular matrix of cartilage (Schwartz & Domowicz 2002). A significant association has been identified with a SNP found in *CSPCP*, but not *VCAN*, and the trait (Table 7.2).

Comparative aspect

The young (human) female athlete is another cohort that shares characteristics of the CrCL rupture phenotype found in dogs. This cohort experiences anterior cruciate ligament (ACL) injuries 2 to 8 times more frequently than their counterpart young athletic males (Arendt & Dick 1995; Gwinn et al. 2000; Lohmander et al. 2004). Usually, the most common cause of ACL tears in people is trauma. However, in this select population the injury usually occurs via noncontact mechanisms (Arendt & Dick 1995).

Several recent studies have evaluated the potential genetic contribution to ACL injuries in humans. The first was a case control study that found those with an ACL injury to be twice as likely to have had a family member with an ACL injury as those study participants that did not have an ACL injury (Flynn et al. 2005). Their findings support a familial predisposition to ACL injuries. Further research

Table 7.1 Microsatellite marker χ^2 results for validation of the four microsatellites found to be significantly associated with CrCL rupture

CFA, location Mb	MSAT name	Allele by status		Genotype by status	
		χ^2 value	Probability	χ^2 value	Probability
3, 68.3	03_068_CT	21.292	**<.0001**	18.917	**0.002**
5, 32.7	05_032_B_CAAA	7.571	**0.0227**	8.274	0.1418
5, 32.9	05_032F_CT	4.086	0.2523	5.961	0.5443
5, 33.2	05_033A_CA	8.448	0.0765	15.072	0.089
13, 32.6	13_032F_CT	6.792	0.1473	10.639	0.3013
13, 32.7	13_032I_CA	6.574	0.0868	10.599	0.1571
13, 33	13_032K_CA	6.866	**0.0323**	6.898	0.1414
13, 33.1	13_033A_CA	5.011	**0.0252**	4.844	0.0887
24, 3.5	24_003B_CA	2.972	0.3959	8.161	0.518
24, 3.7	24_003C_CT	0.461	0.7943	1.807	0.8751
24, 3.8	24_003D_CT	0.032	0.8578	0.748	0.6879
24, 3.8	24_003D_CA	12.234	0.0569	14.836	0.2505

Note: Significant results are highlighted in bold. Reproduced from Wilke et al. (2009), with permission from the American Veterinary Medical Association.

Table 7.2 Pearson Chi-square probability results for single nucleotide polymorphisms (SNPs) identified in positional candidate genes located on chromosome 3

Gene	Status	1,1 genotype (no.) animals	1,2 genotype (no.) animals	2,2 genotype (no.) animals	χ^2 value, probability	1 allele (no.) animals	2 allele (no.) animals	χ^2 value, probability
CSPCP	Normal	33	10	0	2.16, 0.34	76	10	1.95, 0.38
SNP1	Affected	39	5	0		83	5	
CSPCP	Normal	22	18	3	7.8, **0.05**	62	24	7.57, **0.02**
SNP2	Affected	35	8	1		78	10	
VCAN	Normal	23	10	11	0.923, 0.82	56	32	0.58, 0.75
SNP1	Affected	24	6	9		54	24	
VCAN	Normal	20	18	3	2.32, 0.51	58	24	2.05, 0.36
SNP2	Affected	27	15	1		69	17	
VCAN	Normal	3	27	9	3.38, 0.34	33	45	0.007, 0.997
SNP3	Affected	7	21	14		35	49	

Note: Significant results are highlighted in bold.

has targeted mutations in collagen genes as risk factors for ACL injuries. Two separate studies have evaluated a mutation (G1023T; rs1800012) in intron 1 of *Collagen Type 1 alpha 1* (*COL1A1*), the binding site for the transcription factor Sp1, in relation to ACL injury (Khoschnau et al. 2008; Posthumus et al. 2009a). Although the homozygous thymine (TT) genotype was rare, both studies concluded that the TT genotype seemed to have a protective effect on development of ACL rupture. It is proposed that the increased binding of the Sp1 transcription factor increases expression of alpha 1 chain; however it is unknown how this protects against ACL injury. More recently, female study participants with an ACL injury were found to be 2.4 times more likely to have the homozygous adenine (AA) genotype for the SNP (rs970547, S3058G) in exon 65 of *Collagen Type 12 alpha 1* (*COL12A1*; Posthumus et al. 2009b). These studies highlight the recent advances toward our understanding of the underlying genetic mechanisms involved in CrCL rupture.

Summary and future recommendations

In a population of Newfoundland dogs with a 22.4% incidence of CrCL rupture (N = 411, 53 females, 39 males), an autosomal recessive mode of inheritance with 51% penetrance for CrCL rupture was detected. Biological candidate gene analyses ruled out *COMP*, *COL9A1*, *COL9A2*, and *COL9A3*, and *FBN1* as associated with the CrCL rupture trait. A genome-wide association analysis identified and validated an association with regions located on CFA 3, 5, and 13. Some potential comparative candidate genes that warrant further investigation include *COL1A1* and *COL12A1*. A phenotypic screening test that has a strong correlation with genotype can and should be developed. The other potential application for which the above work lays a foundation is a genotype-based diagnostic screening test that would allow early detection of individuals with an increased risk of developing CrCL rupture.

References

Aiken SW, Kass PH, Toombs JP. Intercondylar notch width in dogs with and without cranial cruciate liga-

ment injuries. Vet Comp Orthop Traumatol 1995;8: 128–132.

Arendt E, Dick R. Knee injury patterns among men and women in collegiate basketball and soccer. NCAA data and review of literature. Am J Sports Med 1995; 23:694–701.

Flynn RK, Pedersen CL, Birmingham TB, et al. The familial predisposition toward tearing the anterior cruciate ligament: a case control study. Am J Sports Med 2005;33:23–28.

Galloway RH, Lester SJ. Histopathological evaluation of canine stifle joint synovial membrane collected at the time of repair of cranial cruciate ligament rupture. J Am Anim Hosp Assoc 1995;3:289–294.

Gwinn DE, Wilckens JH, McDevitt ER, et al. The relative incidence of anterior cruciate ligament injury in men and women at the United States Naval Academy. Am J Sports Med 2000;28:98–102.

Khoschnau S, Melhus H, Jacobson A, et al. Type 1 collagen α1 Sp1 polymorphism and the risk of cruciate ligaments ruptures or shoulder dislocations. Am J Sports Med 2008;36:2432–2436.

Lawrence D, Bao S, Canfield PJ, et al. Elevation of immunoglobulin deposition in the synovial membrane of dogs with cranial cruciate ligament rupture. Vet Immunol Immunopathol 1998;65:89–96.

Lohmander LS, Ostenberg A, Englund M, et al. High prevalence of knee osteoarthritis, pain, and functional limitations in female soccer players twelve years after anterior cruciate ligament injury. Arthritis Rheum 2004;50:3145–3152.

Macrossan PE, Kinghorn BP, Wilke VL, et al. Selective genotyping for determination of a major gene associated with cranial cruciate ligament disease in the Newfoundland dog. Proc Assoc Adv Anim Breed Genet 2005;16:346–349.

Niebauer GW, Wolf B, Bashey RI, Newton CD. Antibodies to canine collagen types I and II in dogs with spontaneous cruciate ligament rupture and osteoarthritis. Arthritis Rheum 1987;30:319–327.

Posthumus M, September AV, Keegan M, et al. Genetic risk factors for anterior cruciate ligament ruptures: COL1A1 gene variant. Br J Sports Med 2009a;43: 352–356.

Posthumus M, September AV, O'Cuinneagain D, et al. The association between the COL12a1 gene and anterior cruciate ligament ruptures. Br J Sports Med 2009b; epub.

Reif U, Probst CW. Comparison of tibial plateau angles in normal and cranial cruciate deficient stifles of Labrador retrievers. Vet Surg 2003;32:385–389.

Rooney MB, Kudnig ST, Frankel DJ, et al. Determination of the association between tibial plateau angle and cranial cruciate ligament rupture in the dog. *Proceedings of the 29th Annual Conference of the Veterinary Orthopaedic Society*. The Canyons, UT, 2002, p. 64.

Schwartz NB, Domowicz M. Chondrodysplasias due to proteoglycan defects. Glycobiology 2002;12:57–68.

Shelbourne KD, Davis TJ, Klootwyk TE. The relationship between intercondylar notch width of the femur and the incidence of anterior cruciate ligament tears: A prospective study. Am J Sports Med 1998;26:402–408.

Storey JD, Tibshirani R. Statistical significance for genomewide studies. Proc Natl Acad Sci U S A 2003;100:9440–9445.

Temwichitr J, Hazewinkel HAW, van Hangen MA, Legwater, PAJ. Polymorphic microsatellite markers for genetic analysis of collagen genes in suspected collagenopathies in dogs. J Vet Med A 2007;54:522–526.

Vasseur PB, Pool RR, Arnoczsky SP, Lau RE. Correlative biomechanical and histologic study of the cranial cruciate ligament in dogs. Am J Vet Res 1985;46:1842–1854.

Whitehair JG, Vasseur PB, Willits NH. Epidemiology of cranial cruciate ligament rupture in dogs. J Am Vet Med Assoc 1993;203:1016–1019.

Wilke VL, Conzemius MC, Rothschild MF. SNP detection and association analyses of candidate genes for rupture of the cranial cruciate ligament in the dog. Anim Genet 2005;36:519–521.

Wilke VL, Conzemius MG, Kinghorn BP, et al. Predicting the inheritance of rupture of the cranial cruciate ligament in the Newfoundland dog. J Am Vet Med Assoc 2006;228:61–64.

Wilke VL, Zhang S, Evans RB, et al. Chromosomal regions associated with cranial cruciate ligament rupture in a population of Newfoundland dogs. Am J Vet Res 2009;70:1013–1017.

8 Cruciate Ligament Matrix Metabolism and Development of Laxity

Eithne Comerford

Introduction

Cruciate ligaments are comprised of cells and extracellular matrix (ECM). Most skeletal ligaments contain approximately 60%–80% water, while nearly 70%–80% of the dry weight of ligament is collagen (Frank et al. 1985). Up to 90% of the ligamentous collagens is type I collagen, the principal tensile-resistant fiber, but smaller quantities of types III, V, and VI are also present (Waggett et al. 1996). Smaller proportions of matrix are composed of elastin, proteoglycans, and other biochemical substances such as DNA from cells, enzymes, glycoproteins, lipoproteins, and integrins (Frank et al. 1985; Amiel et al. 1995).

The majority of cells in ligaments are fibroblasts (sometimes referred to as ligamentocytes; Vasseur et al. 1985), although fibrocartilage cells are present at attachment sites. The fibroblasts have multiple small cellular processes, or microvilli. The cells are linked both within the same row and in adjacent rows by connexins allowing a three-dimensional communicating network that extends throughout the ligament (Benjamin & Ralphs 1997).

Advances in the Canine Cranial Cruciate Ligament,
Edited by Peter Muir, © 2010 ACVS Foundation, This Work is a co-publication between the American College of Veterinary Surgeons Foundation and Wiley-Blackwell.

The mechanical properties of cruciate ligaments are dependent on the composition and structure of the ECM, in particular collagen. Collagen turnover is a balance between synthesis and degradation (Cawston 1998). To date, most of the interest in cruciate ligament ECM metabolism has centered on degradation. However, there has been some research into the synthesis of ECM components (e.g., collagen) in ligament, by measuring terminal propeptide levels (Sluss et al. 2001). Levels of the terminal C propeptide of collagen type I (CICP) have been measured in guinea pig cranial cruciate ligament (CrCL; Quasnichka et al. 2005), but this has yet to be evaluated in canine CrCLs.

Proteases, such as the cathepsins (Muir et al. 2002; Barrett et al. 2005; Muir et al. 2005a,b) and matrix metalloproteinases (MMP), including collagenases, stromelysins, and gelatinases (Muir et al. 2005a,b; Comerford et al. 2006), have been mainly implicated in ECM degradation.

Cruciate ligament metabolism and laxity in human beings and other species

Ligament metabolism may affect ligament strength, and it has been suggested that up-regulated anterior cruciate ligament (ACL) remodeling may predispose women to ACL injury

(Foos et al. 2001). Hormonal factors have been shown to play an important role in ligament metabolism and increased anterior knee laxity. In a recent systematic review (Hewett et al. 2007), it was demonstrated that women were at risk for ACL injuries in the first half or preovulatory phase of their menstrual cycle. Estrogen and progesterone appear to influence collagen metabolism in both animal models and human beings. Estrogen (i.e., estradiol) has been shown to decrease fibroblast proliferation and type I pro-collagen, whereas progesterone counterbalances the inhibitory effect of estrogen on female ACLs (Yu et al. 1999).

Most of the work done concerning knee laxity has been done on the ACL, and most studies involve *in vitro* cadaveric testing. *In vitro*, varus–valgus laxity and angulation is increased greatly by sectioning the collateral ligaments (Markolf et al. 1976). Anterior–posterior stability is affected by transection of most ligaments, with ACL sectioning showing the greatest increase at full joint extension (Markolf et al. 1976). Varus–valgus and anteroposterior laxity is thought to be an important contributor in the pathogenesis of human knee arthritis (Sharma et al. 1999). Increased laxity may contribute to abnormal knee biomechanics and abnormally distributed joint loads that likely lead to or accelerate arthritis.

Increased knee laxity was demonstrated in the ovulatory or post-ovulatory phases of the female menstrual cycle (Zazulak et al. 2006). A significantly higher anterior–posterior joint laxity and hyperextension has been identified in noncontact ACL injury in females compared with males (Uhorchak et al. 2003). Although studies have examined the effects of sex hormones on ACL metabolism, there are few reports of normal ACL ECM remodeling/degradation and its relationship to joint laxity.

It has been suggested that increased collagen remodeling of the guinea pig CrCL by gelatinases (MMP-2 and MMP-9) may contribute to ligament and therefore knee joint laxity (Quasnichka et al. 2005). Increased remodeling was demonstrated in CrCLs from a strain of guinea pigs predisposed to the development of spontaneous arthritis (i.e., Dunkin Hartley) at 12 weeks compared with a control strain (i.e., Bristol Strain-2). All of the biochemical and mechanical changes

in the predisposed CrCLs occurred before subchondral bone and cartilage changes at 24 weeks (Anderson-MacKenzie et al. 2005). These studies suggest that increased remodeling of the CrCL may contribute to ligament and therefore knee joint laxity.

Canine cruciate ligament metabolism and laxity

Introduction

Most of the interest in ECM degradation of canine articular tissue has centered on the matrix metalloproteinases (collagenases, stromelysins, and gelatinases), cathepsins (serine, cysteine, and aspartic proteases), and the ADAMTs family of enzymes. The MMPs are controlled by several natural inhibitors, such as the tissue inhibitors of metalloproteinases (TIMPs) and α_2-macroglobulin, in order to prevent excessive activity and associated matrix degradation.

The collagenases (MMP-1, MMP-8, and MMP-13), which cleave the fibrillar collagens at a specific site within their helical domain, generating 3/4 and 1/4 fragments, have been demonstrated in normal and in experimental arthritic canine cartilage (Fernandes et al. 1998). The stromelysins (MMP-3 and MMP-10) (Spreng et al. 1999), and gelatinases (MMP-2 and MMP-9) have been identified in canine synovial fluid in experimentally induced and rheumatoid arthritis, respectively (Coughlan et al. 1998, Panula et al. 1998). However, little attention has been centered on the presence and expression of these proteases in the normal canine CrCL.

The role that the CrCL plays in the mechanical integrity of the canine stifle has been well described (Stouffer et al. 1983, Vasseur 1993, Wingfield et al. 2000). Excessive motion of the canine stifle joint is prevented by ligamentous constraints (the CrCL primarily resisting cranial displacement) and a complex system of reflex arcs from surrounding muscle groups (Vasseur 1993). Although the joint capsule has also been shown to contribute significantly to craniocaudal stability in the canine stifle, the role of the CrCL surpasses this contribution (Lopez et al. 2003).

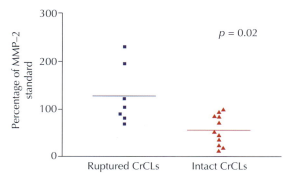

Figure 8.1 Dot diagram of the pro-form of matrix metalloproteinase 2 (pro-MMP-2) as a percentage of the MMP-2 standard indicative of collagen remodeling in 7 ruptured and 11 intact CrCLs from 18 dogs. Horizontal lines represent the mean values of each data set. Reproduced from Comerford et al. (2004), with permission from the American Veterinary Medical Association.

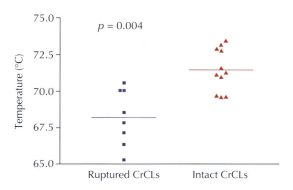

Figure 8.2 Dot diagram of the maximum temperature of denaturation determined via differential scanning calorimetry in 8 ruptured and 11 intact CrCLs from 19 dogs. Horizontal lines represent the mean values of each data set. Reproduced from Comerford et al. (2004), with permission from the American Veterinary Medical Association.

Metabolism in ruptured canine cruciate ligaments

ECM metabolism in ruptured canine CrCLs has been recently investigated (Muir et al. 2002, Comerford et al. 2004). We examined the CrCLs from normal cadaveric Labrador retrievers (breed at high risk of CrCL rupture) and from Labrador retrievers with CrCL rupture. Ruptured CrCLs had significantly higher amounts of immature cross-links, total and sulfated glycosaminoglycans (GAGs), and water content, compared with that of the intact ligaments. Compared with intact CrCLs, the concentration of pro-MMP-2 (inactive MMP-2) was significantly higher and the maximum temperature of collagen denaturation was significantly lower in the ruptured CrCLs (Figures 8.1 and 8.2; Comerford et al. 2004). This work suggested that the ECM of ruptured CrCLs had an increased matrix turnover indicated by higher collagen and GAG synthesis, compared with that of intact CrCLs. It is likely that the ECM changes may have occurred before ligament rupture. However, it is possible that these observed changes may be part of a reparative process after rupture. Ruptured CrCLs also contain greater numbers of cells with the proteinases tartrate-resistant protein (TRAP) and cathepsin K, when compared with CrCLs from healthy, young, or aged dogs (Muir et al. 2002). Therefore, cell-signaling pathways that regulate expression of these proteinases may form part of the mechanism that leads to up-regulation of collagen remodeling within the CrCL (Muir et al. 2002). Levels of cathepsin K and TRAP expression in the canine synovium and CrCL were also found to be significantly correlated in dogs with CrCL rupture (Muir et al. 2005a,b).

The relationship between cruciate ligament metabolism and stifle laxity

Detailed comparisons of joint laxity and other mechanical parameters in stifles with normal CrCL with other ligament parameters (e.g., collagen and extracellular matrix biochemistry) have been reported infrequently in the literature (Vasseur et al. 1985). Vasseur et al. compared the biomechanical and histological properties in dogs and found a positive relationship with age, increasing weight, and degenerative changes in the canine CrCL (Vasseur et al. 1985). However, this study only examined a mixed population of dogs of different breeds, ages, genders, and weights.

This void in the literature contributed to the hypothesis of the author's thesis (Comerford 2002), which was to determine whether increased craniocaudal stifle joint laxity would be present

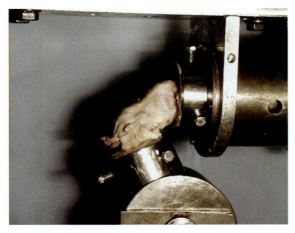

Figure 8.3 Photograph of a canine stifle joint positioned in a materials testing machine (Instron 1122, Instron Ltd, High Wycombe, UK) for craniocaudal mechanical testing. The tibia is positioned in the uppermost stainless steel pot and the load cell is positioned to the top of the picture.

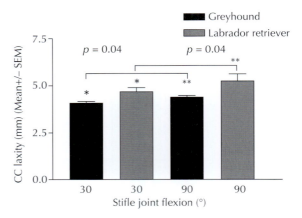

Figure 8.4 Craniocaudal (CC) laxity testing in greyhounds ($n = 11$) and Labrador retrievers ($n = 11$) at 100 N with the joint in 30 and 90° of flexion. Reproduced from Comerford et al. (2005), with permission from Wiley & Sons.

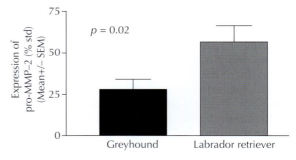

Figure 8.5 Levels of pro-MMP-2 (% inactive zymogen) in Labrador retriever and greyhound cranial cruciate ligaments. std: standard. Reproduced from Comerford et al. (2005), with permission from Wiley & Sons.

in normal stifle joints from a breed that is at a high risk of developing CrCL rupture (Labrador retriever), compared with a low-risk breed (greyhound). We also hypothesized that the stifle joints with increased craniocaudal laxity (high-risk breeds) would demonstrate increased ECM metabolism of their CrCLs. This increased ECM metabolism could result in reduced ligament strength and increased joint laxity, contributing to eventual ligament rupture.

We used mechanical, biochemical, and thermal analyses to test the above hypothesis (Comerford 2002; Comerford et al. 2005). Mechanical analyses involved measurement of craniocaudal laxity and tensile testing of the CrCL. *Ex vivo* mechanical testing of the stifles from both high- and low-risk breeds was performed as previously described (Amis & Dawkins 1991). The stifle joints were mounted in two different test positions (30° and 90° of flexion) (Figure 8.3). CrCL dimensions were measured and the ligaments tested to failure (Woo et al. 1991). Biochemical and thermal analyses to assess ECM metabolism, such as collagen cross-link analysis, gelatin and reverse gelatin zymography (to measure MMPs and TIMPs respectively), total and sulphated GAGS, and differential scanning calorimetry (DSC), were performed on the CrCLs from the stifles which had undergone mechanical testing. Craniocaudal laxity measurement showed the mean tibial displacements of the Labrador retriever stifle joints to be significantly greater than those of the greyhound stifle joints at 30° and 90° of flexion, indicating increased laxity within the high-risk stifle joints (Figure 8.4; Comerford et al. 2005). There was significantly higher expression of pro-MMP-2 in the high-risk CrCLs (Labrador retrievers) compared with the low-risk (greyhound) CrCLs (Figure 8.5). Higher pro-MMP-2 levels can be associated with increased collagen turnover, although this was not confirmed by changes in immature collagen cross-links in this study. The concentrations of

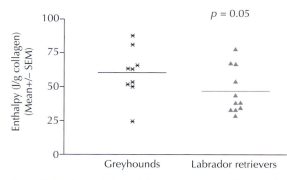

Figure 8.6 The enthalpy of denaturation (J/g collagen) of the differential scanning calorimetry (DSC) thermograms from Labrador retriever and greyhound cranial cruciate ligaments. Reproduced from Comerford et al. (2005), with permission from Wiley & Sons.

pro-MMP-2 had a positive correlation ($r = 0.5$, $p = 0.02$) with craniocaudal laxity at 90°, once both dog groups were combined. The enthalpy of collagen denaturation (indicating the amount of heat required to denature the collagen triple helices) was significantly lower in the Labrador CrCLs than in the greyhounds (Figure 8.6). This implies the presence of partially degraded collagen triple helices in Labrador CrCLs. Increased collagen degradation as indicated by the high levels of MMP-2 is consistent with the thermal properties of the collagenous matrix of the Labrador CrCL, as well as the increased stifle joint laxity within this breed. Interestingly, gender or bodyweight did not correlate significantly with any of the mechanical, biochemical, or thermal analyses in this study.

Conclusion

Differences in cruciate ligament metabolism (ACL and CrCL) indicated by greater MMP-2 expression and collagen denaturation are consistent with identified mechanical properties in guinea pigs and dogs. The ligaments examined in these studies had no apparent pathology, and therefore the changes identified may be intrinsic to ligament metabolism. This may be related to genetics (influencing factors such as stifle joint morphology) and may account for the differing breed predisposition to CrCL rupture within these two species. Therefore, subtle changes in cruciate ligament metabolism and its influence on joint mechanics may play a role in canine (CrCL) and possibly human (ACL) rupture.

References

Amiel D, Chu CR, Lee J. Effect of loading on metabolism and repair of tendons and ligaments. In: *Repetitive Motion Disorders of the Upper Extremity*, Gordon SL, Blair SJ, Fine LJ (eds). Rosemont, IL: American Academy of Orthopaedic Surgeons, 1995, pp. 217–230.

Amis AA, Dawkins GP. Functional anatomy of the anterior cruciate ligament. Fibre bundle actions related to ligament replacements and injuries. J Bone Joint Surg Br 1991;73:260–267.

Anderson-MacKenzie JM, Quasnichka HL, Starr RL, et al. Fundamental subchondral bone changes in spontaneous knee osteoarthritis. Int J Biochem Cell Biol 2005;37:224–236.

Barrett JG, Hao Z, Graf BK, et al. Inflammatory changes in ruptured canine cranial and human anterior cruciate ligaments. Am J Vet Res 2005;66:2073–2080.

Benjamin M, Ralphs JR. Tendons and ligaments—An overview. Histol Histopathol 1997;12:1135–1144.

Cawston T. Matrix metalloproteinases and TIMPs: Properties and implications for the rheumatic diseases. Mol Med Today 1998;4:130–137.

Comerford E. Evaluation of extracellular matrix composition, metabolism, joint mechanics and joint conformation as potential predisposing factors of cranial cruciate ligament rupture in three dog breeds. PhD Thesis, School of Clinical Veterinary Science, University of Bristol, Bristol, 2002.

Comerford EJ, Innes JF, Tarlton JF, et al. Investigation of the composition, turnover, and thermal properties of ruptured cranial cruciate ligaments of dogs. Am J Vet Res 2004;65:1136–1141.

Comerford EJ, Tarlton JF, Innes JF, et al. Metabolism and composition of the canine anterior cruciate ligament relate to differences in knee joint mechanics and predisposition to ligament rupture. J Orthop Res 2005;23:61–66.

Comerford EJ, Tarlton JF, Avery NC, et al. Distal femoral intercondylar notch dimensions and their relationship to composition and metabolism of the canine anterior cruciate ligament. Osteoarthritis Cartilage 2006;14:273–278.

Coughlan AR, Robertson DHL, Bennett D, et al. Matrix metalloproteinases 2 and 9 in canine rheumatoid arthritis. Vet Rec 1998;143:219–223.

Fernandes JC, Martel Pelletier J, Lascau Coman V, et al. Collagenase-1 and collagenase-3 synthesis in normal and early experimental osteoarthritic canine cartilage: An immunohistochemical study. J Rheumatol 1998;25:1585–1594.

Foos MJ, Hickox JR, Mansour PG, et al. Expression of matrix metalloprotease and tissue inhibitor of metalloprotease genes in human anterior cruciate ligament. J Orthop Res 2001;19:642–649.

Frank CB, Amiel D, Woo SL, et al. Normal ligament properties and ligament healing. Clin Orthop Rel Res 1985;196:15–25.

Hewett TE, Zazulak BT, Myer GD. Effects of the menstrual cycle on anterior cruciate ligament injury risk: A systematic review. Am J Sports Med 2007;35:659–668.

Lopez MJ, Kunz D, Vanderby R, Jr. et al. A comparison of joint stability between anterior cruciate intact and deficient knees: A new canine model of anterior cruciate ligament disruption. J Orthop Res 2003;21:224–230.

Markolf KL, Mensch JS, Amstutz HC. Stiffness and laxity of the knee—The contributions of the supporting structures. A quantitative *in vitro* study. J Bone Joint Surg Am 1976;58A:583–594.

Muir P, Hayashi K, Manley PA, et al. Evaluation of tartrate-resistant acid phosphatase and cathepsin K in ruptured cranial cruciate ligaments in dogs. Am J Vet Res 2002;63:1279–1284.

Muir P, Schamberger GM, Manley PA, et al. Localization of cathepsin K and tartrate-resistant acid phosphatase in synovium and cranial cruciate ligament in dogs with cruciate disease. Vet Surg 2005a;34:39–246.

Muir P, Danova NA, Argyle DJ, et al. Collagenolytic protease expression in cranial cruciate ligament and stifle synovial fluid in dogs with cranial cruciate ligament rupture. Vet Surg 2005b;34:482–490.

Panula HE, Lohmander LS, Ronkko S, et al. Elevated levels of synovial fluid PLA(2), stromelysin (MMP-3) and TIMP in early osteoarthrosis after tibial valgus osteotomy in young beagle dogs. Acta Orthop Scand 1998;69:152–158.

Quasnichka HL, Anderson-MacKenzie JM, Tarlton JF, et al. Cruciate ligament laxity and femoral intercondylar notch narrowing in early-stage knee osteoarthritis. Arthritis Rheum 2005;52:3100–3109.

Sharma L, Lou C, Felson DT, et al. Laxity in healthy and osteoarthritic knees. Arthritis Rheum 1999;42:861–870.

Sluss JR. Liberti JP, Jiranek WA, et al. pN collagen type III within tendon grafts used for anterior cruciate ligament reconstruction. J Orthop Res 2001;19:852–857.

Spreng D, Sigrist N, Busato A, et al. Stromelysin activity in canine cranial cruciate ligament rupture. Vet Comp Orthop Traumatol 1999;12:159–165.

Stouffer DC, Butler DL, Kim H. Tension-torsion characteristics of the canine anterior cruciate ligament—Part I: Theoretical framework. J Biomech Eng 1983;105:154–159.

Uhorchak JM, Scoville CR, Williams GN, et al. Risk factors associated with noncontact injury of the anterior cruciate ligament: a prospective four-year evaluation of 859 West Point cadets. Am J Sports Med 2003;31:31–842.

Vasseur PB. Stifle joint. In: *Textbook of Small Animal Surgery*, Slatter D (ed.), second edition. New York: WB Saunders, 1993, pp. 1817–1867.

Vasseur PB, Pool RR, Arnoczky SP, et al. Correlative biomechanical and histologic study of the cranial cruciate ligament in dogs. Am J Vet Res 1985;46:1842–1854.

Waggett AD, Kwan APL, Woodnutt DJ, et al. Collagens in fibrocartilages at the Achilles tendon insertion—A biochemical, molecular biological and immunohistochemical study. Trans Orthop Res Soc 1996;21:25.

Wingfield C, Amis AA, Stead AC, et al. Comparison of the biomechanical properties of rottweiler and racing greyhound cranial cruciate ligaments. J Small Anim Pract 2000;41:303–307.

Woo SL, Hollis JM, Adams DJ, et al. Tensile properties of the human femur-anterior cruciate ligament-tibia complex. The effects of specimen age and orientation. Am J Sports Med 1991;19:217–225.

Yu WD, Liu SH, Hatch JD, et al. Effect of estrogen on cellular metabolism of the human anterior cruciate ligament. Clin Orthop 1999;366:229–238.

Zazulak BT, Paterno M, Myer GD, et al. The effects of the menstrual cycle on anterior knee laxity: a systematic review. Sports Med 2006;36:847–862.

9 Stifle Morphology

Eithne Comerford

Introduction

Biologists use the term morphology to describe the size, shape, and structure of an organism or one of its parts. The morphology and function of the cruciate ligaments has been discussed in Chapter 1. This chapter will describe the morphology of the bones involved in stifle joint articulation in dogs, and highlight comparative aspects of knee joint morphology in noncontact anterior cruciate ligament (ACL) injury in human beings.

Stifle joint morphology may play a causative role in canine cranial cruciate ligament (CrCL) degeneration and rupture. Conformational variation of canine pelvic limbs such as a straight stifle joint, narrow intercondylar notch (ICN), and steep tibial plateau slope, and the resultant abnormal stress and microinjury of the CrCL have been hypothesized to cause progressive ligament rupture and arthritis (Aiken et al. 1995; Comerford et al. 2006; Duerr et al. 2007).

Advances in the Canine Cranial Cruciate Ligament,
Edited by Peter Muir, © 2010 ACVS Foundation, This Work is a co-publication between the American College of Veterinary Surgeons Foundation and Wiley-Blackwell.

Distal femur

The distal femoral ICN contains both the CrCL and the caudal cruciate ligament, as they twist around each other from their femoral origin to their tibial insertion sites. The distal femoral ICN is narrowed in dogs and human beings with CrCL/ACL rupture and arthritis because of increased osteophyte formation (Aiken et al. 1995; Wada et al. 1996). Stenotic or narrowed ICNs have been implicated as a risk factor in large studies of human ACL injuries (LaPrade & Burnett 1994; Shelbourne et al. 1998). Radiographic comparison of other morphological features of the distal femur did not identify anatomic differences in dogs with and without CrCL rupture (Guerrero et al. 2007).

A stenotic ICN causes impingement by the medial aspect of the lateral femoral condyle or the intercondylar roof on the CrCL/ACL (Aiken et al. 1995). If a normal-sized ACL passes through a narrowed ICN, the reduced space could impede the normal function of the ACL, causing impingement and therefore damage to the ACL (Muneta et al. 1997). A recent study suggested that ACL impingement may occur at the anterior and posterior roof of the notch during tibia external rotation and abduction, resulting in ligament microinjury (Dienst et al. 2007). This study also found a significant correlation between ACL cross-sectional area to notch surface area, with a smaller notch being associated with a smaller mid-substance cross-sectional area of the ACL. Some patients with congenital stenosis who sustained an ACL tear by noncontact means were found to be young, with small ICN width index measurements (Souryal et al. 1988). It is also thought that knee laxity may contribute to ICN narrowing and then result in further ACL impingement and damage (Wada et al. 1996).

To date, notch width (NW) and notch width index (NWI) have been the parameters used to determine the width of the human and canine ICN. The shape of the notch is also thought to be a critical factor in the role of the ICN in ACL injury. ICN shapes have been described as bell- or inverted U-shaped, A-shaped, or wave/crest-shaped (Anderson et al. 2001). In dogs, the ICN is bell-shaped (Fitch et al. 1995). Normal ICNs tend to be inverted U-shaped, whereas narrower notches tend to more wave- or crest-shaped (Anderson et al. 2001). A recent study on ICN shape has shown that this categorization does not correlate with ACL injured and noninjured patients. It suggested that determining the notch shape index (NSI; Tillman et al. 2002) may be a more useful measurement as it is a relative measure of the notch width in a medial–lateral direction to the notch height in the anterior–posterior direction. A low NSI will cause the ACL to be pushed into a smaller anterior outlet of the ICN, with the joint in extension. The NSI was also found to be lower in women than in men, suggesting that notch shape may help to explain gender differences in the risk for ACL rupture (Figure 9.1; Tillman et al. 2002).

Until recently, differences in the ICN and its width had not been investigated in normal stifle joints from dog breeds with differing predispositions to CrCL rupture. We hypothesized that dogs at a high risk for CrCL rupture, such as Labradors and golden retrievers, may have smaller ICNs than dogs at a low risk, for example, greyhounds (Comerford et al. 2006). The smaller ICN may cause ligament impingement with associated biochemical changes within the extracellular matrix (ECM), leading to CrCL degeneration. Tendons and ligaments that pass through or around bony structures are subjected to compressive as well tensile forces, and this reflects in changes in biochemical composition in that they become more

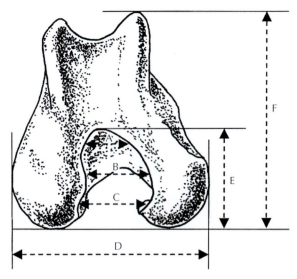

Figure 9.1 Measurements of the canine intercondylar notch (ICN; adapted from Fitch et al. 1995). A: cranial notch width, B: central notch width; C: caudal notch width; D: condylar width; E: ICN height; F: femoral condyle height. The cranial notch width index (NWI) is A/D, the central NWI is B/D, and the caudal NWI is C/D; the notch shape index (NSI) is B/E and ICN height index is E/F. Reproduced from Comerford et al. (2006), with permission from Elsevier.

fibrocartilaginous in compressed regions (Benjamin & Ralphs 1998). To date, it is not known whether alterations in the biochemical composition of ligaments in areas of impingement are adaptive or degenerative.

Cranial NWIs were significantly greater in the low-risk breed (greyhounds) than in high-risk breeds (retrievers) in a cadaveric study (Comerford et al. 2006). However, there was no significant difference in the NSI between high- and low-risk dog breeds (Figure 9.2). As part of this study, the stifle joints of the three dog breeds were placed in full extension, and the areas of the CrCLs impinged by the ICN were marked and removed (Comerford et al. 2006). Analyses for biochemical parameters such as collagen content and cross-links, matrix metalloproteinases (MMPs), tissue inhibitors of metalloproteinases (TIMPs), and sulfated and total glycosaminoglycans (GAGs) were then performed as previously described (Comerford et al. 2004). Expression of pro- and active MMP-2 was significantly increased in CrCLs of the high-

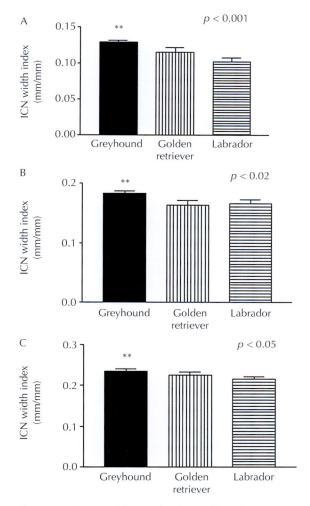

Figure 9.2 Intercondylar notch (ICN) width indices: (A) cranial, (B) central, and (C) caudal in greyhound ($n = 60$), golden retriever ($n = 23$), and Labrador retriever ($n = 26$). **denotes stated statistical significance to the other two groups. Reproduced from Comerford et al. (2006), with permission from Elsevier.

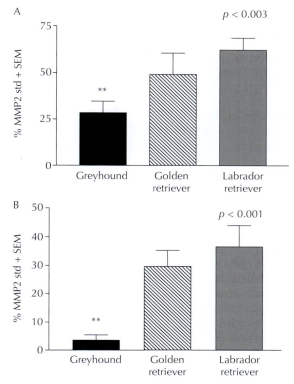

Figure 9.3 The levels of pro-MMP-2 (A) and active (B) MMP-2 (% of standard) in the impinged parts of greyhound ($n = 10$), golden retriever ($n = 8$), and Labrador retriever ($n = 10$) cranial cruciate ligaments. **denotes stated statistical significance to the other two groups. SEM: standard error of the mean. Reproduced from Comerford et al. (2006), with permission from Elsevier.

risk breed, compared with the low-risk breed, suggesting increased collagen remodeling (Figure 9.3). There were significantly more sulfated GAGs in the impinged areas of the high-risk CrCLs, compared with those of the low-risk breed (Figure 9.4). Interestingly, the bodyweight of the Labrador retrievers was correlated with a decrease in the central NWI ($p = 0.004$, $r = 0.50$), while age did not correlate with any of the ICN parameters. It is possible that increased load on the Labrador retriever stifle joints alters joint mechanics and that this may contribute to ICN remodeling and narrowing. Gender was only shown to have an influence on greyhound NSIs, with narrower NSIs in female greyhounds. NSI was not a factor in the predisposed dogs. Taken together, these data suggest that impingement by the ICN on the CrCLs of the high-risk breeds may result in reduced structural integrity of the ligament, predisposing the ligament to increased laxity and eventual joint degeneration. A recent computed tomography study confirmed these findings. Cranial ICN measurements were significantly narrower in unilateral and bilateral CrCL rupture group, when compared with the normal population (Lewis et al. 2008).

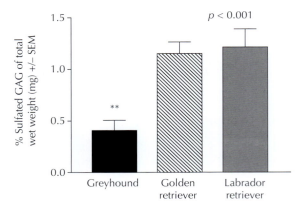

Figure 9.4 Levels of sulfated GAG (% total weight) in the impinged parts of Greyhound (*n* = 10), golden retriever (*n* = 8) and Labrador retrievers (*n* = 10) cranial cruciate ligaments. **denotes stated statistical significance to the other two groups. Reproduced from Comerford et al. (2006), with permission from Elsevier.

Tibia

The stifle joint is subjected to external ground reaction forces during weight-bearing and internal forces generated by muscular contraction. These forces not only compress the femoral and tibial articular surfaces, but also generate a cranially directed shear force in the tibia known as cranial tibial thrust (CTT). CTT is present in the stifle as the tibial plateau is not perpendicular to a line drawn between the center of motion of the stifle and hock joints, but is directed caudodistally (Slocum & Devine 1983). There have been numerous studies evaluating the association of tibial plateau angle (TPA) and CrCL rupture (Read & Robbins 1982; Macias et al. 2002; Duerr et al. 2007). Although anatomical differences in the shape of the proximal tibia have been documented in dogs with CrCL rupture, its role in the rupture mechanism is unclear (Wilke et al. 2002; Guastella et al. 2008). The mean TPA in dogs varies between 23° and 25°, while a wide range of TPA has been reported (13° to 34°) in normal dogs. A study by Wilke et al. (2002) revealed that the functional TPA is approximately parallel to the ground in most dogs. Although pathological increases in TPA (>55°) have been correlated with CrCL rupture (Read & Robins 1982; Macias et al. 2002), whether a general association between TPA and CrCL rupture exists in dogs remains controversial. Studies have shown that the TPAs are not significantly different in Labrador retrievers with and without CrCL rupture, and in a comparison between greyhounds and Labrador retrievers (Wilke et al. 2002; Reif & Probst 2003). Interestingly, German shepherd dogs have an increased TPA, when compared with dogs of high-risk breeds, such as the Rottweiler (Guastella et al. 2008). The true effect of TPA on CrCL stresses *in vivo* is currently unknown, as muscular force, body size, obesity, rapid weight gain, relative inactivity, and exercise can all modify the amount of stress sustained by CrCL in addition to the TPA (Colborne et al. 2005).

Development of the tibial tuberosity and the shape (convexity) of tibial condyles may also be relevant in the pathogenesis of CrCL rupture (Guerrero et al. 2007). Smaller tibial tuberosity widths are thought to increase CTT and promote CrCL degeneration, thus leading to rupture in a younger population of dogs (Inauen et al. 2009). In another study in Labrador retrievers, cranial angulation of the proximal portion of the tibia, excessive steepness of the tibial plateau, and distal femoral torsion appeared more likely to be associated with CrCL deficiency than femoral angulation, tibial torsion, ICN stenosis, and increased inclination of the patellar ligament (Mostafa et al. 2009).

In human beings, controversy also exists over whether posterior tibial slope is an anatomical risk factor for ACL injuries. Meister et al. (1998) demonstrated no relationship between noncontact ACL injuries and the posterior tibia slope. However, in more recent work, Stijak et al. (2008) found that ACL-injured patients had a significantly greater slope of the lateral tibial plateau and a nonsignificant lower slope of the medial tibial plateau compared with a control group.

Patella/quadriceps mechanism and Q angle

Conformational abnormalities of the distal femur, such as genu varum and malalignment of the quadriceps mechanism, associated with medial patellar luxation (MPL), can cause increased internal stress on the CrCL (Duval et al. 1999). In human beings, the quadriceps (Q angle) may contribute to an increased risk of ACL injury (Shambaugh et al. 1991). However, its role in non-contact ACL injuries is unclear. The Q angle is the angle formed by a line directed from the insertion of the *m. rectus femoris* on the ilium to the middle to the trochlear groove and a second line from the tibial tuberosity to the trochlear groove mirroring the course of the patella tendon. In normal dogs, the Q angle is reported to be 10.5° medially, increasing with a greater severity of MPL (up to 36.6° for a grade III MPL). The average Q angle in dogs with isolated CrCL rupture was reported to be 19.3°, because of loss of CrCL restraint on the internal rotation of the tibia (Kaiser et al. 2001).

The angles between the patellar ligament and the tibial plateau have also been measured in humans (Nisell 1985) and in healthy dogs (Dennler et al. 2006), as a function of stifle joint flexion. Dogs with partially torn CrCLs, anatomically, have marginally larger angles between the patellar ligament and tibial plateau compared with joints with intact CrCLs (Schwandt et al. 2006).

Fabella

A recent study found that 70% of West Highland white terriers had a mediodistal position of their medial fabella, compared with other small and large breed dogs. This finding was not associated with MPL or CrCL ruptures and is considered a normal anatomical finding for this breed (Stork et al. 2009).

Conclusion

Stifle joint morphology, in particular the distal femoral ICN and the TPA, may play a contributing role to CrCL degeneration and rupture in dogs. The ICN has been shown to be smaller in dog breeds with an increased predisposition to ligament rupture, resulting in altered ECM turnover. However, the role of these factors *in vivo*, along with neuromuscular forces, has yet to be elucidated.

References

Aiken SW, Kass PH, Toombs JP. Intercondylar notch width in dogs with and without cranial cruciate ligament injuries. Vet Comp Orthop Traumatol 1995; 8:128–132.

Anderson AF, Dome DC, Gautam S, et al. Correlation of anthropometric measurements, strength, anterior cruciate ligament size, and intercondylar notch characterisitics to sex differences in anterior cruciate ligament tear rates. Am J Sports Med 2001;29:58–65.

Benjamin M, Ralphs JR. Fibrocartilage in tendons and ligaments—An adaptation to a compressive load. J Anat 1998;193:481–484.

Colborne GR, Innes JF, Comerford EJ, et al. Distribution of power across the hind limb joints in Labrador retrievers and greyhounds. Am J Vet Res 2005; 66:1563–1571.

Comerford EJ, Innes JF, Tarlton JF, et al. Investigation of the composition, turnover, and thermal properties of ruptured cranial cruciate ligaments of dogs. Am J Vet Res 2004;65:1136–1141.

Comerford EJ, Tarlton JF, Avery NC, et al. Distal femoral intercondylar notch dimensions and their relationship to composition and metabolism of the canine anterior cruciate ligament. Osteoarthritis Cartilage 2006;14: 273–278.

Dennler R, Kipfer NM, Tepic S, et al. Inclination of the patellar ligament in relation to flexion angle in stifle joints of dogs without degenerative joint disease. Am J Vet Res 2006;67:1849–1854.

Dienst M, Schneider G, Altmeyer K, et al. Correlation of intercondylar notch cross sections to the ACL size: A high resolution MR tomographic in vivo analysis. Arch Orthop Traumatol Surg 2007;127:253–260.

Duerr FM, Duncan CG, Savicky RS, et al. Risk factors for excessive tibial plateau angle in large-breed dogs with cranial cruciate ligament disease. J Am Vet Med Assoc 2007;231:1688–1691.

Duval JM, Budsberg SC, Flo GL, et al. Breed, sex, and body weight as risk factors for rupture of the cranial cruciate ligament in young dogs. J Am Vet Med Assoc 1999;215:811–814.

Fitch RB, Montgomery RD, Milton JL, et al. The intercondylar fossa of the normal canine stifle an anatomic and radiographic study. Vet Surg 1995;24:148–155.

Guastella DB, Fox DB, Cook JL. Tibial plateau angle in four common canine breeds with cranial cruciate ligament rupture, and its relationship to meniscal tears. Vet Comp Orthop Traumatol 2008;21:125–128.

Guerrero TG, Geyer H, Hassig M, et al. Effect of conformation of the distal portion of the femur and proximal portion of the tibia on the pathogenesis of cranial cruciate ligament disease in dogs. Am J Vet Res 2007;68:1332–1337.

Inauen R, Koch D, Bass M, et al. Tibial tuberosity conformation as a risk factor for cranial cruciate ligament rupture in the dog. Vet Comp Orthop Traumatol 2009;22:16–20.

Kaiser S, Cornely D, Golder W, et al. Magnetic resonance measurements of the deviation of the angle of force generated by contraction of the quadriceps muscle in dogs with congenital patellar luxation. Vet Surg 2001;30:552–558.

LaPrade RF, Burnett QM. Femoral intercondylar notch stenosis and correlation to anterior cruciate ligament injuries. A prospective study. Am J Sports Med 1994; 22:198–203.

Lewis BA, Allen DA, Henrikson TD, et al. Computed tomographic evaluation of the canine intercondylar notch in normal and cruciate deficient stifles. Vet Comp Orthop Traumatol 2008;21:119–124.

Macias C, McKee WM, May C. Caudal proximal tibial deformity and cranial cruciate ligament rupture in small-breed dogs. J Small Anim Pract 2002;43:433–438.

Meister K, Talley MC, Horodyski MB, et al. Caudal slope of the tibia and its relationship to noncontact injuries to the ACL. Am J Knee Surg 1998;11:217–219.

Mostafa AA, Griffon DJ, Thomas MW, et al. Morphometric characteristics of the pelvic limbs of Labrador retrievers with and without cranial cruciate ligament deficiency. Am J Vet Res 2009;70:498–507.

Muneta T, Takakuda K, Yamamoto H. Intercondylar notch width and its relation to the configuration and cross-sectional area of the anterior cruciate ligament. A cadaveric knee study. Am J Sports Med 1997; 25:69–72.

Nisell R. Mechanics of the knee. A study of joint and muscle load with clinical applications. Acta Orthop Scand 1985;216:S1–S42.

Read RA, Robins GM. Deformity of the proximal tibia in dogs. Vet Rec 1982;111:295–298.

Reif U, Probst CW. Comparison of tibial plateau angles in normal and cranial cruciate deficient stifles of Labrador retrievers. Vet Surg 2003;32:385–389.

Schwandt CS, Bohorquez-Vanelli A, Tepic S, et al. Angle between the patellar ligament and tibial plateau in dogs with partial rupture of the cranial cruciate ligament. Am J Vet Res 2006;67:1855–1860.

Shambaugh JP, Klein A, Herbert JH. Structural measures as predictors of injury basketball players. Med Sci Sports Exerc 1991;23:522–527.

Shelbourne KD, Davis TJ, Klootwyk TE. The relationship between intercondylar notch width of the femur and the incidence of anterior cruciate ligament tears. A prospective study. Am J Sports Med 1998;26: 402–408.

Slocum B, Devine T. Cranial tibial thrust: A primary force in the canine stifle. J Am Vet Med Assoc 1983; 183:456–459.

Souryal TO, Moore HA, Evans JP. Bilaterality in anterior cruciate ligament injuries: Associated intercondylar notch stenosis. Am J Sports Med 1988;16: 449–454.

Stijak L, Herzog RF, Schai P. Is there an influence of the tibial slope of the lateral condyle on the ACL lesion? A case-control study. Knee Surg Sports Traumatol Arthrosc 2008;16:112–117.

Stork CK, Petite AF, Norrie RA, et al. Variation in position of the medial fabella in West Highland white terriers and other dogs. J Small Anim Pract 2009;50:236–240.

Tillman MD, Smith KR, Bauer JA, et al. Differences in three intercondylar notch geometry indices between males and females: A cadaver study. Knee 2002;9: 41–46.

Wada M, Imura S, Baba H, et al. Knee laxity in patients with osteoarthritis and rheumatoid arthritis. Br J Rheumatol 1996;35:560–563.

Wilke VL, Conzemius MG, Besancon MF, et al. Comparison of tibial plateau angle between clinically normal greyhounds and Labrador retrievers with and without rupture of the cranial cruciate ligament. J Am Vet Med Assoc 2002;221:1426–1429.

10 Role of Nitric Oxide Production and Matrix Protease Activity in Cruciate Ligament Degeneration

David E. Spreng

NO overview

Nitric oxide (NO) is an important mediator in physiologic and pathophysiologic pathways in the body. In addition to its effect as one of the major vasodilators, it also plays a role in platelet function, inflammation, and pain perception. Pro-inflammatory mediators such as NO, interleukin 1 (IL-1), tumor necrosis factor (TNF), and prostaglandins are all overproduced in chondrocytes from patients with ostheoarthritis (OA; Weinberg et al. 2007).

NO is a nonpolar, diffusible, highly reactive gas that targets oxygen, iron, and sulfhydril groups. It has been identified as the small-molecular-weight mediator released from endothelial cells that promotes relaxation of adjacent vascular smooth muscle. This explains its earlier acronym "endothelium-derived relaxing factor." Generation of NO occurs when nitric oxide synthase (NOS) catalyzes the conversion of L-arginine into NO and citrulline (Figure 10.1; Marletta 1988).

Three isoforms of NOS with characteristic tissue distribution have been described. Endothelial

NOS (cNOS) and neuronal NOS (nNOS) are calcium-dependent and constitutively produce relatively low levels of NO. Inducible NOS (iNOS) is synthesized *de novo* upon appropriate cell or tissue stimulation. iNOS is expressed by a variety of cell types, including activated macrophages, hepatocytes, synovial cells, and smooth muscle cells. In contrast to cNOS and nNOS, activation of iNOS is calcium-independent and long lasting, thereby promoting the production of large amounts of NO over extended periods of time (Weinberg et al. 2007).

With regard to its biologic effects, NO is a major regulator of blood flow, blocks platelet aggregation, and has been identified as a neurotransmitter of certain non-adrenergic, non-cholinergic nerve cells within cardiac muscle and the colon in the dog. In addition, NO is a mediator of antimicrobial and antitumoral activity in host defense through inactivation of enzymes of the cell cycle and of the respiratory chain. It inhibits synthesis of acute phase and other proteins in the liver, is immunosuppressive, regulates inflammation, is implicated in autoimmune processes, and is mutagenic. In addition to signaling by NO alone, reactive oxygen species (ROS) are generated by the combination of NO and superoxide to form peroxynitrite, contributing to a number of destructive events including chondrocyte apoptosis (Del Carlo & Loeser 2002).

Advances in the Canine Cranial Cruciate Ligament, Edited by Peter Muir, © 2010 ACVS Foundation, This Work is a co-publication between the American College of Veterinary Surgeons Foundation and Wiley-Blackwell.

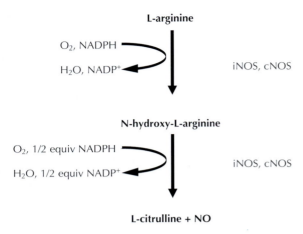

Figure 10.1 Production of nitric oxide via the oxidation of L-arginine by a family of NOS enzymes.

NO activity in articular tissues

NO, iNOS, cNOS, nNOS, and peroxynitrite have all been detected in different healthy and osteoarthritic joint tissues (Amin et al. 1995; Pelletier et al. 2000; Di Mauro et al. 2006). There is good evidence that articular joint NO production originates mainly through iNOS-derived NO production in chondrocytes. NO production in synovial membrane is generally low in normal as well as osteoarthritic joints (Spreng et al. 2000). Assessment of NO production in ligament tissue, especially in partially or totally ruptured cranial cruciate ligament (CrCL), is difficult. Specimens of naturally diseased CrCL are usually retrieved from canine patients during surgical repair, leading to the problem that highly traumatized tissue is examined without knowing if measured production of NO and NO metabolites is triggered by the original CrCL pathology, or is only a consequence of the mechanical trauma of ligament disruption. Interestingly, normal CrCL produces more NO compared with normal cartilage or normal medial collateral ligaments of the stifle in dogs. Inhibition of canine CrCL NO production by a specific iNOS inhibitor demonstrated that NO in the ligament is mainly derived from the inducible NOS pathway (Spreng et al. 2000). Additionally, *in vitro* activation of ligaments with an inflammatory cocktail of LPS/IL1/TNF leads to increased NO production and iNOS activity in the CrCL, compared with the medial collateral ligament and the ligament of the head of the femur, indicating that ligamentocytes in the CrCL indeed produce substantial amounts of NO under a specific stimulus (Louis et al. 2006).

Role of NO in the joint

NO is believed to be mainly a catabolic player in joint physiology (Figure 10.2). Chondrocytes from patients with OA express iNOS in the superficial zone of articular cartilage, reflecting an increase in NO during OA (Häuselmann et al. 1998). NO inhibits the synthesis of proteoglycans and collagen in cartilage culture and up-regulates the synthesis of matrix metalloproteinases (MMP), with both contributing to extracellular matrix destruction. It has also been shown that NO mediates the expression of pro-inflammatory cytokines such as IL-18 and IL-1 converting enzyme (Boileau et al. 2002).

In addition to contributing to the degradation of extracellular matrix, NO is also known to mediate apoptosis in joint tissues. *In vitro* experiments have shown that articular chondrocytes treated with the NO donor sodium nitroprusside induce apoptosis, and treatment with a NO scavenger significantly decreases cell damage. Apoptosis has also been detected in canine ligamentocytes with a moderate but significant correlation to NO (Gyger et al. 2007). There are indications that apoptosis in ligamentocytes is present before mechanical disruption of the ligament (Krayer et al. 2008). Interestingly, it has been shown in other studies that NO alone does not induce apoptotic death. However, incubation of chondrocytes with NO donors and the reactive nitrogen oxide compound peroxynitrite induced apoptotic cell death (Del Carlo & Loeser 2002). Peroxynitrite is an unstable species, formed by the reaction of NO with the superoxide radical (O_2^-). Peroxynitrite is a powerful oxidant that damages tissue through degradation of proteins, lipids, and nucleic acids.

These facts demonstrate the catabolic action of NO in joints. However, recently, it has been shown that this approach is too simplistic (Xia et al. 2006; Shi et al. 2007; Hancock & Riegger-Krugh 2008). Chondrocytes can respond differently to NO based on their location in the cartilage, and they can also act in a differentiated way depending on the mode of activation. For example, in a zymosan-

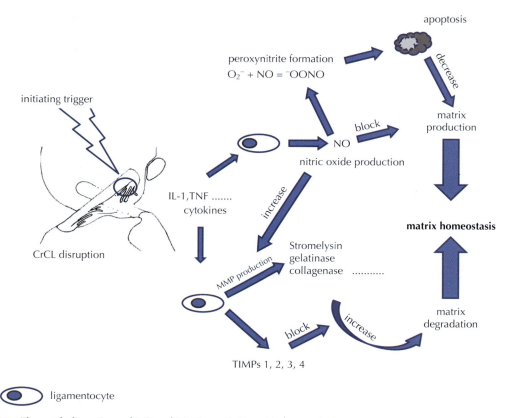

Figure 10.2 The catabolic actions of NO and MMPs on CrCL matrix homeostasis.

induced arthritis model, NO and peroxynitrite induced inflammation and proteoglycan loss. Addition of a selective iNOS inhibitor ameliorated inflammation but increased glycosaminoglycan loss. However, by adding uric acid, a peroxynitrite scavenger, the inflammation and proteglycan loss was ameliorated, suggesting that targeting peroxynitrite might be more effective for protection against OA (Bezzera et al. 2004).

MMP overview

Matrix metalloproteinases (MMPs) are a group of endopeptidases that have been detected in almost every disease process in which inflammation is present. Broad functions in defense, injury, inflammation, and repair have been attributed to MMPs (Manicone & McGuire 2008). The role of MMPs in matrix degradation and remodeling is considered to be most important in the context of CrCL rupture and stifle arthritis. The precise balance of tissue remodeling and synthesis is controlled by MMPs and their natural tissue inhibitors (TIMPs; Nagase et al. 2006). The TIMPs comprise a four-member family of homologous MMP inhibitors. TIMP concentrations generally far exceed the concentrations of MMPs in tissue, thereby limiting their proteolytic activity in the pericellular matrix.

MMPs in the articular environment are produced by synovial cells, cartilage, ligamentocytes, and leukocytes. MMPs can be divided into collagenases, gelatinases, stromelysins, and membrane-type MMPs, based mainly on their substrate specificity. For example, collagen type I is degraded by MMP-8, collagen type II by MMP-13, and collagen type III by MMP-1. On the other hand, stromelysin-1 (MMP-3) has a broader specificity including collagen type IV, V, VII, IX, and XI, as well as proteoglycans, elastin, laminin, and fibronectin. MMP-2, also termed gelatinase A, is another important MMP that cleaves collagen type IV and V, and degrades collagen type I and III (Manicone & McGuire 2008).

MMPs can be detected in joint tissue specimens as well as in synovial fluids. As with other components of synovial fluid, it is not possible to differentiate the origin of MMP production measured in synovial fluid. Therefore, MMP measurement in synovial fluid is only of limited value in understanding the pathophysiologic pathways of a specific disease (Fujita et al. 2006; Salinardi et al 2006; Tang et al. 2009).

The role of MMPs in the stifle joint

Joint diseases all include an inflammatory component and a matrix degrading component. MMPs play a role in both parts of the disease. Most actions of MMPs in the joint are catabolic in nature (Figure 10.2). They are associated with increased extracellular matrix degeneration of cartilage or ligaments, as well as with marked inflammation of synovial tissue (Foos et al. 2001; Muir et al. 2005; Doom et al. 2008; Tang et al. 2009). However, some MMPs have opposite roles in the development of specific diseases. For example, MMP-2 and MMP-9 (gelatinase A and B) have very similar substrate specificity for matrix proteins, but they have opposite non-matrix-related actions: MMP-2 is important for degradation of inflammatory factors, whereas MMP-9 is an important product of macrophages and neutrophils. Experimentally, this leads to exacerbated arthritis by MMP-2 deficiency, and reduced arthritis by MMP-9 deficiency (Itoh et al. 2002).

MMPs have been detected in CrCL tissue and have been correlated to CrCL injury. Expression of MMP-2, MMP-9, and MMP-13 genes was significantly increased in ruptured CrCL, and there was also a tendency for MMP-3 to be elevated all compared with intact canine CrCL (Spreng et al. 1999; Muir et al. 2005).

Influence of NO and MMPs on cranial cruciate ligament structure

The pathogenesis of canine CrCL rupture is poorly understood. One of the main reasons for this fact is that it is difficult to study the early phase of the CrCL rupture condition. One of the general pathways used to explain CrCL disruption involves a triggering event that leads to processes that slowly weaken the matrix of the ligament until mechanical rupture of the matrix components (Figure 10.2). This event is followed by clinical manifestation of lameness and partial or total rupture of the ligament with formation of arthritis. There is good evidence that NO and MMPs modulate the consequences of CrCL rupture, for example, OA (Abramson 2008). On the other hand, almost all scientific information specifically from the CrCL on NO and MMP involvement in the early and subclinical stages of the cruciate rupture arthropathy is only descriptive and fragmented and does not allow definite conclusions on the exact pathway of CrCL disruption. Some of these data concerning direct actions of NO and MMP on the ligament are described below.

External stimuli induce NO and MMP in ligaments

CrCL tissue responds to transection of the ligament, that is, trauma, by releasing MMP-2 (Tang et al. 2009). Synoviectomy of the synovial membrane covering the CrCL of rabbits induces a significant increase in collagenase activity within the ligament, indicating the protective role of the synovial sheath in intact CrCL. The released collagenase after synoviectomy may reflect the reaction of the CrCL to synovial fluid mediators released during inflammatory arthropathies (Amiel et al. 1990). Canine CrCL explant cultures, as well as fibroblastic monolayer cultures derived from CrCL activated with an inflammatory stimulus, produce significantly more NO and MMP compared with non-stimulated cultures over a period of 48 hours (Riitano et al. 2002). The same stimulus induces a significantly higher iNOS expression in CrCL, compared with medial collateral ligaments and femoral head ligaments (Louis et al. 2006). This could be an indication that CrCLs react differently to an inflammatory stimulus compared with other ligaments, with much higher NO production and subsequently more substrate available to produce reactive peroxynitrite.

High NO levels inhibit collagen synthesis in ligamentocytes

It has been shown that the CrCL produces more NO compared with other ligaments (Cao et al. 2000; Spreng et al. 2000). There is evidence that upon stimulation of ligamentocytes, levels of iNOS-induced NO increase and inhibit normal collagen synthesis (Cao et al. 2000). High NO concentrations could, therefore, be a reason for the insufficient healing capacities of ruptured CrCL in humans and in dogs. It can also be concluded that high NO concentrations inhibit normal matrix homeostasis, leading to intrinsic weakness of the ligament.

NO combined with peroxynitrite induces apoptosis in the ligament

Upon stimulation with nitroprusside, a NO donor, ligamentocytes from the CrCL were more prone to apoptosis compared with cells from the medial collateral ligament. DNA fragmentation and apoptosis were completely inhibited with a caspase-3 inhibitor (Murakami et al. 2005). On the other hand, oral treatment with L-N6-(1-iminoethyl)-lysine (L-NIL), a specific iNOS inhibitor, did not have a direct influence on the amount of apoptotic ligamentocytes in dogs with CrCL rupture (Hofer et al. 2009). Therefore, NO alone is not responsible for increased levels of apoptosis in the CrCL. This corresponds to other literature on chondrocytes indicating that only the combination of NO and ROS induces apoptosis (Del Carlo & Loeser 2002). Increased NO production could be an early step in CrCL rupture and may contribute to induction of cell death followed by catabolic derangement of the homeostasis of the ligament.

Conclusion

All these observations correspond with the theory that an initial incident is leading to inflammation of the CrCL (Hayashi et al. 2004). Ligamentocytes develop a dysregulation of matrix homeostasis as a reaction to the inflammatory stimulus, including up-regulation of matrix degrading enzymes,

down-regulation of matrix production, and peroxynitrite-induced premature ligamentocyte death (Figure 10.2). The role of NO, however, is not so simple. By extrapolating data from cartilage experiments, it seems that inhibition of NOS generation is able to decrease inflammation but has little effect of protecting the joint from cartilage loss. On the other hand, peroxynitrite inhibition with systemic uric acid application reduces intra-articular inflammation and loss of articular cartilage (Bezzera et al. 2004). Other studies, however, have shown the opposite: OA dogs treated with a specific iNOS inhibitor showed a reduction in osteophyte formation, decrease in the severity of histologic cartilage lesions, and reduced levels of apoptosis in cartilage compared with untreated dogs (Pelletier et al. 2000). And still other recent results show some evidence of protective effects of NO in tenocytes and human chronic OA (Xia et al. 2006; Hancock et al. 2008; Wallace et al. 2009). These conflicting results show that the role of NO in OA is not clear at the moment.

References

Abramson SB. Nitric oxide in inflammation and pain associated with osteoarthritis. Arthritis Res Ther 2008;10:S2.

Amiel D, Billings E, Jr., Harwood FL. Collagenase activity in anterior cruciate ligament: Protective role of the synovial sheath. J Appl Physiol 1990;69:902–906.

Amin AR, Di Cesare PE, Vyas P, et al. The expression and regulation of nitric oxide synthase in human osteoarthritis-affected chondrocytes: Evidence for up-regulated neuronal nitric oxide synthase. J Exp Med 1995;182:2097–2102.

Bezerra MM, Brain SD, Greenacre S, et al. Reactive nitrogen species scavenging, rather than nitric oxide inhibition, protects from articular cartilage damage in rat zymosan-induced arthritis. Br J Pharmacol 2004;141:172–182.

Boileau C, Martel-Pelletier J, Moldovan F, et al. The in situ up-regulation of chondrocyte interleukin-1-converting enzyme and interleukin-18 levels in experimental osteoarthritis is mediated by nitric oxide. Arthritis Rheum 2002;46:2637–2647.

Cao M, Stefanovic-Racic M, Georgescu HI, et al. Does nitric oxide help explain the differential healing capacity of the anterior cruciate, posterior cruciate, and medial collateral ligaments? Am J Sports Med 2000;28:176–182.

Del Carlo M, Jr., Loeser RF. Nitric oxide-mediated chondrocyte cell death requires the generation of additional reactive oxygen species. Arthritis Rheum 2002;46:394–403.

Di Mauro D, Bitto L, D'Andrea L, et al. Behaviour of nitric oxide synthase isoforms in inflammatory human joint diseases: An immunohistochemical study. Ital J Anat Embryol. 2006;111:111–123.

Doom M, de Bruin T, de Rooster H, et al. Immunopathological mechanisms in dogs with rupture of the cranial cruciate ligament. Vet Immunol Immunopathol 2008;125:143–161.

Foos MJ, Hickox JR, Mansour PG, et al. Expression of matrix metalloprotease and tissue inhibitor of metalloprotease genes in human anterior cruciate ligament. J Orthop Res 2001;19:642–649.

Fujita Y, Hara Y, Nezu Y, et al. Pro-inflammatory cytokine activities, matrix metalloproteinase-3 activity, and sulfated glycosaminoglycan content in synovial fluid of dogs with naturally acquired cranial cruciate ligament rupture. Vet Surg 2006;35:369–376.

Gyger O, Botteron C, Doherr M, et al. Detection and distribution of apoptotic cell death in normal and diseased canine cranial cruciate ligaments. Vet J 2007;174:371–377.

Hancock CM, Riegger-Krugh C. Modulation of pain in osteoarthritis: The role of nitric oxide. Clin J Pain 2008;24:353–365.

Hayashi K, Manley PA, Muir P. Cranial cruciate ligament pathophysiology in dogs with cruciate disease: A review. J Am Anim Hosp Assoc 2004;40:385–390.

Häuselmann HJ, Stefanovic-Racic M, Michel BA, Evans CH. Differences in nitric oxide production by superficial and deep human articular chondrocytes: Implications for proteoglycan turnover in inflammatory joint diseases. J Immunol 1998;160:1444–1448.

Hofer D, Forterre S, Schweighauser A, et al. Selective iNOS-inhibition does not influence apoptosis in ruptured canine cranial cruciate ligaments. Vet Comp Orthop Traumatol 2009;22:198–203.

Itoh T, Matsuda H, Tanioka M, et al. The role of matrix metalloproteinase-2 and matrix metalloproteinase-9 in antibody-induced arthritis. J Immunol 2002;169: 2643–2647.

Krayer M, Rytz U, Oevermann A, et al. Apoptosis of ligamentous cells of the cranial cruciate ligament from stable stifle joints of dogs with partial cranial cruciate ligament rupture. Am J Vet Res 2008;69:625–630.

Louis E, Remer KA, Doherr MG, et al. Nitric oxide and metalloproteinases in canine articular ligaments: A comparison between the cranial cruciate, the medial genual collateral and the femoral head ligament. Vet J 2006;172:466–472.

Manicone AM, McGuire JK. Matrix metalloproteinases as modulators of inflammation. Semin Cell Dev Biol 2008;19:34–41.

Marletta MA. Mammalian synthesis of nitrite, nitrate, nitric oxide, and N-nitrosating agents. Chem Res Toxicol 1988;1:249–257.

Muir P, Danova NA, Argyle DJ, et al. Collagenolytic protease expression in cranial cruciate ligament and stifle synovial fluid in dogs with cranial cruciate ligament rupture. Vet Surg 2005;34:482–490.

Murakami H, Shinomiya N, Kikuchi T, et al. Differential sensitivity to NO-induced apoptosis between anterior cruciate and medial collateral ligament cells. J Orthop Sci 2005;10:84–90.

Nagase H, Visse R, Murphy G. Structure and function of matrix metalloproteinases and TIMPs. Cardiovasc Res 2006;69:562–573.

Pelletier JP, Jovanovic DV, Lascau-Coman V, et al. Selective inhibition of inducible nitric oxide synthase reduces progression of experimental osteoarthritis in vivo: Possible link with the reduction in chondrocyte apoptosis and caspase 3 level. Arthritis Rheum 2000;43:1290–1299.

Riitano MC, Pfister H, Engelhardt P, et al. Effects of stimulus with pro-inflammatory mediators on nitric oxide production and matrix metalloproteinase activity in explants of cranial cruciate ligaments obtained from dogs. Am J Vet Res 2002;63:1423–1428.

Salinardi BJ, Roush JK, Schermerhorn T, Mitchell KE. Matrix metalloproteinase and tissue inhibitor of metalloproteinase in serum and synovial fluid of osteoarthritic dogs. Vet Comp Orthop Traumatol 2006;19: 49–55.

Shi HP, Wang SM, Zhang GX, et al. Supplemental L-arginine enhances wound healing following trauma/hemorrhagic shock. Wound Repair Regen 2007;15:66–70.

Spreng D, Sigrist N, Busato A, et al. Stromelysin activity in canine cranial cruciate ligament rupture. Vet Comp Orthop Traumatol 1999;12:159–165.

Spreng D, Sigrist N, Jungi T, et al. Nitric oxide metabolite production in the cranial cruciate ligament, synovial membrane, and articular cartilage of dogs with cranial cruciate ligament rupture. Am J Vet Res 2000;61:530–536.

Tang Z, Yang L, Wang Y, et al. Contributions of different intraarticular tissues to the acute phase elevation of synovial fluid MMP-2 following rat ACL rupture. J Orthop Res 2009;27:243–248.

Wallace JL, Viappiani S, Bolla M. Cyclooxygenase-inhibiting nitric oxide donators for osteoarthritis. Trends Pharmacol Sci 2009;30:112–117.

Weinberg JB, Fermor B, Guilak F. Nitric oxide synthase and cyclooxygenase interactions in cartilage and meniscus: Relationships to joint physiology, arthritis, and tissue repair. Subcell Biochem 2007;42:31–62.

Xia W, Szomor Z, Wang Y, Murrell GA. Nitric oxide enhances collagen synthesis in cultured human tendon cells. J Orthop Res 2006;24:159–172.

11 Role of Antibodies to Type I and II Collagen

Hilde de Rooster, Tanya de Bruin, and Eric Cox

Introduction

One of the major limitations in many investigations on the ethiopathogenesis of cruciate rupture in dogs is that most studies have focused on the affected stifle joint after rupture, the end-stage of the condition. Recently, studies on humoral and cellular immunopathological mechanisms in predisposed dogs before clinical rupture of the contralateral cranial cruciate ligament (CrCL) have been carried out (de Bruin et al. 2007a,b).

Antigenicity of collagen

The CrCL has a microstructure of collagen bundles of multiple types, but mostly type I. The menisci are also composed mainly of type I collagen, whereas the articular cartilage is composed mainly of type II collagen (van Sickle et al. 1993).

The cruciate ligaments are covered by a fold of synovial membrane, and although they have an intra-articular position, they are extrasynovial (Alm & Strömberg 1974; Arnoczky et al. 1979). Recently, scanning electron microscopy ascertained the presence of many small holes in the enveloping membrane, allowing infiltration of the cruciate ligaments by synovial fluid (Kobayashi et al. 2006). Local inflammatory processes and/or trauma may result in exposure of macromolecules such as collagen that trigger immune-mediated inflammatory responses (Figure 11.1). Once autoantibodies have been produced, newly released type I collagen can enhance joint inflammation by forming immune complexes with these antibodies, resulting in activation of complement and of phagocytes (Bari et al. 1989; Carter et al. 1999).

Prevalence of antibodies to type I and II collagen

Type I and II anticollagen antibodies have been detected in dogs that sustained a CrCL rupture (Niebauer & Menzel 1982; Niebauer et al. 1987; Bari et al. 1989; de Rooster et al. 2000). Antibodies are present in both sera and synovial fluid aspirated from the affected stifle joint, with a higher incidence in the synovial fluid (Niebauer & Menzel 1982; Niebauer et al. 1987; Bari et al. 1989), thus indicating local antibody production. This is sup-

---

Advances in the Canine Cranial Cruciate Ligament,
Edited by Peter Muir, © 2010 ACVS Foundation, This Work is a co-publication between the American College of Veterinary Surgeons Foundation and Wiley-Blackwell.

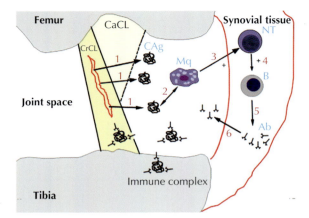

Figure 11.1 Schematic representation of immune-mediated inflammatory responses in dogs with cranial cruciate ligament (CrCL) rupture. Step 1: impaired CrCL with release of type I collagen (CAg); Step 2: collagen uptake by macrophage (Mq); Step 3: antigen presentation to naive T cell (NT); Step 4: B cell (B) activation/differentiation with antibody production (Ab); Step 5: release of antibodies in synovial tissue; Step 6: release of antibodies in the synovial fluid and formation of immune complexes with type I collagen. CaCL: caudal cruciate ligament.

ported by histological studies on synovial tissue from stifle joints of dogs with cruciate rupture (Tirgari 1977;, Galloway & Lester 1995; Lawrence et al. 1998; Hewicker et al. 1999). The main cell types detected in the synovial tissue are macrophages, T lymphocytes, B lymphocytes, and plasma cells belonging predominantly to the IgG isotype (Tirgari 1977; Galloway & Lester 1995; Lawrence et al. 1998; Hewicker et al. 1999; Lemburg et al. 2004). Furthermore, significantly higher amounts of IgG and IgM have been detected in the synovial tissue of stifle joints of dogs with cruciate rupture compared with normal stifle joints (Lawrence et al. 1998). In addition, one study reported that 67% of the dogs had distinct lymphoplasmacytic nodules within the synovial tissue (Galloway & Lester 1995).

Studies on cellular immune mechanisms suggest that there is an inflammatory process in the contralateral joints of predisposed dogs preceding detectable joint instability (de Bruin et al. 2007a). Type I anticollagen antibodies have been measured sequentially in the synovial fluid aspirated from multiple joints. In predisposed dogs, higher type I anticollagen titers were found in the stifle joints that eventually sustained a CrCL rupture, compared with the titers in a remote joint (de Bruin et al. 2007a).

Relevance of antibodies to type I and II collagen

It remains uncertain whether antibodies play an active role in the initiation of CrCL rupture. Prospective studies on dogs initially presented with unilateral CrCL rupture did not provide evidence for this since not all dogs with high antibodies developed a contralateral CrCL rupture (de Bruin et al. 2007a). Nevertheless, it is possible that anticollagen antibodies perpetuate chronic joint inflammation in some dogs with cruciate degeneration, even if collagen is not the primary arthritogenic agent. The finding of higher type I anticollagen titers in the stifle joints that did not yet have a clinically detectable cruciate rupture at the time of measurement, compared with the titers in a remote joint, suggests that there was an inflammatory process with production of collagen-specific antibodies in these contralateral stifle joints (de Bruin et al. 2007a).

Histological studies on synovial tissue from stifle joints of dogs with a cruciate rupture detected plasma cells belonging predominantly to the IgG isotype (Tirgari 1977; Galloway & Lester 1995; Lawrence et al. 1998; Hewicker et al. 1999; Lemburg et al. 2004) and lymphoplasmacytic nodules (Galloway & Lester 1995). However, to date, no synovial tissue cells from cruciate patients have been cultured to discover if they effectively produce antibodies and, if so, against which antigens.

Type I and II anticollagen antibodies have also been detected in the synovial fluid of stifle joints with arthritis secondary to arthropathies other than CrCL rupture (Niebauer et al. 1987; Bari et al. 1989), suggesting that these antibodies are not specific for the type of joint disorder (de Rooster et al. 2000). However, in dogs with complete rupture, unexpectedly low or undetectable type I anticollagen antibody titers were found in the synovial fluid of dogs with complete rupture (de Bruin et al. 2007a). This suggests either that the autoimmune response stops after the rupture or that antibodies cannot be detected since they are all present in immune complexes of these antibodies and collagen.

References

Alm A, Strömberg B. Vascular anatomy of the patellar and cruciate ligaments. A microangiographic and histologic investigation in the dog. Acta Chir Scand Suppl 1974;445:25–35.

Arnoczky SP, Rubin RM, Marshall JL. Microvasculature of the cruciate ligaments and its response to injury. An experimental study in dogs. J Bone Joint Surg Am 1979;61:1221–1229.

Bari AS, Carter SD, Bell SC, et al. Anti-type II collagen antibody in naturally occurring canine joint diseases. Br J Rheumatol 1989;28:480–486.

Carter SD, Barnes A, Gilmore WH. Canine rheumatoid arthritis and inflammatory cytokines. Vet Immunol Immunopathol 1999;69:201–214.

de Bruin T, de Rooster H, van Bree H, Cox E. Evaluation of anticollagen type I antibody titers in synovial fluid of both stifle joints and the left shoulder joint of dogs with unilateral cranial cruciate disease. Am J Vet Res 2007a;68:283–289.

de Bruin T, de Rooster H, van Bree H, et al. Lymphocyte proliferation to collagen type I in dogs. J Vet Med A Physiol Pathol Clin Med 2007b;54:292–296.

de Rooster H, Cox E, van Bree H. Prevalence and relevance of antibodies to type-I and -II collagen in synovial fluid of dogs with cranial cruciate ligament damage. Am J Vet Res 2000;61:1456–1461.

Galloway RH, Lester SJ. Histopathological evaluation of canine stifle joint synovial membrane collected at the time of repair of cranial cruciate ligament rupture. J Am Anim Hosp Assoc 1995;31: 289–294.

Hewicker TM, Carter SD, Bennett D. Immunocytochemical demonstration of lymphocyte subsets and MHC class II antigen axpression in synovial membranes from dogs with rheumatoid arthritis and degenerative joint disease. Vet Immunol Immunopathol 1999; 67:341–357.

Kobayashi S, Baba H, Uchida K, et al. Microvascular system of anterior cruciate ligament in dogs. J Orthop Res 2006;24:1509–1520.

Lawrence D, Bao S, Canfield PJ, Allanson M, Husband AJ. Elevation of immunoglobulin deposition in the synovial membrane of dogs with cranial cruciate ligament rupture. Vet Immunol Immunopathol 1998;65:89–96.

Lemburg AK, Meyer-Lindenberg A, Hewicker-Trautwein M. Immunohistochemical characterization of inflammatory cell populations and adhesion molecule expression in synovial membranes from dogs with spontaneous cranial cruciate ligament rupture. Vet Immunol Immunopathol 2004;97:231–240.

Niebauer GW, Menzel EJ. Immunological changes in canine cruciate ligament rupture. Res Vet Sci 1982;32: 235–241.

Niebauer GW, Wolf B, Bashey RI, Newton CD. Antibodies to canine collagen types I and II in dogs with spontaneous cruciate ligament rupture and osteoarthritis. Arthritis Rheum 1987;30:319–327.

Tirgari M. Changes in the canine stifle joint following rupture of the anterior cruciate ligament. J Small Anim Pract 1977;19:17–26.

van Sickle DC, Delleman DH, Brown EM 1993. Connective and supportive tissues. In: *Textbook of Veterinary Histology*, Dellmann H, van Sickle DC, Brown EM (eds). Philadelphia: Lea & Febiger, 1993, pp. 29–53.

12 Synovitis or Stifle Instability, Which Comes First?

Jason A. Bleedorn and Peter Muir

Introduction

Cranial cruciate ligament (CrCL) rupture in the dog is historically considered a degenerative process with progressive mid-substance rupture of the ligament. Many etiologic factors have been proposed, including age-related deterioration, joint conformation, and synovial inflammation leading to degradation of the ligament (Vasseur et al. 1985; Slocum & Slocum 1993; Comerford et al. 2006). It is well understood that inflammation of the synovium develops in association with the cruciate rupture arthropathy in dogs, although its role in the pathogenesis of the condition remains unclear.

Immune complex formation and anticollagen antibodies were identified in the synovial fluid and sera of dogs with naturally occurring CrCL rupture by Niebauer and Menzel in the early 1980s, and it was hypothesized that an immunological mechanism promotes the development of CrCL rupture (Niebauer & Menzel 1982). Similarly, histologic features of lymphoplasmacytic synovitis with distinct, nodular aggregates were

identified in the synovial membranes of two thirds of dogs with cruciate rupture at the time of surgery to stabilize the stifle joint (Galloway & Lester 1995). Further investigations have identified elevation in biomarkers of joint inflammation in association with the cruciate rupture arthropathy in dogs (Doom et al. 2008). Recent evidence supports the argument that persistent synovitis and development of an inflammatory arthritis is likely a significant factor promoting degenerative rupture of the CrCL (Fujita et al. 2006). Clinical, radiographic, and arthroscopic evidence of stifle synovitis and arthritis can be found in dogs with stable stifle joints, with similar severity to the contralateral unstable stifles with complete CrCL rupture (Bleedorn et al. 2009). These findings are significant because they challenge the historical dogma of degenerative CrCL rupture in dogs and raise the question: which comes first, synovitis or joint instability?

Synovitis

The synovial membrane is a specialized collagenous tissue lining the interior and all structures within a synovial joint. Synovium has two layers: an inner synovial intima containing a rich vascular, nerve, and lymphatic network with villous

---

Advances in the Canine Cranial Cruciate Ligament, Edited by Peter Muir, © 2010 ACVS Foundation, This Work is a co-publication between the American College of Veterinary Surgeons Foundation and Wiley-Blackwell.

projections, and an outer supportive layer that is continuous with the fibrous joint capsule (Sutton et al. 2009). Synoviocytes are loosely arranged within the membrane and have an integral function in maintaining joint health (Iwanaga et al. 2000).

Synovitis is characterized by infiltration of the synovial membrane with inflammatory cells resulting in vascularisation and hyperplasia of the synovium. The cellular distribution is typically a mononuclear leukocyte infiltrate, with a predominance of T cells (Sutton et al. 2009; Figure 12.1).

Pro-inflammatory cytokines synthesized in the synovium potentiate the cascade of biologically active substances that contribute to the degradation of the joint (Doom et al. 2008). Whether the morphologic changes within the synovial membrane are a primary, rheumatoid-like, inflammatory process, or secondary to cruciate rupture and joint inflammation remains unclear.

Synovitis is believed to contribute to the development of pain, joint inflammation, and progression of osteoarthritis (Sutton et al. 2009). Induction of an immune synovitis has been shown to cause significant reduction in CrCL strength and leads to structural failure and mid-substance rupture in experimental animals (Goldberg et al. 1982). Objective evaluation of the synovial membrane in the stifle joint of dogs is not routine in clinical practice. Ultrasound and magnetic resonance imaging (MRI) have been used to evaluate synovial membrane pathology and joint effusion severity in the human knee, but lack clinical validation in dogs (Tarhan & Unlu 2003). Stifle arthroscopy enhances macroscopic evaluation of the synovial membrane with increased access and magnification, and is considered the gold standard for assessment of articular cartilage and synovium in human joints (Ayral 1996). Arthroscopic features of synovitis are well described in the human knee and defined by three baseline parameters: intensity, extent, and location (Ayral 1996). Scoring systems have been described to provide objective evaluation of disease severity; arthroscopic scoring of disease severity correlates well with noninvasive imaging modalities (Fernandez-Madrid et al. 1995; Tarhan & Unlu 2003; Karim et al. 2004). Arthroscopic assessment also correlates well with histologic characteristics of disease severity, particularly in rheumatoid arthritis

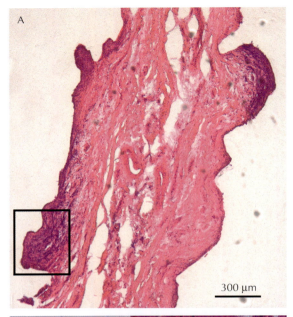

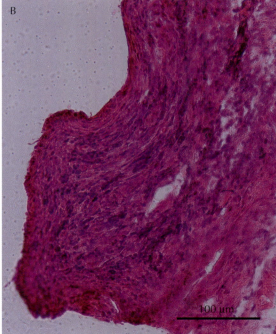

Figure 12.1 Biopsy of synovial membrane from the stable contralateral stifle joint of a dog with CrCL rupture. (A) Distinct cellular aggregates forming nodules along the margin of the synovial membrane. (B) Higher magnification of area designated by box showing dense mononuclear infiltration of the synovial intima and subintimal tissues. Frozen section with hematoxylin and eosin stain. (A)–bar = 300 μm, (B)–bar = 100 μm.

patients (Lindblad & Hedfors 1985). Similar arthroscopic features of synovitis can be identified in the stifle joints of dogs with CrCL rupture arthropathy. Increased vascularity and proliferation of the synovium occur with some global variation within affected joints (Bleedorn et al. 2009). Arthroscopic assessment using a similar scoring system is significantly correlated with radiographic arthritis severity (Bleedorn et al. 2009).

Joint instability

Stifle joint instability develops secondary to CrCL rupture in the dog, with various degrees of severity based on several factors. Mild cruciate tears can result in minimal instability limited to only flexion and/or extension based on percentage of torn fibers (Heffron & Campbell 1978). Concurrent joint pathology, such as meniscal injury and periarticular fibrosis, can also impact stifle joint stability (Scavelli et al. 1990).

Clinical examination of the stifle joint using cranial drawer and cranial tibial thrust provides subjective evaluation of stifle stability in dogs (see Chapter 15). Stress radiography (Chapter 18) provides an additional objective assessment of stifle stability, which may be helpful to differentiate between intact or stable partial rupture and complete CrCL rupture (de Rooster et al. 1998; de Rooster & van Bree 1999; Figure 12.2A–D). Arthroscopic evaluation of the stifle joint in dogs is becoming more common in veterinary practice and allows for direct examination of the cruciate ligaments and probing of their integrity (van Gestel 1985; Beale et al. 2003). A substantial proportion of the population of dogs with naturally occurring cruciate rupture have a partial CrCL tear and a clinically stable stifle at the time of surgery (Scavelli et al. 1990; Ralphs & Whitney 2002). However, these findings likely underestimate the true incidence since these reports only describe patients that were treated surgically.

Surgical treatment for dogs with the cruciate rupture arthropathy has historically focused on elimination of joint instability. Despite stifle stabilization, synovitis may persist and arthritis is progressive with varying degrees of associated lameness (Vasseur & Berry 1992; Girling et al.

2006; Sanderson et al. 2009). In addition, the incidence of CrCL rupture in the contralateral stifle in affected dogs is between 37% and 48% within 10–17 months of initial diagnosis (Doverspike et al. 1993; Buote et al. 2009). These findings question conventional thinking regarding the relationship between development of joint instability and development of stifle synovitis in affected dogs.

Synovitis in stable stifles

Although it is clear that experimental CrCL transection leads to joint instability and synovitis in dogs (Gardner et al. 1984; Lipowitz et al. 1985; Myers et al. 1990), recent work has highlighted the fact that development of joint inflammation before development of CrCL rupture and stifle instability is common (Bleedorn et al. 2009). Clinical findings may include lameness, joint effusion, and discomfort upon passive range-of-motion and hyperextension of the stifle, but no cranial drawer or cranial tibial thrust instability. The presence of radiographic stifle joint effusion and varying degrees of osteophytosis provide supportive evidence for development of stifle arthritis and early stifle joint degeneration. Although it has been suggested that surgical treatment of this type of patient with tibial plateau leveling osteotomy (TPLO) may help preserve stifle stability by unloading the CrCL, prospective clinical trial data are lacking.

The synovium in stable stifle joints with early clinical or radiographic evidence of arthritis is inflamed (Bleedorn et al. 2009). In a recent case series, synovitis was present without arthroscopically apparent fraying the CrCL in dogs with lameness and stifle arthritis (Figure 12.3A); in the remaining dogs, superficial fraying of the CrCL, and occasionally the caudal cruciate ligament, was seen together with synovitis (Figure 12.3B; Bleedorn et al. 2009). Interestingly, the severity of arthroscopic changes in stable stifles is comparable to those with complete CrCL rupture and joint instability (Figure 12.2C,D). These observations support the hypothesis that development of synovitis induces degeneration of CrCL matrix and eventual progressive fraying and rupture of the ligament in dogs.

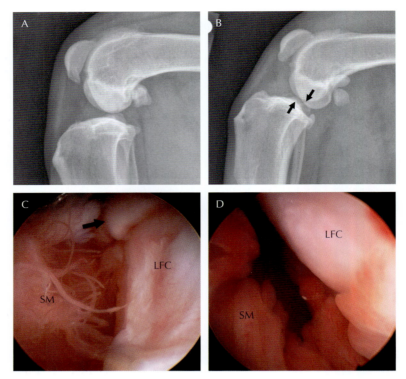

Figure 12.2 Lateral stress radiographic projections and arthroscopic images from stable (A,C) and unstable (B,D) stifle joints of dogs with cranial cruciate ligament (CrCL) rupture. (A,B) There is moderate degenerative joint disease with marked joint effusion and osteophytosis of the patella, femoral trochlear ridges, fabellae, and tibial plateau in both stifle joints. In (B), the intercondylar eminences of the tibia are translated cranial in relation to the femoral condyles, resulting in cranial tibial subluxation (arrows) because of CrCL rupture. (C) There is increased circulation and marked filamentous proliferation of the synovial membrane in the lateral joint compartment. Osteophytes are present along the lateral trochlear ridge of the femur (arrow). (D) There is marked increased capillary hyperemia and club-like villous proliferation of the synovial membrane in the lateral joint compartment. LFC: lateral femoral condyle, SM: synovial membrane.

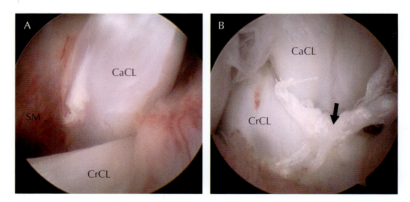

Figure 12.3 Arthroscopic images from the contralateral stable stifle joints of dogs with cranial cruciate ligament (CrCL) rupture. (A) Mild synovitis is present in both joints with normal appearing cruciate ligaments, and (B) mild mid-substance fraying of the caudolateral bulk of the CrCL along the intercondylar notch (arrow). CrCL: cranial cruciate ligament, CaCL: caudal cruciate ligament, SM: synovial membrane.

Conclusion

In conclusion, recent research suggests that stifle synovitis precedes the development of CrCL rupture in dogs affected with the cruciate rupture arthropathy. The underlying etiopathogenesis of stifle synovitis and its contribution to the development of cruciate rupture remains an important research question. Future studies should focus on the immunologic mechanism that induces chronic synovitis, as well as disease-modifying therapies to reduce joint inflammation.

References

Ayral X. Diagnostic and quantitative arthroscopy: Quantitative arthroscopy. Baillieres Clin Rheumatol 1996;10:477–494.

Beale BS, Hulse DA, Schulz KS, Whitney WO. *Small Animal Arthroscopy*. Philadelphia: W.B. Saunders, 2003, pp. 117–157.

Bleedorn JA, Greuel E, Manley PA, et al. Synovitis precedes development of joint instability in dogs with degenerative cranial cruciate ligament rupture. Vet Surg 2009;38:E26.

Buote N, Fusco J, Radasch R. Age, tibial plateau angle, sex, and weight as risk factors for contralateral rupture of the cranial cruciate ligament in labradors. Vet Surg 2009;38:481–489.

Comerford EJ, Tarlton JF, Avery NC, et al. Distal femoral intercondylar notch dimensions and their relationship to composition and metabolism of the canine anterior cruciate ligament. Osteoarthritis Cartilage 2006;14: 273–278.

de Rooster H, van Ryssen B, van Bree H. Diagnosis of cranial cruciate ligament injury in dogs by tibial compression radiography. Vet Rec 1998;142:366–368.

de Rooster H, van Bree H. Radiographic measurement of craniocaudal instability in stifle joints of clinically normal dogs and dogs with injury of a cranial cruciate ligament. Am J Vet Res 1999;60:1567–1570.

Doom M, de Bruin T, de Rooster H, et al. Immunopathological mechanisms in dogs with rupture of the cranial cruciate ligament. Vet Immunol Immunopathol 2008;125:143–161.

Doverspike M, Vasseur PB, Harb MF, Walls CM. Contralateral cranial cruciate ligament rupture: Incidence in 114 dogs. J Am Anim Hosp Assoc 1993;29: 167–170.

Fernandez–Madrid F, Karvonen RL, Teitge RA, et al. Synovial thickening detected by MR imaging in osteoarthritis of the knee confirmed by biopsy as synovitis. Magn Reson Imaging 1995;13:177–183.

Fujita Y, Hara Y, Ochi H, et al. Proinflammatory cytokine activities, matrix metalloproteinase-3 activity, and sulfated glycosaminoglycan content in synovial fluid of dogs with naturally acquired cranial cruciate ligament rupture. Vet Surg 2006;35:369–376.

Galloway RH, Lester SJ. Histopathological evaluation of canine stifle joint synovial membrane collected at the time of repair of cranial cruciate ligament rupture. J Am Anim Hosp Assoc 1995;31:289–294.

Gardner DL, Bradley WA, O'Connor P, et al. Synovitis after surgical division of the anterior cruciate ligament of the dog. Clin Exp Rheumatol 1984;2:11–15.

Girling SL, Bell SC, Whitelock RG, et al. Use of biochemical markers of osteoarthritis to investigate the potential disease-modifying effect of tibial plateau levelling osteotomy. J Small Anim Pract 2006;47: 708–714.

Goldberg VM, Burstein A, Dawson M. The influence of an experimental immune synovitis on the failure mode and strength of the rabbit anterior cruciate ligament. J Bone Joint Surg Am 1982;64:900–906.

Heffron LE, Campbell JR. Morphology, histology, and functional anatomy of the canine cranial cruciate ligament. Vet Rec 1978;102:280–283.

Iwanaga T, Shikichi M, Kitamura H, et al. Morphology and functional roles of synoviocytes in the joint. Arch Histol Cytol 2000;63:17–31.

Karim Z, Wakefield RJ, Quinn M, et al. Validation and reproducibility of ultrasonography in the detection of synovitis in the knee: A comparison with arthroscopy and clinical examination. Arthritis Rheum 2004;50: 387–394.

Lindblad S, Hedfors E. Intraarticular variation in synovitis. Local macroscopic and microscopic signs of inflammatory activity are significantly correlated. Arthritis Rheum 1985;28:977–986.

Lipowitz AJ, Wong PL, Stevens JB. Synovial membrane changes after experimental transection of the cranial cruciate ligament in dogs. Am J Vet Res 1985;46: 1166–1170.

Myers SL, Brandt KD, O'Connor BL, et al. Synovitis and osteoarthritic changes in canine articular cartilage after anterior cruciate ligament transection. Effect of surgical hemostasis. Arthritis Rheum 1990;33: 1406–1415.

Niebauer GW, Menzel EJ. Immunological changes in canine cruciate ligament rupture. Res Vet Sci 1982; 32:235–241.

Ralphs SC, Whitney WO. Arthroscopic evaluation of menisci in dogs with cranial cruciate ligament injuries: 100 cases (1999–2000). J Am Vet Med Assoc 2002;221:1601–1604.

Sanderson RO, Beata C, Filipo RM, et al. Systematic review of the management of canine osteoarthritis. Vet Rec 2009;164:418–424.

Scavelli TD, Schraeder SC, Matthiesen DT, Skorup DE. Partial rupture of the cranial cruciate ligament of the stifle in dogs: 25 cases (1982–1988). J Am Vet Med Assoc 1990;96:1135–1138.

Slocum B, Slocum TD. Tibial plateau leveling osteotomy for repair of cranial cruciate ligament rupture in the canine. Vet Clin North Am Small Anim Pract 1993;23:777–795.

Sutton S, Clutterbuck A, Harris P, et al. The contribution of the synovium, synovial derived inflammatory cytokines and neuropeptides to the pathogenesis of osteoarthritis. Vet J 2009;179:10–24.

Tarhan S, Unlu Z. Magnetic resonance imaging and ultrasonographic evaluation of the patients with knee osteoarthritis: A comparative study. Clin Rheumatol 2003;22:181–188.

van Gestel MA. Arthroscopy of the canine stifle. Vet Q 1985;7:237–239.

Vasseur PB, Berry CR. Progression of stifle osteoarthrosis following reconstruction of the cranial cruciate ligament in 21 dogs. J Am Anim Hosp Assoc 1992;28: 129–136.

Vasseur PB, Pool RR, Arnoczky SP, Lau RE. Correlative biomechanical and histologic study of the cranial cruciate ligament in dogs. Am J Vet Res 1985;46: 1842–1854.

13 Role of Synovial Immune Responses in Stifle Synovitis

Peter Muir

Introduction

The historical paradigm for the cranial cruciate ligament (CrCL) rupture mechanism has been that ligament rupture is largely a consequence of trauma, with arthritis developing secondary to joint instability. However, a growing body of evidence suggests that this relationship is incorrect and that in dogs with naturally occurring cruciate rupture, synovitis and arthritis typically precede the development of ligament rupture and associated stifle instability. In dogs with CrCL rupture, epidemiologic studies suggest that if subtle radiographic change is present in the contralateral stifle, the risk of contralateral rupture at 16 months is as high as 65% (Doverspike et al. 1993). While it is clear that CrCL transection and associated stifle instability contributes to the development of synovitis (Lipowitz et al. 1985), the growing use of arthroscopy for stifle evaluation in the dog and the use of tibial plateau leveling osteotomy surgery to treat dogs with partial CrCL ruptures and a stable stifle has led to a greater appreciation that synovitis is typically present in stable stifles of affected

---

Advances in the Canine Cranial Cruciate Ligament, Edited by Peter Muir, © 2010 ACVS Foundation, This Work is a co-publication between the American College of Veterinary Surgeons Foundation and Wiley-Blackwell.

dogs (Bleedorn et al. 2009). The cruciate ligaments are intra-articular, but extra synovial and are covered in synovium. Experimentally, persistent synovitis induces substantial degradation of CrCL tensile strength (Goldberg et al. 1982). The deleterious effects of chronic joint inflammation on the tissue matrix of the cruciate ligaments is likely due to the blood–cruciate barrier in the ligament microvasculature, such that cruciate ligament metabolism is closely related to changes in synovial fluid (Kobayashi et al. 2006).

A logical extension of this shift in thinking is to focus on understanding the disease mechanism that leads to the development of stifle arthritis in dogs. Much work has demonstrated that stifle arthritis in dogs has a substantial inflammatory component, suggesting that synovial immune responses may be an important factor promoting joint inflammation and progressive degradation of intra-articular structures over time, including the cruciate ligaments (Doom et al. 2008).

Inflammatory cell populations within the stifle joint

Synovitis involves the intima of the CrCL epiligament. The inflammatory cell population is typically a mixed mononuclear population and includes activated tartrate-resistant acid

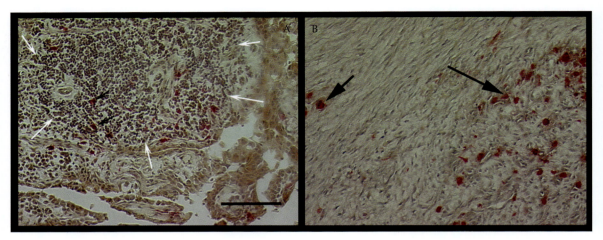

Figure 13.1 Photomicrographs of frozen sections of (A) synovium and (B) ruptured cranial cruciate ligament (CrCL) from a 5-year-old dog with CrCL rupture. (A) In this specimen, aggregates of mononuclear cells are present in the synovial intima (white arrows), including activated macrophages stained red for tartrate-resistant acid phosphatase (TRAP) (black arrows). (B) In ruptured CrCL from the same dog, aggregates of TRAP⁺-activated macrophages can also be seen infiltrating the CrCL. TRAP histochemical stain, with Mayer's hematoxylin counterstain. Bar = 100 µm. Reproduced from Muir et al. (2005), with permission from Wiley-Blackwell.

phosphatase-positive (TRAP) macrophages (Figure 13.1), T and B lymphocytes (Figure 13.2), plasma cells, and major histocompatibility complex (MHC) class II-positive dendritic cells (Faldyna et al. 2004; Lemburg et al. 2004; Klocke et al. 2005; Muir et al. 2005, 2007a,b, 2009). In dogs with stifle arthritis, the proportion of T lymphocytes within synovial tissues is increased in dogs with CrCL rupture (Faldyna et al. 2004). Expression of the T cell antigen receptor complex is also increased in synovium and synovial fluid in affected dogs (Muir et al. 2009). While lymphocytes play a key role in antigen-specific immunity, activated macrophages and their inflammatory products play a key role in innate immunity and the pathogenesis of tissue inflammation.

Antigen-specific immune responses within joint tissues

Recruitment and proliferation of T lymphocytes within joint tissue is a key pro-inflammatory feature of arthritis, including arthropathies that have traditionally been considered to be associated with little joint inflammation (Sakkas & Platsoucas 2007). Identification of large populations of lymphocytes within synovial tissues of affected dogs suggests that activation of antigen-specific immune responses is an important component of the disease mechanism for the cruciate rupture arthropathy. An MHC class II genetic susceptibility has been identified in many immune-mediated arthritides in humans, and recent work suggests that similar genetic susceptibility to inflammatory arthritis exists in dogs (Ollier et al. 2001). At present, a major unanswered question is the identity of the immunologic trigger that induces and promotes chronic stifle synovitis. Several studies have explored the hypothesis that neoepitopes of type I and type II collagen may be important in this regard (Niebauer et al. 1987; de Bruin et al. 2007a,b; see Chapter 11). Translocation of bacterial material to the stifle joint is a common event in dogs (Muir et al. 2007c). A polymicrobial population of bacteria that are not recognized joint pathogens is typically present, particularly Gram-negative organisms (Muir et al. 2010). Similar microbial populations are found in human arthritic joints (Kempsell et al. 2000). Therefore, it remains a possibility that the primary triggering antigen in the cruciate rupture arthropathy may be derived from small amounts of microbial mate-

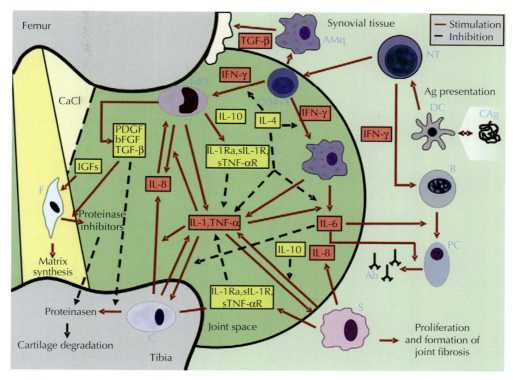

Figure 13.2 Schematic representation of the possible cytokine cascade in dogs with CrCL rupture (begin at antigen presentation in the synovial tissue; black lines: stimulation; red lines: inhibition; yellow boxes: pro-inflammatory; red boxes: anti-inflammatory). Antigen-stimulated dendritic cells present antigen to naive T lymphocytes. Activated CD4+ T lymphocytes can then stimulate different cells (macrophages, monocytes, B lymphocytes, fibroblasts, and synoviocytes) by cytokine release to produce antibodies, osteophytes, ligament degeneration, and synovial tissue proliferation (black lines). Next to the pro-inflammatory reactions, anti-inflammatory responses are seen (red lines). Ab: antibodies; Ag: antigen; AMq: activated macrophage; B: B lymphocyte, bFGF: basic fibroblast growth factor; C: chondrocyte; CaCL: caudal cruciate ligament; CAg: collagen antigen; CD4+T: CD4+ T lymphocyte; DC: dendritic cell, IFN-γ: interferon gamma; IGFs: insulin-like growth factors; IL: interleukin; IL-1Ra: interleukin 1 receptor antagonist, F: fibroblast, Mo: monocyte, NT: naive T lymphocyte, PC: plasma cell, PDGF: platelet-derived growth factor; S: synoviocyte, sIL–1R: soluble IL-1 receptor; sTNF-αR: soluble TNF-α receptor; TGF-β: transforming growth factor beta; TNF-α: tumor necrosis factor alpha. Reproduced from Doom et al. (2008), with permission from Elsevier.

rial that have translocated to the stifle synovium from the circulation.

Innate immune responses within joint tissues

Although it is increasingly clear that activation of antigen-specific immune responses within the stifle is important for the development of synovial inflammation, activation of innate immune responses is also likely important. Pattern recognition receptors (PRR) are expressed by leukocytes and epithelial cells and are used by the innate immune system to detect the presence of infection (Akira et al. 2006). Activation of PRR also appears to contribute to disease pathology in inflammatory and autoimmune conditions (e.g., Bryant & Fitzgerald 2009). Activation of PRR, such as toll-like receptors (TLR) and nucleotide-binding oligomerization domain (NOD) containing proteins, leads to activation of nuclear factor kappa B (NFκβ) and up-regulation of immune response genes and pro-inflammatory cytokines. Innate

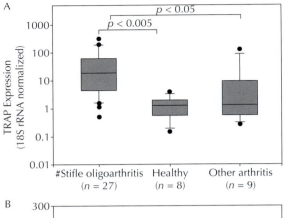

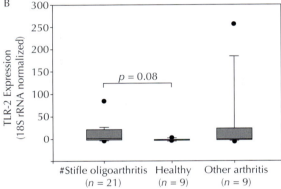

Figure 13.3 (A) Relative expression of tartrate-resistant acid phosphatase (TRAP) and (B) toll-like receptor 2 (TLR-2) in synovial fluid cells collected from dogs with stifle arthritis and degenerative CrCL, healthy dogs, and dogs with other forms of osteoarthritis (OA), characterized by cartilage loss. Gene expression was normalized to peripheral blood mononuclear cells (PBMC) as an internal control using the $-\Delta\Delta C_t$ method. 18S rRNA was used as the house-keeping gene. # indicates a significant difference from internal PBMC controls ($p < 0.05$). Boxes represent median and the 25th and 75th percentiles. Whiskers represent 10th and 90th percentiles. Outliers are also plotted. Significant differences between groups are as indicated. Reproduced from Muir et al. (2007b), with permission from Elsevier.

immune responses to PRR also regulate subsequent adaptive immune responses via dendritic cell signaling (Iwasaki & Medzhitov 2010). Defective PRR function has been implicated in various chronic inflammatory conditions, such as Crohn's disease in human beings and perianal fistulae in dogs (House et al. 2008). Analysis of synovial fluid cells from dogs with stifle arthritis and degenerative cruciate rupture suggests that expression of TRAP is increased relative to healthy dogs and dogs with osteoarthritis (Figure 13.3A; Muir et al. 2007b). Higher expression of TLR-2 in arthritic joints was also found (Figure 13.3B; Muir et al. 2007b). Collectively, these findings suggest that macrophage activation is also an important factor in the development of chronic synovitis in the cruciate rupture arthropathy.

Conclusion

In conclusion, activation of both antigen-specific and innate immune responses within the stifle appears important to the development of synovitis and joint degeneration over time. Further research into the mechanisms that lead to the development of chronic stifle synovitis should be a focus of future research. Evidence of an immunogenetic susceptibility would suggest that immune responses are dysregulated. T lymphocytes and activated macrophages also likely represent important therapeutic targets for amelioration of joint inflammation in this arthropathy. If joint degeneration can be successfully blocked with medical therapy, then such a treatment may ameliorate the development of cruciate rupture and associated joint instability in affected dogs.

References

Akira S, Uematus S, Takeuchi O. Pathogen recognition and innate immunity. Cell 2006;124:783–801.

Bleedorn JA, Greuel E, Manley PA, et al. Synovitis precedes development of joint instability in dogs with degenerative cranial cruciate ligament rupture. Vet Surg 2009;38:E26.

de Bruin T, de Rooster H, van Bree H, Cox E. Evaluation of anticollagen type I antibody titers in synovial fluid of both stifles and the left shoulder of dogs with unilateral cranial cruciate disease. Am J Vet Res 2007a;68:283–289.

de Bruin T, de Rooster H, van Bree H, Waelbers T, Cox E. Lymphocyte proliferation to collagen type I in dogs. J Vet Med A Physiol Pathol Clin Med 2007b;54: 292–296.

Bryant C, Fitzgerald KA. Molecular mechanisms involved in inflammasome activation. Trends Cell Biol 2009;19:455–464.

Doom M, de Bruin T, de Rooster H, et al. Immunopathological mechanisms in dogs with rupture of the cranial cruciate ligament. Vet Immunol Immunopathol 2008;125:143–161.

Doverspike M, Vasseur PB, Harb MF, Walls CM. Contralateral cranial cruciate ligament rupture: Incidence in 114 dogs. J Am Anim Hosp Assoc 1993;29:167–170.

Faldyna M, Zatloukal J, Leva L, Kohout P, et al. Lymphocyte subsets in stifle joint synovial fluid of dogs with spontaneous rupture of the cranial cruciate ligament. Acta Vet Brno 2004;73:79–84.

Goldberg VM, Burstein A, Dawson M. The influence of an experimental immune synovitis on the failure mode and strength of the rabbit anterior cruciate ligament. J Bone Joint Surg Am 1982;64:900–906.

House AK, Gregory SP, Catchpole B. Pattern-recognition receptor mRNA expression and function in canine monocyte/macrophages and relevance to canine anal furunculosis. Vet Immunol Immunopathol 2008;124:230–240.

Iwasaki A, Medzhitov R. Regulation of adaptive immunity by the innate immune system. Science 2010;327:291–295.

Kempsell KE, Cox CJ, Hurle M, et al. Reverse transcriptase—PCR analysis of bacterial rRNA for detection and characterization of bacterial species in arthritis synovial tissue. Infect Immun 2000;68:6012–6026.

Klocke NW, Snyder PW, Widmer WR, Zhong W, et al. Detection of synovial macrophages in the joint capsule of dogs with naturally occurring rupture of the cranial cruciate ligament. Am J Vet Res 2005;66:493–499.

Kobayashi S, Baba H, Uchida K, Negoro K, et al. Microvascular system of the anterior cruciate ligament in dogs. J. Orthop Res 2006;24:1509–1520.

Lemburg AK, Meyer-Linenberg A, Hewicker-Trautwein M. Immunohistochemical characterization of inflammatory cell populations and adhesion molecule expression in synovial membranes from dogs with spontaneous cranial cruciate ligament rupture. Vet Immunol Immunopathol 2004;97:231–240.

Lipowitz AJ, Wong PL, Stevens JB. Synovial membrane changes after experimental transection of the cranial cruciate ligament in dogs. Am J Vet Res 1985;46:1166–1170.

Muir P, Schamberger GM, Manley PA, Hao Z. Localization of cathepsin K and tartrate-resistant acid phosphatase in synovium and cranial cruciate ligament in dogs with cruciate disease. Vet Surg 2005;34:239–246.

Muir P, Kelly JL, Suresh M, et al. Synovium and ruptured ligament contain activated CD4+ and CD8+ T lymphocytes in dogs with chronic knee synovitis and degenerative anterior cruciate ligament rupture. Trans Orthop Res Soc 2007a;53:718.

Muir P, Schaefer SL, Manley PA, Svaren JP, et al. Expression of immune response genes in the stifle joint of dogs with oligoarthritis and degenerative cranial cruciate ligament rupture. Vet Immunol Immunopathol 2007b;119:214–221.

Muir P, Oldenhoff WE, Hudson AP, Manley PA, et al. Detection of DNA from a range of bacterial species in the knee joints of dogs with inflammatory knee arthritis and associated degenerative anterior cruciate ligament rupture. Microb Pathog 2007c;42:47–55.

Muir P, Schaefer SL, Manley PA, et al. T Lymphocyte antigen receptor expression in dogs with inflammatory stifle arthritis and degenerative cranial cruciate ligament rupture. Vet Surg 2009;38:E40.

Muir P, Rox R, Wu Q, Hudson AP, et al. Seasonal variation in detection of bacterial DNA in the stifle joints of dogs with inflammatory arthritis and degenerative cranial cruciate ligament rupture. Vet Microbiol 2010;141:127–133.

Niebauer GW, Wolf B, Bashey RI, Newton CD. Antibodies to canine collagen types I and II in dogs with spontaneous cruciate ligament rupture and osteoarthritis. Arthritis Rheum 1987;30:319–327.

Ollier WER, Kennedy LJ, Thomson W, et al. Dog MHC alleles containing the human RA shared epitope confer susceptibility to canine rheumatoid arthritis. Immunogenetics 2001;53:669–673.

Sakkas LI, Platsoucas CD. The role of T cells in the pathogenesis of osteoarthritis. Arthritis Rheum 2007;56:409–424.

Section III

Clinical Features

Introduction

Over the last 20 years, veterinarians have become increasingly aware that it is difficult to relate the typical clinical features of the cruciate rupture arthropathy in dogs with the paradigm that stifle arthritis is a consequence of ligament rupture. Moderate to severe arthritis is often identified at initial presentation. Advances in diagnostic imaging, including development of methods for stress radiography of the stifle, have also helped to more thoroughly determine the extent of cranial cruciate ligament (CrCL) disruption during patient evaluation. Clinically, it is also important to relate knowledge of ligament biomechanics to assessment of the status of the CrCL in dogs with stifle arthritis. Recent research findings have also shed new light on which components of stifle pathology contribute to joint pain and lameness in affected dogs.

This section provides a detailed discussion of the clinical features of the cruciate rupture arthropathy.

14 Epidemiology of Cranial Cruciate Ligament Rupture

James L. Cook

Cranial cruciate ligament (CrCL) rupture is an extremely common musculoskeletal disorder that causes lameness in dogs (Witsberger et al. 2008). As such, the epidemiologic aspects of CrCL rupture are diverse and, to date, largely uncharacterized. What is clear is that there is no "poster child" for CrCL rupture and that dogs of nearly any age, reproductive status, breed, size, body condition, and intended function can be affected. Therefore, we should consider CrCL rupture as a spectrum of disease with various subcategories of primary etiology, specific disease mechanisms, pathology, and progression. The clinical implications of this spectrum of disease are critical and include preventative strategies through breeding and training, diagnostic approach, treatment strategies, and client education. Each of these components should be addressed through a patient- and client-based approach to optimize outcomes for each specific patient.

Peak incidence of CrCL rupture is reported to most commonly fall in the age range of 2–10 years (Whitehair et al. 1993; Duval et al. 1999; Powers et al. 2005; Harasen 2008; Witsberger et al. 2008).

Advances in the Canine Cranial Cruciate Ligament, Edited by Peter Muir, © 2010 ACVS Foundation, This Work is a co-publication between the American College of Veterinary Surgeons Foundation and Wiley-Blackwell.

In a recent study examining medical records data from over 1 million cases, we reported that dogs less than 4 years of age were significantly less likely to be diagnosed with CrCL rupture, compared with dogs greater than 4 years of age (Witsberger et al. 2008; Table 14.1). Multiple studies have examined gender and reproductive status differences in dogs with and without CrCL rupture with variable results, again highlighting the spectrum of disease. The largest studies published to date have agreed that neutered males and spayed females have significantly increased odds for having CrCL rupture compared with intact dogs of both genders (Whitehair et al. 1993; Duval et al. 1999; Witsberger et al. 2008; Table 14.1). In addition, early neutering (before 6 months of age) was reported to be a significant risk factor for development of excessive tibial plateau angles in large-breed dogs with CrCL rupture in one study (Duerr et al. 2007). These findings implicate a direct or indirect role of hormonal influences on mechanisms of disease. With respect to breed, those that are consistently at highest risk for CrCL rupture are medium, large, and giant breeds and include Newfoundlands, Rottweilers, Labrador retrievers, bulldogs, and boxers (Witsberger et al. 2008; Table 14.1). Breeds protected against being diagnosed with CrCL rupture are in the small, hound, and chondrodystrophoid breed categories (e.g., Miniature Dachshund, Dachshund, Miniature

Table 14.1 Potential risk factors for cranial cruciate ligament rupture in dogs based on current evidence

Category	Potential risk factors
Age	>4 years
Reproductive status	Neutered (before 6 months may increase further)
Breed	Newfoundland Rottweiler Labrador retriever Bulldog Boxer Chow Chow American Staffordshire Terrier
Weight	>22 kg
Body condition	Unknown (small thigh and crus muscle mass)
Intended function	Unknown
Stifle anatomy	Narrow intercondylar notch Excessive tibial plateau angle (degree varies among reports: >28°, >32°, >35°) Relatively small proximal tibial width Cranial angulation of the proximal tibia Distal femoral torsion

Schnauzer, Greyhound, Shih Tzu, and Pekingnese; Witsberger et al. 2008). The overall prevalence at which these breeds are consistently affected suggests a genetic component to etiopathogenesis at least in this subcategory in the spectrum of CrCL rupture. Importantly, canine hip dysplasia is a genetic disorder that also has a reportedly high prevalence in many of these same breeds, often concurrent with CrCL rupture, giving further credence to genetic factors being involved in this spectrum of disease (Powers et al. 2005; Wilke et al. 2006; Witsberger et al. 2008). The genetics of CrCL rupture are discussed in Chapter 7.

A critical factor to consider in the epidemiology of CrCL rupture in dogs is the occurrence of bilateral disease. This has profound ramifications for understanding etiopathogenesis and, more impor-

tantly, for honestly and thoroughly communicating with clients regarding expectations and commitment to treatment. The contralateral stifle is reported to be affected with CrCL rupture concurrent with or subsequent to initial diagnosis in 22%–61% of cases (Doverspike et al. 1993; Moore & Read 1995;, de Bruin et al. 2007; Cabrera et al. 2008; Buote et al. 2009; Table 14.2). Subsequent diagnosis can be made within days to years of the initial diagnosis of CrCL rupture. Buote et al. reported that approximately 50% of Labradors will have contralateral CrCL rupture within 5.5 months of initial diagnosis but that age, weight, gender, and tibial plateau angle were not good predictors for occurrence of contralateral CrCL rupture. The relatively high occurrence of bilateral disease among studies supports etiopathogeneses other than overt trauma or athletic injury and should be clearly communicated to clients at the time of initial diagnosis.

Body condition has not been studied comprehensively as it relates to CrCL rupture in dogs. The studies that have examined this factor reported that higher body weights are associated with increased risk of CrCL rupture (Table 14.1) and that the thigh and crus musculature of CrCL rupture limbs weighed less than in normal limbs (Whitehair et al. 1993; Duval et al. 1999; Ragetly et al. 2008). Another study reported that muscle atrophy associated with CrCL deficiency appears to predominantly affect the quadriceps muscles (Mostafa et al. 2010). However, no study has examined body condition score, body mass index, or bone, muscle, or fat contents or ratios with respect to CrCL rupture. Similarly, overall conformation of dogs affected and unaffected by CrCL rupture has received little attention in the literature. Conformation, or more appropriately, relative anatomy of the stifle joint has received tremendous attention recently. The most recent theories that have been advocated by many as causes of CrCL rupture revolve around intercondylar notch dimensions (Comerford EJ et al. 2006; Lewis et al. 2008), overall limb alignment (Dismukes et al. 2008; Mostafa et al. 2009), and proximal tibial conformation (Selmi et al. 2001; Macias et al. 2002; Dennler et al. 2006; Osmond et al. 2006; Schwandt et al. 2006; Guerrero et al. 2007; Cabrera et al. 2008; Inauen et al. 2009). Anatomic factors that are associated with a pre-

Table 14.2 Risk of contralateral rupture concurrent with or subsequent to initial diagnosis of cranial cruciate ligament disease in dogs based on current evidence

Study	
	Risk of bilateral rupture at diagnosis
Cabrera et al. (2008)	17% (25 of 150 dogs)
Buote et al. (2009)	10.6% (10 of 94 dogs)
	Risk of subsequent contralateral rupture after diagnosis of unilateral rupture
Doverspike et al. (1993)	37% at mean of 17 months with normal stifle radiographs
	59% at mean of 16 months with abnormal stifle radiographs
Moore & Read (1995)	22% at mean of 14 months
de Bruin et al. (2007)	43% at 12 months
	(risk of contralateral rupture increased with signs of arthritis radiographically)
Cabrera et al. (2008)	45% at mean of 13 months
Buote et al. (2009)	48% within 5.5 months
	Combined risk of contralateral rupture concurrent or subsequent to diagnosis
Cabrera et al. (2008)	61.3% (92 of 150 dogs)
Buote et al. (2009)	58.5% (55 of 94 dogs)

disposition to CrCL rupture include a narrow intercondylar notch, excessive or pathologic (i.e., outside the 95% confidence intervals for the population) tibial plateau angle, a relatively small proximal tibial width, cranial angulation of the proximal tibia, and distal femoral torsion (Table 14.1). While a great number of studies have focused on the effects of tibial plateau angle and, more recently, patellar tendon–tibial plateau angle, no study definitively shows either of these as significant risk factors for CrCL rupture in dogs. Theories and *ex vivo* research suggest increased CrCL strain and an increased shear component of total joint force when each of these angles is considered high based on reference ranges in dogs (Warzee et al. 2001; Reif et al. 2002; Kowaleski et al. 2005; Shahar & Milgram 2006; Apelt et al. 2007; Duerr et al. 2007; Kim et al. 2008; Kipfer et al. 2008). Therefore, these components may be contributory in some way but do not appear to be primary causal factors based on current best evidence (Wilke et al. 2002; Conzemius et al. 2005; Guerrero et al. 2007; Havig et al. 2007; Guastella et al. 2008).

No studies were found in the peer-reviewed literature that determined the epidemiological aspects of dogs' activity levels and/or intended function with respect to CrCL rupture. This is another area that begs for comprehensive assessment in order for real progress to be made in prevention, diagnosis, treatment, and client communication for CrCL rupture in dogs.

Prevalence of CrCL rupture in dogs has been steadily increasing over the past four decades (Witsberger et al. 2008). Relatively little is known regarding the epidemiologic aspects of this pervasive problem, but what is known suggests that CrCL rupture involves a spectrum of etiopathogeneses, clinical presentations, and treatment indications (Table 14.1). It is likely that genetic, hormonal, conformational, and activity-related factors are involved in initiation, development, and progression of CrCL rupture in dogs. It is unlikely that single preventative, diagnostic, or therapeutic approaches will be applicable to all dogs affected by this disorder. A comprehensive understanding of epidemiology forms the foundation for determining etiologies, disease mechanisms, diagnostic, therapeutic, and prognostic protocols, and the basis for accurate and thorough communication to our clients. It is vital that we pursue this understanding with vigor.

References

Apelt D, Kowaleski MP, Boudrieau RJ. Effect of tibial tuberosity advancement on cranial tibial subluxation in canine cranial cruciate-deficient stifle joints: An *in vitro* experimental study. Vet Surg 2007;36:170–177.

Buote N, Fusco J, Radasch R. Age, tibial plateau angle, sex, and weight as risk factors for contralateral rupture of the cranial cruciate ligament in Labradors. Vet Surg 2009;38:481–489.

Cabrera SY, Owen TJ, Mueller MG, Kass PH. Comparison of tibial plateau angles in dogs with unilateral versus bilateral cranial cruciate ligament rupture: 150 cases (2000–2006). J Am Vet Med Assoc 2008;232: 889–892.

Conzemius MG, Evans RB, Besancon MF, et al. Effect of surgical technique on limb function after surgery for rupture of the cranial cruciate ligament in dogs. J Am Vet Med Assoc 2005;226:232–236.

Comerford EJ, Tarlton JF, Avery NC, et al. Distal femoral intercondylar notch dimensions and their relationship to composition and metabolism of the canine anterior cruciate ligament. Osteoarthritis Cartilage 2006;14: 273–278.

de Bruin T, de Rooster H, van Bree H, et al. Radiographic assessment of the progression of osteoarthrosis in the contralateral stifle joint of dogs with a ruptured cranial cruciate ligament. Vet Rec 2007;161: 745–750.

Dennler R, Kipfer NM, Tepic S, et al. Inclination of the patellar ligament in relation to flexion angle in stifle joints of dogs without degenerative joint disease. Am J Vet Res 2006;67:1849–1854.

Dismukes DI, Fox DB, Tomlinson JL, et al. Determination of pelvic limb alignment in the large-breed dog: A cadaveric radiographic study in the frontal plane. Vet Surg 2008;37:674–682.

Doverspike M, Vasseur PB, Harb MF, Walls CM. Contralateral cranial cruciate ligament rupture: Incidence in 114 dogs. J Am Anim Hosp Assoc 1993;29: 167–170.

Duerr FM, Duncan CG, Savicky RS, et al. Risk factors for excessive tibial plateau angle in large-breed dogs with cranial cruciate ligament disease. J Am Vet Med Assoc 2007;231:1688–1691.

Duval JM, Budsberg SC, Flo GL, Sammarco JL. Breed, sex, and body weight as risk factors for rupture of the cranial cruciate ligament in young dogs. J Am Vet Med Assoc 1999;215:811–814.

Guastella DB, Fox DB, Cook JL. Tibial plateau angle in four common canine breeds with cranial cruciate ligament rupture, and its relationship to meniscal tears. Vet Comp Orthop Traumatol 2008;21:125–128.

Guerrero TG, Geyer H, Hässig M, Montavon PM. Effect of conformation of the distal portion of the femur and proximal portion of the tibia on the pathogenesis of cranial cruciate ligament disease in dogs. Am J Vet Res 2007;68:1332–1337.

Harasen G. Canine cranial cruciate ligament rupture in profile: 2002–2007. Can Vet J 2008;49:193–194.

Havig ME, Dyce J, Kowaleski MP, et al. Relationship of tibial plateau slope to limb function in dogs treated with a lateral suture technique for stabilization of cranial cruciate ligament deficient stifles. Vet Surg 2007;36:245–251.

Inauen R, Koch D, Bass M, Haessig M. Tibial tuberosity conformation as a risk factor for cranial cruciate ligament rupture in the dog. Vet Comp Orthop Traumatol 2009;22:16–20.

Kim SE, Pozzi A, Kowaleski MP, Lewis DD. Tibial osteotomies for cranial cruciate ligament insufficiency in dogs. Vet Surg 2008;37:111–125.

Kipfer NM, Tepic S, Damur DM, et al. Effect of tibial tuberosity advancement on femorotibial shear in cranial cruciate-deficient stifles. An *in vitro* study. Vet Comp Orthop Traumatol 2008;21:385–290.

Kowaleski MP, Apelt D, Mattoon JS, Litsky AS. The effect of tibial plateau leveling osteotomy position on cranial tibial subluxation: An in vitro study. Vet Surg 2005;34:332–336.

Lewis BA, Allen DA, Henrikson TD, Lehenbauer TW. Computed tomographic evaluation of the canine intercondylar notch in normal and cruciate deficient stifles. Vet Comp Orthop Traumatol 2008;21:119–124.

Macias C, McKee WM, May C. Caudal proximal tibial deformity and cranial cruciate ligament rupture in small-breed dogs. J Small Anim Pract 2002;43:433–438.

Moore KW, Read RA. Cranial cruciate ligament rupture in the dog — a retrospective study comparing surgical techniques. Aust Vet J 1995;72:281–285.

Mostafa AA, Griffon DJ, Thomas MW, Constable PD. Morphometric characteristics of the pelvic limbs of Labrador retrievers with and without cranial cruciate ligament deficiency. Am J Vet Res 2009;70: 498–507.

Mostafa AA, Griffon DJ, Thomas MW, Constable PD. Morphometric characteristics of the pelvic limb musculature of Labrador retrievers with and without cranial cruciate ligament deficiency. Vet Surg 2010;39:380–389.

Osmond CS, Marcellin-Little DJ, Harrysson OL, Kidd LB. Morphometric assessment of the proximal portion of the tibia in dogs with and without cranial cruciate ligament rupture. Vet Radiol Ultrasound 2006;47: 136–141.

Powers MY, Martinez SA, Lincoln JD, et al. Prevalence of cranial cruciate ligament rupture in a population of dogs with lameness previously attributed to hip dysplasia: 369 cases (1994–2003). J Am Vet Med Assoc 2005;227:1109–1111.

Ragetly CA, Griffon DJ, Thomas JE, et al. Noninvasive determination of body segment parameters of the hind limb in Labrador retrievers with and without cranial cruciate ligament disease. Am J Vet Res 2008;69:1188–1196.

Reif U, Hulse DA, Hauptman JG. Effect of tibial plateau leveling on stability of the canine cranial cruciate-deficient stifle joint: An *in vitro* study. Vet Surg 2002;31:147–154.

Schwandt CS, Bohorquez-Vanelli A, Tepic S, et al. Angle between the patellar ligament and tibial plateau in dogs with partial rupture of the cranial cruciate ligament. Am J Vet Res 2006;67:1855–1860.

Selmi AL, Padilha Filho JG. Rupture of the cranial cruciate ligament associated with deformity of the proximal tibia in five dogs. J Small Anim Pract 2001;42:390–393.

Shahar R, Milgram J. Biomechanics of tibial plateau leveling of the canine cruciate-deficient stifle joint: A theoretical model. Vet Surg 2006;35:144–149.

Warzee CC, Dejardin LM, Arnoczky SP, Perry RL. Effect of tibial plateau leveling on cranial and caudal tibial thrusts in canine cranial cruciate-deficient stifles: An in vitro experimental study. Vet Surg 2001;30: 278–286.

Whitehair JG, Vasseur PB, Willits NH. Epidemiology of cranial cruciate ligament rupture in dogs. J Am Vet Med Assoc 1993;203:1016–1019.

Wilke VL, Conzemius MG, Besancon MF, et al. Comparison of tibial plateau angle between clinically normal greyhounds and Labrador retrievers with and without rupture of the cranial cruciate ligament. J Am Vet Med Assoc 2002;221:1426–1429.

Wilke VL, Conzemius MG, Kinghorn BP, et al. Inheritance of rupture of the cranial cruciate ligament in Newfoundlands. J Am Vet Med Assoc 2006;228: 61–64.

Witsberger TH, Villamil JA, Schultz LG, et al. Prevalence of and risk factors for hip dysplasia and cranial cruciate ligament deficiency in dogs. J Am Vet Med Assoc 2008;232:1818–1824.

15 History and Clinical Signs of Cruciate Ligament Rupture

Peter Muir

Introduction

The cruciate rupture arthropathy has been recognized since the early part of the twentieth century. Although this condition was initially considered a traumatic injury, in the last 20 years it has become more widely appreciated that it is a degenerative or pathological condition in the majority of patients (Bennett et al. 1988). It is also important to exclude the cruciate rupture arthropathy before making recommendations about management of hip dysplasia because of the high prevalence of stifle arthritis in dogs with pelvic limb lameness and hip dysplasia (Powers et al. 2005).

History

Although owners will often provide a history suggestive of trauma, careful analysis will usually reveal either that the onset of lameness was insidious or that lameness was observed by the owner to develop after an incident of minor trauma typi-cally associated with normal daily activity. In a proportion of patients, owners will provide a clear history of major trauma, such as injury from a motor vehicle accident, suggesting traumatic rupture of the cranial cruciate ligament (CrCL) has occurred. Further investigation of such patients will often reveal avulsion fracture of a cruciate ligament attachment site. Epidemiologically, this proportion is not clearly documented, although in medium to large breed dogs, this incidence is likely to be less than 5% of patients; a large majority of dogs do not have a history of obvious trauma. Therefore, CrCL rupture is considered pathological and is associated with a pre-existing stifle arthropathy. Lameness in affected dogs is usually weight-bearing and is typically worse after exercise. Duration of lameness described by owners is highly variable. Occasionally owners may report an audible clicking during walking.

It is also common for dogs to be presented for treatment because of more subtle pelvic lameness, which is usually continuous and fairly unresponsive to medical therapy with nonsteroidal anti-inflammatory drugs. Observant owners may notice that bilateral lameness is common, with the dog exhibiting a stiff pelvic limb gait. Such patients typically have stifle arthritis, but a stable stifle with a partial CrCL rupture on further investigation.

Advances in the Canine Cranial Cruciate Ligament,
Edited by Peter Muir, © 2010 ACVS Foundation, This Work is a co-publication between the American College of Veterinary Surgeons Foundation and Wiley-Blackwell.

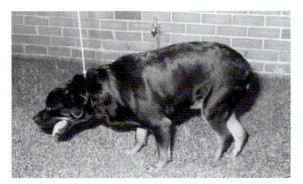

Figure 15.1 Photograph of a female Rottweiler with bilateral pelvic limb lameness and bilateral cranial cruciate ligament rupture. Notice that she is leaning forward to unload the pelvic limbs.

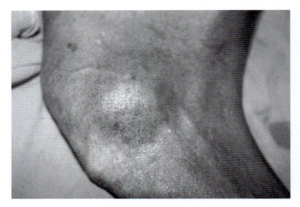

Figure 15.2 Photograph of the medial aspect of the right stifle. Prominent fibrosis of the stifle is evident. It is important to check for firm swelling of the medial aspect of the stifle. This sign is typical of chronic cranial cruciate ligament rupture.

Clinical signs

On physical examination, affected dogs typically exhibit unilateral or bilateral weight-bearing pelvic limb lameness. If the lameness is bilateral, dogs will usually lean forward and alter their stance to unload the pelvic limbs (Figure 15.1). Occasionally, a non-weight-bearing lameness may be evident. In dogs with unilateral lameness, external rotation of the affected limb may be evident when walking. Similarly, during sitting affected dogs will often position the affected limb so that limb is externally rotated and stifle flexion is reduced, compared with a normal symmetric sitting posture. This is sometimes referred to as the "sit test." In this posture, the calcaneus is not directly underneath the tuber ischii, because the stifle is not fully flexed. On general examination, atrophy of pelvic limb musculature in the affected limb(s) is usually evident. Occasionally, an audible clicking may be heard during walking, and is usually indicative of meniscal damage, most commonly a bucket handle tear. Careful physical examination is important, as neurological disease may initially be suspected in dogs that have difficulty rising from a sitting to a standing position because of bilateral CrCL rupture.

During examination of the stifle, effusion is typically found, with the lateral and medial margins of the patella tendon feeling indistinct on palpation. Subtle effusion can be hard to detect on physical examination. Stifle radiography is a more sensitive diagnostic test for this pathological change. As the cruciate rupture arthropathy is so prevalent, if there is any uncertainty about this aspect of stifle physical examination, bilateral stifle radiographs should be made in dogs with pelvic limb lameness and examined for effusion and arthritic change. Radiographs underestimate pathological change, so an obvious stifle synovitis may be present, with only subtle change radiographically.

Palpation of the medial side of the stifle will often reveal a firm thickening, indicative of peri-articular fibrosis (Figure 15.2). This pathological change is almost always indicative of CrCL rupture.

Cranial–caudal instability between the tibia and femur may be identified by use of the cranial drawer test or the cranial tibial thrust test (Figures 15.3 and 15.4, respectively; Henderson & Milton 1978; Muir 1997). During application of these tests to the stifle, it is important to place the examining fingers directly on the bony prominences of the stifle, to avoid interpreting movement of the skin and overlying soft tissues as indicative of translation of the tibia relative to the femur. It is often helpful to repeat these tests after sedation or general anesthesia of the patient to ensure that subtle instability has not been missed on physical examination. This is particularly important in dogs with chronic stifle arthritis. Here, periarticu-

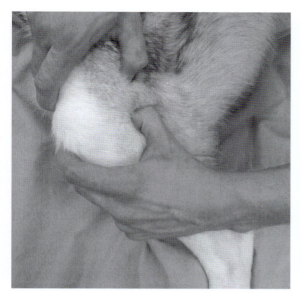

Figure 15.3 Photograph of the left pelvic limb of a Siberian Husky. When checking for cranial drawer motion in the stifle, it is important to place the fingertips on the tibial crest, the fibular head, the patella, and the lateral fabella to avoid interpreting compression of soft tissue or internal rotation as cranial drawer motion.

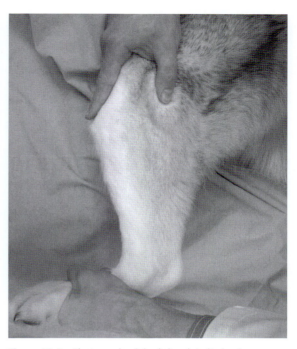

Figure 15.4 Photograph of the left pelvic limb of a Siberian Husky. With the stifle extended, an index finger is placed on the tibial crest to determine whether cranial displacement of the tibia occurs when the hock is flexed. If cranial translation of the tibia relative to the femur is identified, this is a positive cranial tibial thrust test (tibial compression test) and is indicative of cranial cruciate ligament rupture.

lar fibrosis may reduce, but not eliminate, cranial translation of the tibia relative to the femur. It is also important in nervous dogs with tense muscles, where stifle instability may be less apparent. Rupture of the CrCL may also lead to excessive internal rotation of the tibia relative to the femur, which may be apparent on physical examination.

The cranial drawer and cranial tibial thrust tests are best performed with dog in lateral recumbency and the stifle in partial flexion at a normal standing angle. Crepitation and pain may also be found on flexion and extension of the stifle as these tests are performed. Medial and lateral stress to the stifle should also be applied during physical examination to assess the stability of the collateral ligaments of the stifle, as collateral ligament rupture combined with cruciate ligament rupture can be a consequence of traumatic injury to the stifle.

Detection of stifle instability and cranial translation of the tibia relative to the femur is indicative of complete biomechanical disruption of the CrCL. In immature dogs, a small degree of cranial translation of the tibia relative to the femur of a few millimeters is normal and is indicative of slight laxity in the ligament. Here, during the cranial drawer maneuver the small amount of tibiofemoral translation will come to an abrupt stop. In contrast, in dogs with incipient CrCL rupture, the small degree of tibiofemoral translation will end in a soft or spongy stop.

During physical examination, the clinician should also palpate the stifle carefully for caudal drawer motion. Here the cranial drawer test will elicit an abrupt stop with minimal translation, whereas caudal drawer motion will be elicited. Isolated rupture of the caudal cruciate ligament (CaCL) is rare, but can occur. Also, a small proportion of dogs with CrCL rupture will also have rupture of the CaCL. In dogs with rupture of both cruciate ligaments, it can be particularly difficult to recognize that both cruciate ligaments are ruptured during physical examination of the stifle.

Conclusion

Detection of cranial drawer and cranial tibial thrust on physical examination remains a key part of patient investigation in dogs with CrCL rupture. However, detection of stifle instability can often be difficult to distinguish from mild laxity, which might be normal in puppies. These limitations will likely change in the future as knowledge of stifle kinematics improves, as discussed elsewhere in this book. In future work, development of a stifle arthrometer that objectively measures subtle translation of the tibia relative to the femur would also be advantageous for early identification of dogs with partial CrCL rupture.

References

Bennett D, Tennant B, Lewis DG, et al. A reappraisal of anterior cruciate ligament disease in the dog. J Small Anim Pract 1988;29:275–297.

Henderson RA, Milton JL. The tibial compression mechanism: A diagnostic aid in stifle injuries. J Am Anim Hosp Assoc 1978;14:474–479.

Muir P. Physical examination of lame dogs. Compend Cont Ed Pract Vet 1997;19:1149–1161.

Powers MY, Martinez SA, Lincoln JD, et al. Prevalence of cranial cruciate ligament rupture in a population of dogs with lameness previously attributed to hip dysplasia: 369 cases (1994–2003). J Am Vet Med Assoc 2005;227:1109–1111.

16 Partial versus Complete Rupture of the Cranial Cruciate Ligament

Peter Muir

Introduction

Ligament injuries are classified as Grade I through III, depending on the severity of the injury. Grade I injuries do not affect joint instability and are associated with sub-failure damage to the ligament tissue (Provenzano et al. 2002). However, historically, rupture of the cranial cruciate ligament (CrCL) has been classified as partial or complete based on an anatomic definition. In human beings, identification and grading of partial anterior cruciate ligament injuries is controversial, as these lesions may or may not be associated with joint instability, and may involve a variable amount of the cross-section of the ligament during arthroscopic evaluation (Hong et al. 2003).

Partial CrCL rupture

In dogs, the CrCL has a craniomedial and a caudolateral component containing bundles of longitudinally orientated collagen fibers (Heffron &

Campbell 1978). The craniomedial component is taut in both flexion and extension, whereas the caudolateral component is only taut in extension (Arnoczky & Marshall 1977). Biomechanically, *ex vivo* sectioning of either the craniomedial component or the caudolateral component of the CrCL induces the development of mild joint instability in partial flexion, with ≤3 mm of cranial drawer motion (Heffron & Campbell 1978). This small amount of cranial drawer motion may be difficult to detect on physical examination (Table 16.1; Heffron & Campbell 1978). These findings suggest that if cranial drawer instability is detected clinically on physical examination, then the majority of the CrCL has been disrupted biomechanically (Heffron & Campbell 1978). In human patients, joint translation can be measured using an arthrometer (Bach et al. 1990). Development of an arthrometer for the dog stifle that can objectively measure cranial–tibial translation would likely be valuable for improving early diagnosis of a stable partial CrCL rupture in dogs.

Clinically, partial rupture of the CrCL may or may not be associated with the presence of joint instability and cranial drawer motion on physical examination (Scavelli et al. 1990). Detection of cranial drawer motion in only partial flexion is not a reliable indicator of disruption to only the craniomedial component of the CrCL (Scavelli et al. 1990). Although it has been previously questioned

---

Advances in the Canine Cranial Cruciate Ligament, Edited by Peter Muir, © 2010 ACVS Foundation, This Work is a co-publication between the American College of Veterinary Surgeons Foundation and Wiley-Blackwell.

Table 16.1 Results of partial and total sectioning of the canine cranial cruciate ligament (CrCL)

	Degree of stifle flexion from maximal extension			
	0°	20°	40°	60°
Craniomedial component cut (n = 5)	1.5 (0,2)	2 (2,3)	1 (1,2.5)	1 (0.5,1.5)
Caudolateral component cut (n = 5)	0 (0,1.5)	1 (1,1)	0.5 (0,1)	0 (0,0)
Whole CrCL cut (n = 10)	7.7 ± 3.4	13.0 ± 1.4	10.4 ± 2.0	7.6 ± 1.5

Note: Results represent cranial translation of the tibia relative to the femur in millimeters. For the whole CrCL cut, data represent mean ± standard deviation. For the other two experiments, data represent median (range). (Reproduced and modified from Heffron & Campbell 1978, with permission from the British Veterinary Association).

whether a lack of cranial drawer motion during physical examination of dogs with partial CrCL rupture may be a consequence of periarticular fibrosis (Scavelli et al. 1990), the increasing use of arthroscopy to examine the stifle joint of dogs with very mild arthritis suggests that incipient rupture of the CrCL is often associated with fraying of the ligament during arthroscopic examination of the stifle in joints that are clinically stable (Figure 16.1; Bleedorn et al. 2009).

Conclusion

In conclusion, if stifle joint instability is detected clinically, this is indicative of substantial disruption to the CrCL biomechanically, even if there is only a partial rupture anatomically. In dogs with partial anatomic ruptures, the remaining ligament tissue is often found to be stretched out and slack during surgical treatment. The definition of partial rupture is best limited to stifles that are clinically stable. In future work, increased recognition of partial CrCL rupture in dogs with stifle arthritis and a stable stifle will be important for the development of disease-modifying therapy aimed at preventing further deterioration in the biomechanical properties of the CrCL and associated development of stifle instability.

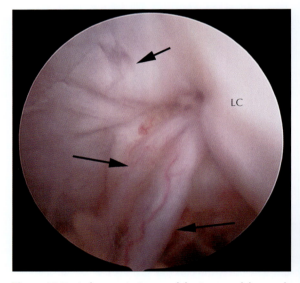

Figure 16.1 Arthroscopic image of the intercondylar notch region of the distal femur of the right stifle of a 5-year-old female golden retriever with a stable stifle and mild stifle arthritis radiographically. Disruption of some of the fibers of the cranial cruciate ligament and inflammation of the overlying synovial intima is visible (arrows). LC: lateral femoral condyle.

References

Arnoczky SP, Marshall JL. The cruciate ligaments of the canine stifle: An anatomical and functional analysis. Am J Vet Res 1977;38:1807–1814.

Bach BR Jr., Warren RF, Flynn WM, et al. Arthrometric evaluation of knees that have a torn anterior cruciate ligament. J Bone Joint Surg Am 1990;72:1299–1306.

Bleedorn JA, Greuel E, Manley PA, et al. Synovitis precedes development of joint instability in dogs with degenerative cranial cruciate ligament rupture. Vet Surg 2009;38:E26.

Heffron LE, Campbell JR. Morphology, histology, and functional anatomy of the canine cranial cruciate ligament. Vet Rec 1978;102:280–283.

Hong SH, Choi J-Y, Lee GK, Choi J-A, et al. Grading of anterior cruciate ligament injury. Diagnostic efficacy of oblique coronal magnetic resonance imaging of the knee. J Comput Assist Tomogr 2003;27:814–819.

Provenzano PP, Heisey D, Hayashi K, Lakes R, Vanderby R, Jr. Subfailure damage in ligament: A structural and cellular evaluation. J Appl Physiol 2002;92:362–371.

Scavelli TD, Schrader SC, Matthiesen DR, Skorup DE. Partial rupture of the cranial cruciate ligament in the stifle in dogs (1982–1988). J Am Vet Med Assoc 1990;196:1135–1138.

17 Caudal Cruciate Ligament Rupture

Peter Muir

Introduction

Rupture of the caudal cruciate ligament (CaCL) is thought to be much less common than rupture of the cranial cruciate ligament (CrCL) and isolated disruption of the CaCL is found in less than 2% of stifle surgery patients (Harari 1993). Experimentally, transection of the CaCL does not cause an obvious lameness and only leads to mild internal rotation of the tibia relative to the femur (Harari et al. 1987). Although caudal drawer motion was detectable during a 6-month study period, minimal degeneration of the articular cartilage with very little osteophyte formation was found experimentally (Pournas et al. 1983; Harari et al. 1987). Meniscal disruption was not found after experimental transection of the CaCL (Pournas et al. 1983; Harari et al. 1987). Therefore, whether naturally occurring isolated disruption of the CaCL causes lameness clinically in the dog is unclear.

Rupture of the CaCL often involves avulsion fracture of an attachment site and affected dogs usually have a history of trauma and may have other complicating injuries (Johnson & Olmstead

---

Advances in the Canine Cranial Cruciate Ligament, Edited by Peter Muir, © 2010 ACVS Foundation, This Work is a co-publication between the American College of Veterinary Surgeons Foundation and Wiley-Blackwell.

1987). Complete disruption of the CaCL is also seen in dogs with stifle luxation, in combination with rupture of the CrCL and the medial collateral ligament, secondary to stifle trauma (Hulse & Shires 1986; Aron 1988). However, mild disruption of the CaCL is underappreciated clinically. CaCL fraying is often observed during arthroscopic treatment of dogs affected with CrCL rupture (Figures 17.1 and 17.2).

Clinical presentation

Mid-substance tears

Dogs with isolated mid-substance tears usually have a history and clinical signs that are similar to dogs affected with the cruciate rupture arthropathy. In some patients, a history of trauma may be described by the owner. Although stifle instability is often appreciated on physical examination, caudal drawer motion is difficult to recognize specifically, and may be interpreted as cranial drawer motion. Consequently, it is easy to misdiagnose patients as having CrCL rupture. Radiographic signs are also similar to dogs with the cruciate rupture arthropathy. Caudal displacement of the tibia relative to the femur may be evident on a lateral radiograph of the stifle (Soderstrom et al. 1998). Unless magnetic resonance imaging (MRI)

110   Clinical Features

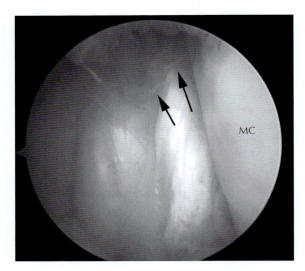

Figure 17.1   Arthroscopic image of the intercondylar notch region of the distal femur of the right stifle of a 7-year-old neutered female mixed-breed dog with a stable stifle and very mild stifle arthritis radiographically. Mild disruption of some of the fibers of the caudal cruciate ligament is evident, particularly adjacent to the femoral attachment site (arrows). Use of an arthroscopic probe will facilitate detection of deeper tearing within the core region of the ligament. MC: medial femoral condyle.

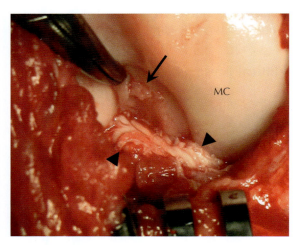

Figure 17.2   Photograph of the intercondylar notch region of the distal femur of the right stifle of a 1-year-old neutered male Labrador with an unstable stifle, moderate arthritis, and rupture of the cranial cruciate ligament. Complete disruption of the cranial cruciate ligament (arrowheads), together with partial rupture of the caudal cruciate ligament, with disruption of ligament fascicles was found at surgery (arrow). MC: medial femoral condyle.

of the stifle is performed, a specific diagnosis is most likely to be made during arthroscopy or arthrotomy of the stifle (Johnson & Olmstead 1987). In dogs with CaCL rupture, it is presently unclear whether degeneration or disruption of the CrCL is also present in affected dogs and that these dogs are essentially affected with the cruciate rupture arthropathy, albeit with a less common pattern of cruciate disruption. Menisci are often intact in dogs with CaCL rupture (Johnson & Olmstead 1987).

Avulsion fracture

Dogs with an avulsion fracture of the proximal or distal attachment site of the CaCL are usually young dogs, presented with a clear history of trauma and a persistent lameness (Reinke 1982). Stifle swelling and instability is often detected on physical examination. Avulsion fracture fragments are usually evident radiographically, with careful examination of high-quality radiographs. However, if an avulsion fracture fragment is identified radiographically, it can be difficult to determine which cruciate ligament it is associated with.

Multiple ligamentous injuries to the stifle

In dogs with severe stifle trauma and disruption to multiple stifle ligaments, the CaCL is ruptured in more than 80% of patients (Aron 1988). The presence of CaCL rupture is often masked by stifle instability because of disruption to other supporting structures, such as the CrCL and the medial collateral ligament (Hulse & Shires 1986; Aron 1988).

Treatment

In dogs with isolated tearing of the CaCL, the need for surgical treatment is unclear, particularly because experimental transection of the CaCL does not lead to lameness. Although various extracapsular and intra-articular stabilization methods have been proposed, objective long-term evaluations of these procedures are not available

(Harari 1993). In dogs with the cruciate rupture arthropathy in which tibial plateau level osteotomy (TPLO) surgery is planned, it is particularly important to determine whether caudal drawer motion may be present before surgery, and whether CaCL damage is present during surgery, as this is a contraindication for the TPLO procedure. TPLO increases CaCL stress and is reliant upon a biomechanically intact CaCL being present (Warzee et al. 2001; Zachos et al. 2002).

In dogs with avulsion fractures, if the fracture fragment is sufficiently large, fracture repair with a lag screw is recommended (Reinke 1982; Harari 1993). In patients where the fracture fragment is small, debridement of the fragment is recommended. Again, the need for a stifle stabilization procedure in these patients is unclear (Harari 1993).

In dogs with multiple ligamentous injury, surgical treatment of disruption to the CrCL, the medial collateral ligament, and the menisci should be a priority. Menisci and their supporting structures should be preserved where possible. Collateral ligament rupture should again be repaired with sutures if possible. A number of procedures are available for stifle stabilization, including extracapsular stabilization and use of a trans-articular external skeletal fixator.

Conclusion

In conclusion, disruption to both the CrCL and the CaCL is often found during arthroscopy or arthrotomy in dogs affected with the cruciate rupture arthropathy. Fraying of the CaCL is underappreciated unless a probe is used to specifically examine the ligament during surgery. This is important, as disruption of the CaCL is a contraindication for TPLO.

References

Aron DN. Traumatic dislocation of the stifle joint: Treatment of 12 dogs and one cat. J Am Anim Hosp 1988;24:333–340.

Harari J, Johnson AL, Stein LE, et al. Evaluation of experimental transection and partial excision of the caudal cruciate ligament in dogs. Vet Surg 1987;16:151–154.

Harari J. Caudal cruciate ligament injury. Vet Clin North Am Small Anim Pract 1993;23:821–829.

Hulse DA, Shires P. Multiple ligament injury of the stifle joint in the dog. J Am Anim Hosp Assoc 1986;22:105–110.

Johnson AL, Olmstead ML. Caudal cruciate ligament rupture. A retrospective analysis of 14 dogs. Vet Surg 1987;16:202–206.

Pournaras J, Symeonides PP, Karkavelas G. The significance of the posterior cruciate ligament in the stability of the knee. An experimental study in dogs. J Bone Joint Surg Br 1983;65:204–209.

Reinke JD. Cruciate ligament avulsion injury in the dog. J Am Anim Hosp Assoc 1982;18:257–264.

Soderstrom MJ, Rochat MC, Drost WT. Radiographic diagnosis: Avulasion fracture of the caudal cruciate ligament. Vet Radiol Ultrasound 1998;39:536–538.

Warzee CC, Dejardin LM, Arnoczky SP, Perry RL. Effect of tibial plateau leveling on cranial and caudal tibial thrusts in canine cranial cruciate deficient stifles: an in vitro experimental study. Vet Surg 2001;30:278–286.

Zachos TA, Arnoczky SP, Lavagnino M, Tashman S. The effect of cranial cruciate ligament insufficiency on caudal cruciate ligament morphology: An experimental study in dogs. Vet Surg 2002;31:596–603.

18 Stress Radiography of the Stifle

Henri van Bree, Hilde de Rooster, and Ingrid Gielen

Introduction

Cranial cruciate ligament (CrCL) rupture is a common problem in dogs, and is generally evaluated by physical examination. CrCL rupture often develops without an obvious history of trauma. The most consistent findings are joint swelling and instability of the stifle. To assess the instability, two tests, the cranial drawer test and the tibial compression test, are often used in veterinary practice. CrCL ruptures can be difficult to diagnose by these classical clinical tests alone (Robins 1990). Detection of craniocaudal instability may be masked by factors such as muscle tone caused by pain or stress, effusion, torn menisci, or periarticular fibrosis that develops in chronic cases of cruciate rupture (Flo & DeYoung 1978).

A radiograph shows the spatial relationship between the bones at the joint level. The position of the tibia in relation to the femur will be related directly to the status of the supporting ligaments that originate on one bone, and insert on the other (Jacobsen 1976). On a neutral view of a normal canine stifle in 90° of flexion, the perpendicular on the femoral axis that runs just cranial

to the fabellae, will be almost tangential to the caudal projection of the lateral tibial condyle (Meinen & Verbeek 1980). In a small number of cases, cranial displacement of the proximal tibia may be visible on a standard lateral radiograph, without any special stresses being applied to the leg during the positioning (Singleton 1957; Pond & Campbell 1972; Park 1979; Kirby 1993). This particular sign is called "Cazieux-positive," and always indicates a ruptured CrCL (Meinen & Verbeek 1980). The tibial compression test (Henderson & Milton 1978) mimics the contraction of the gastrocnemius muscles and increases load in the CrCL (Figure 18.1). The tip of the index finger of the hand that immobilizes the femur rests on the tibial tuberosity, and the hock joint is repeatedly flexed and extended with the other hand. This test is positive when a cranial displacement of the tibial tuberosity can be felt under the index finger of the upper hand. A stress radiographic technique, based on the clinical tibial compression test, has been developed to improve the diagnostic accuracy of clinical evaluation of craniocaudal instability.

Tibial compression radiography

A protocol for obtaining a tibial compression radiograph has been designed for dogs. It was devel-

---

Advances in the Canine Cranial Cruciate Ligament, Edited by Peter Muir, © 2010 ACVS Foundation, This Work is a co-publication between the American College of Veterinary Surgeons Foundation and Wiley-Blackwell.

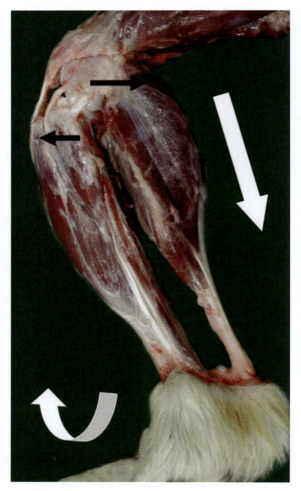

Figure 18.1 The tibial compression test: If cranial cruciate ligament rupture is present, the tibial plateau will slide cranially in relation to the distal femur (black arrows) by the contraction of the gastrocnemius muscles (white strait arrow) when the hock joint is maximally flexed (curved white arrow).

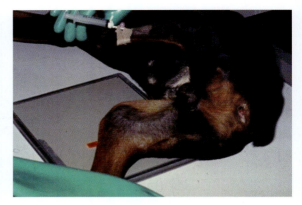

Figure 18.2 To obtain a tibial compression radiograph, the dog is positioned in lateral recumbency. A standard lateral radiographic view of the stifle joint is performed with the joint at 90° of flexion. Care should be taken to perfectly superimpose both femoral condyles.

oped to measure relative displacement of bony landmarks on paired lateral radiographs (neutral and tibial compression). An alternative radiographic method to quantify cranial tibial translation involves use of an external jig (Lopez et al. 2004). Although tibial compression radiography is typically performed without the use of a jig, a jig can be used to control more precisely the stifle flexion angle at which the test is performed (Bhandal et al. 2008).

To perform tibial compression radiography, each dog is positioned in lateral recumbency (Figure 18.2). A standard lateral radiographic view of the stifle joint is obtained with the joint at 90° of flexion (neutral position). While maintaining the angle of flexion of the stifle joint, the tarsal joint is maximally flexed by use of manual pressure, and a second radiograph was obtained (tibial compression position; Figure 18.3). In the case of a positive tibial compression radiograph, when compared with the neutral view, the proximal tibia will move cranially in relation to the distal femur when stress is applied (Figure 18.4). The radiographic test is objective and there is no interposition of soft tissue. Tibial compression radiography is reliable for both complete and partial CrCL ruptures, showing a high sensitivity and a hundred percent specificity (de Rooster et al. 1998; de Rooster & van Bree 1999a). The location of the sesamoid bone of the popliteal muscle on stress radiographs is also a useful and easy parameter in the interpretation of tibial compression radiographs in cases of CrCL rupture in the dog. Distal displacement of the popliteal sesamoid will confirm the presence of CrCL rupture (Figure 18.4b; de Rooster & van Bree 1999b). In a small number of dogs the popliteal sesamoid does not ossify, and therefore remains invisible as a radiographic parameter. A lack of ossification mainly occurs in small-breed dogs. In most of

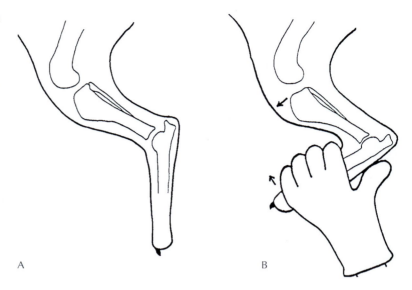

Figure 18.3 Paired lateral radiographs (neutral and tibial compression) are obtained. A standard lateral radiographic view is obtained with the joint at 90° of flexion (neutral position A). While maintaining the angle of flexion, the tarsal joint is maximally flexed by use of manual pressure, and a second radiograph is obtained (tibial compression position B). (Reproduced from de Rooster et al. 1998, with permission from the British Veterinary Association.)

these dogs, however, the craniocaudal displacement of the tibia will already be so obvious on the tibial compression radiograph that no additional parameters need to be assessed to come to a definite diagnosis of CrCL damage. An accuracy of 99% and a specificity of 100% were achieved by assessing the localization of the sesamoid bone in the diagnosis of cruciate rupture (de Rooster & van Bree 1999b).

In partial CrCL rupture, the cranial drawer test demands a certain portion of the CrCL to be torn. All cases of partial rupture in the present study showed a positive tibial compression radiograph (de Rooster & van Bree 1999a). In contrast with the physical tibial compression test (Henderson & Milton 1978), the stifle is held at an angle of 90° while making the tibial compression radiograph. The canine CrCL is formed by a craniomedial and a caudolateral bundle; the former is under tension during the whole range of motion of the stifle, while the latter is loose when the joint is flexed (Arnoczky & Marshall 1977). These features can have an effect in cases of partial rupture of the CrCL. At full extension, a false negative result is likely if only the craniomedial bundle of the ligament has ruptured, because the caudolateral bundle can mask the instability. In flexion, however, the caudolateral bundle of the cranial cruciate will always be slack, regardless of the state of the craniomedial bundle. As a result, fewer cases of incomplete damage will be missed when the tibial compression stress is exerted on a flexed stifle joint. Differences in degree of damage to the ligament and medial meniscus cannot be deduced from the amount of relative displacement measured on radiographs (de Rooster & van Bree 1999c).

Discussion and conclusion

Tibial compression stress radiography is a valuable asset in the diagnosis of canine stifle instability because of CrCL rupture. It is a useful technique to prove (or disprove) a tentative diagnosis of CrCL damage, especially when there is a lack of cranial drawer sign on clinical examination. No false positive results were obtained. Tibial compression stress radiography is able to detect complete or partial tears of the CrCL. It is an easy and reliable technique that does not require expensive equipment or a high level of technical proficiency.

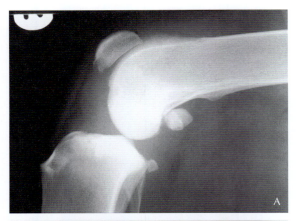
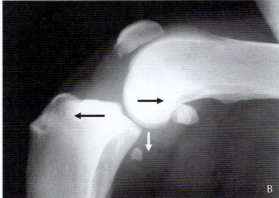

Figure 18.4 Tibial compression radiographs of a dog with a ruptured cranial cruciate ligament: neutral (A) and tibial compression (B). By flexing the hock joint a caudal displacement of the distal femur in relation to the tibial plateau becomes obvious (black arrows). Also notice the ventral displacement of the sesamoid bone of the popliteous muscle (white arrow).

References

Arnoczky SP, Marshall JL. The cruciate ligaments of the canine stifle: An anatomical and functional analysis. Am J Vet Res 1977;38:1807–1814.

Bhandal J, Kuzma A, Schiller T, et al. Application of a tibial compression device to diagnose partial or complete rupture of the cranial cruciate ligament in 129 dogs. *Proceedings of the Veterinary Orthopedic Society Annual Meeting*. Big Sky, MT, 2008, p. 65.

de Rooster H, van Bree H. Use of compression stress radiography for the detection of partial tears of the canine cranial cruciate ligament. J Small Anim Pract 1999a;40:573–576.

de Rooster H, van Bree H. Popliteal sesamoid displacement associated with cruciate rupture in the dog. J Small Anim Pract 1999b;40:316–318.

de Rooster H, van Bree H. Radiographic measurement of craniocaudal instability in stifle joints of clinically normal dogs and dogs with injury of a cranial cruciate ligament. Am J Vet Res 1999c;60:1567–1570.

de Rooster H, Van Ryssen B, van Bree H. Diagnosis of cranial cruciate ligament injuries in dogs by tibial compression radiography. Vet Rec 1998;142:366–368.

Flo GL, DeYoung D. Meniscal injuries and medial meniscectomy in the canine stifle. J Am Anim Hosp Assoc 1978;14:683–689.

Henderson RA, Milton JL. The tibial compression mechanism: A diagnostic aid in stifle injuries. J Am Anim Hosp Assoc 1978;14:474–479.

Jacobsen K. Stress radiographical measurement of the anteroposterior, medial and lateral stability of the knee joint. Acta Orthop Scand 1976;47:335–344.

Kirby BM. Decision-making in cranial cruciate ligament ruptures. Vet Clin North Am Small Anim Pract 1993;23:797–819.

Lopez MJ, Hagquist W, Jeffrey SL, et al. Instrumented measurement of in vivo anterior-posterior translation in the canine knee to assess anterior cruciate integrity. J Orthop Res 2004;22:949–954.

Meinen JJ, Verbeek M. Voorste kruisbandlaesies bij de hond: een evaluatie van therapie, klinisch en röntgenologisch verloop bij 215 patiënten. Referaat. Geneeskunde van het Kleine Huisdier, Vakgroep Radiologie, Rijksuniversiteit te Utrecht 1980.

Park RD. Radiographic evaluation of the canine stifle joint. Comp Cont Ed 1979;1:833–841.

Pond MJ, Campbell JR. The canine stifle joint. I. Rupture of the anterior cruciate ligament. An assessment of conservative and surgical treatment. J Small Anim Pract 1972;13:1–10.

Robins GM. The canine stifle. The diagnosis and management of acquired abnormalities. In: *Canine Orthopaedics*, Whittick WG (ed). Philadelpia: Lea & Febiger, 1990, pp. 724–752.

Singleton WB. The diagnosis and surgical treatment of some abnormal stifle conditions in the dog. Vet Rec 1957;69:1387–1394.

19 Stifle Ultrasonography

Cristi R. Cook

The normal stifle joint

Canine stifle joint disorders have been frequently diagnosed based on physical exam findings, radiographs, and arthrography (Reed et al. 1995; Kramer et al. 1999; Soler et al. 2007). More recently ultrasonography, computed tomography, and magnetic resonance imaging have been used to further evaluate the stifle joint (Gnudi & Bertoni 2001; Samii & Long 2002; Soler et al. 2007). Musculoskeletal ultrasound is commonly performed in humans. Canine stifle ultrasound has recently become a more common diagnostic modality to evaluate the intra-articular stifle joint structures (Kramer et al. 1999; Gnudi & Bertoni 2001; Samii & Long 2002; Soler et al. 2007). It is useful in evaluating the intra-articular soft tissues and the supporting extra-articular structures.

Stifle ultrasound examination is best performed using a 10–14 MHz high resolution, linear transducer (Kramer et al. 1999). To minimize artifacts, the hair along the stifle joint should be clipped and ultrasound coupling gel applied to the skin surface. The linear transducer is most appropriate for imaging superficial structures with high detail while minimizing the artifacts from anisotropy, which occurs when the fibers of the tendon or ligament are not perpendicular to the ultrasound beam (Figure 19.1a,b). This will appear as a hypoechoic area within the tendon or ligament, but when the structure becomes perpendicular to the ultrasound beam, the fibers will reappear (Reed et al. 1995; Kramer et al. 1999). It is important to look at potential lesions in both the longitudinal and transverse planes to confirm that the lesion is real or artifact, while making sure the transducer face is perpendicular to the structure of interest (Reef et al. 1998; O'Connor & Grainger 2005).

The cranial joint space is imaged with the transducer interface along the patellar tendon. The patellar tendon is seen in both transverse and sagittal planes as a superficial structure with low to moderate echogenicity and linear hyperechoic interstitial fibers (Reed et al 1995; Kramer et al. 1999; Soler et al. 2007). On transverse imaging the patellar tendon is an oval appearance with hyperechoic, pinpoint foci of the interstitial fibers. The peritendous tissue should be a thin, hyperechoic line (Kramer et al. 1999; Soler et al. 2007). Deep to the patellar tendon is the infra-patellar fat pad, which is hypoechoic to the patellar tendon and has a coarser echotexture compared with the ligament (Reed et al. 1995; Kramer et al. 1999; Soler et al. 2007). The collateral ligaments are similar in

---

Advances in the Canine Cranial Cruciate Ligament, Edited by Peter Muir, © 2010 ACVS Foundation, This Work is a co-publication between the American College of Veterinary Surgeons Foundation and Wiley-Blackwell.

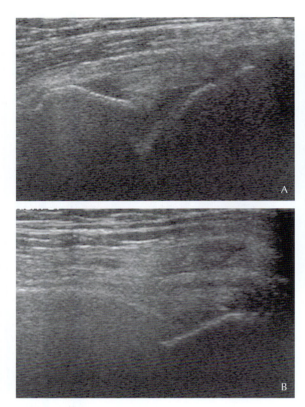

Figure 19.1 Normal tendon anisotropy. (A) The tendon fibers "drop out" when the ultrasound beam is not parallel to the tendon fibers. (B) The tendon fibers reappear when the beam is parallel.

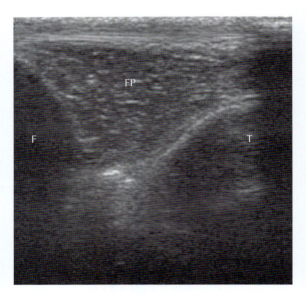

Figure 19.2 Normal cranial joint space of the stifle. The synovium is the very thin, hyperechoic line just cranial to the tibial cortex. F: femur; T: tibia; FP: fat pad.

appearance to the patellar tendon in their echogenicity and echotexture, in contradiction to other reports that state they are not visible (Kramer et al. 1999; Samii & Long 2002; Soler et al. 2007). The lateral collateral ligament can be identified along the lateral joint, caudal to the long digital extensor tendon with the tibial attachment angling caudodistally toward the fibular head (Vasseur & Arnoczky 1981). The medial collateral ligament is seen along the medial joint surface, at the most distal curve of the femoral condyle. The long digital extensor (LDE) tendon is seen along the craniolateral joint space superficial to the lateral meniscus and cranial to the lateral collateral ligament. The thickness of the LDE tendon will increase as the transducer is moved distally, toward the musculotendinous junction (Reed et al.

1995). The stifle ligaments, in general, should maintain a constant width.

The femoral condyles and tibial plateau are defined as hyperechoic lines with distal acoustic shadowing. The cartilage is a very thin, hypoechoic line, superficial to the hyperechoic cortical bone. The cruciate ligaments, being deep intra-articular structures, are the most difficult ligaments of the stifle joint to examine. The cranial cruciate ligament (CrCL) at its tibial attachment is best imaged from the cranial, sagittal plane with the joint in full flexion. In large dogs, the CrCL can be seen in full extension, but in small dogs, the intercondylar space is too narrow, so it is not visible (Kramer et al. 1999). The CrCL appears as a hypoechoic structure compared with the patellar tendon and is lined by the echogenic fat of the infra-patellar fat pad and synovium, which is a discrete, thin, hyperechoic line deep to the infra-patellar fat pad (Figure 19.2). The cruciate ligament becomes hyperechoic when the transducer is perpendicular to the ligament fibers (Gnudi & Bertoni 2001; Seong et al. 2005). In one study, the hyperechoic fibers became hypoechoic when the transducer was angled 3° off perpendicular (i.e., drop-out or off-angle artifact; Reed et al. 1995; O'Connor & Grainger 2005). The caudal cruciate

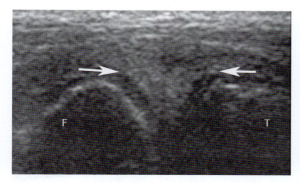

Figure 19.3 Normal meniscus. Note: the abaxial surface of the meniscus positioned along the femoral and tibial cortical margins (arrows). F: femur; T: tibia.

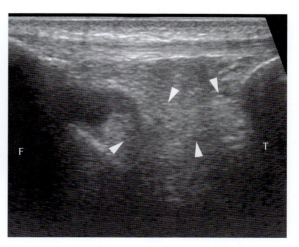

Figure 19.4 Hyperechoic, irregular tissue between the arrowheads associated with synovial thickening. F: femur; T: tibia.

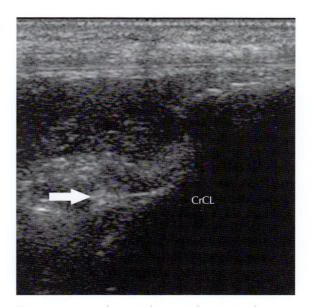

Figure 19.5 Irregular cranial cruciate ligament with irregular ends (arrow) consistent with a complete rupture. CrCL: cranial cruciate ligament rupture.

ligament (CaCL) is not easily visible with any cranial imaging technique (Kramer et al. 1999). The femoral attachment of the CaCL has been imaged in multiple studies with the use of a water bath, with the stifle in extension or full flexion (Reed et al. 1995; Gnudi & Bertoni 2001; Samii & Long 2002; Seong et al. 2005).

The medial and lateral menisci are best seen on sagittal plane images. They appear as a triangular, echogenic structure that is fairly homogenous (Reed et al. 1995; Kramer et al. 1999; Soler et al. 2007). The apex of the triangle points axially, conforming to the femoral condyle and tibial plateau (Figure 19.3). The cranial, central, and caudal regions of the medial meniscus are visible, whereas the different sections of the lateral meniscus are more difficult to identify routinely. The different sections of the menisci are based on their location to the collateral ligaments (i.e., the cranial horn of the meniscus is found cranial to the collateral ligament, the caudal horn, caudal to the ligament and the central region, adjacent to the collateral ligament).

The abnormal stifle joint

The most common abnormality of the stifle joint is CrCL rupture. In acute cases, the joint effusion can be mild to severe. The tear of the ligament may be identified if it is near the tibial attachment and may not be visible if it is closer to the midsection or femoral attachment. In chronic cruciate ruptures the ultrasonographic features seen are thickening of the synovium, minimal effusion, unless complicated by a meniscal tear, and an irregular bone surface because of osteophyte formation (Figure 19.4). In chronic cases, an irregular and thickened ligament may be seen with retraction of the ends at the site of the tear (Figure 19.5). Occa-

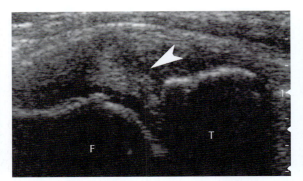

Figure 19.6 Meniscal tear. There is flattening of the tibial side of the meniscus with adjacent fluid. F: femur; T: tibia.

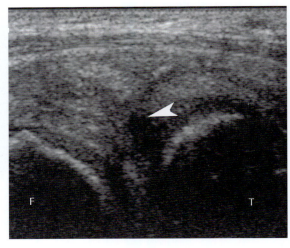

Figure 19.7 Macerated meniscus. The mottled appearance of the meniscal tissue with an abnormal shape (arrowhead). F—femur; T—tibia.

sionally, interstitial tears of the CrCL (i.e., intact epiligament with internal fibers disrupted) can be identified.

Meniscal tears are a common primary injury in the human knee, but rarely occur as a primary stifle injury in dogs and are usually secondary to CrCL rupture. The occurrence of secondary meniscal tears varies between studies, ranging from 20% to 77% (Mahn et al. 2005; Thieman et al. 2006).

The ultrasonographic findings associated with meniscal tears have been previously reported as (1) abnormal shape of the meniscus, (2) increased fluid adjacent to the meniscus, (3) change in the echogenicity of the meniscus, and (4) displacement of the meniscus. The most common abnormal appearance for a meniscal tear is the flattening of the tibial side of the meniscus (Figure 19.6; Mahn et al. 2005). Occasionally, axial splitting of the meniscus is identified in some patients with radial tears. Small radial tears or fraying of the meniscal edges may be too small to see specific changes with ultrasound, but other characteristics of meniscal tears are usually present. The macerated meniscus is usually an irregular, hyperechoic mass of tissue with no specific shape (Figure 19.7). Fluid accumulation is often seen adjacent to the meniscal tear and may be the only visible fluid within the joint. The meniscal echogenicity is relatively hyperechoic to the surrounding muscles with a finer echotexture. With meniscal tears, the meniscus may appear hypoechoic or mottled (Kramer et al. 1999). Occasionally, there may be a hyperechoic appearance adjacent to the tibial side of the meniscus. This has been confirmed with arthroscopy as hypertrophied synovium along the meniscus. Meniscal displacement may be the most difficult stifle feature to evaluate for new musculoskeletal ultrasonographers. There is a faint, hyperechoic line between the medial meniscus and the joint capsule that is used as a reference for the meniscal position. Normally, this line is adjacent to the plane of the femoral and tibial cortices (Figure 19.3; Mahn et al. 2005). Caution should be used if there are large osteophytes adjacent to the joint, as the meniscus can appear falsely displaced (abaxially) when in reality or with further evaluation, the osteophyte is the cause of the apparent displacement. When this interface is truly abaxially displaced, it has been associated with a displaced bucket-handle tear.

Patellar tendon abnormalities are most commonly associated with rupture (incomplete or complete) or desmitis associated with a previous surgical treatment. In acute patellar tendon injuries it will appear hypoechoic and thickened when compared with normal (Kramer et al. 1999). The fibers may be visible, but not parallel, disrupted with a distinct peritenon, disrupted fibers and peritenon, or complete rupture of the ligament and periligament (Figure 19.8). Chronic patellar ligament injuries appear hyperechoic, focally narrowed, with or without dystrophic mineralization

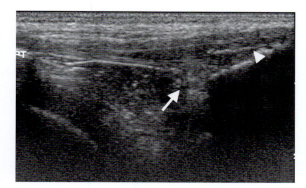

Figure 19.8 Thickening of the distal patellar tendon with irregular margins of ligament (arrow) and interstitial tear (arrowhead) consistent with partial tears.

within the tendon or enthesophytes at the tibial crest.

Conclusion

Ultrasound in general is cost-effective and readily available. But, interest and training in musculoskeletal ultrasound is much less common. Interpretation and diagnosis may rely on the training and experience of the ultrasonographer in musculoskeletal ultrasound. Thorough knowledge of the anatomy of the joint or structures is important, as well as the normal and abnormal ultrasonographic appearance of these structure. When learning the ultrasonographic appearance of a new musculoskeletal area, one is encouraged to evaluate the contralateral limb or image a normal patient for comparison.

References

Gnudi G, Bertoni G. Echography examination of the stifle joint affected by cranial cruciate ligament rupture in the dog. Vet Radiol Ultrasound 2001;42:266–270.

Kramer M, Stengel H, Gerwing M, et al. Sonography of the canine stifle. Vet Radiol Ultrasound 1999;40:282–293.

Mahn MM, Cook JL, Cook CR, Balke MT. Arthroscopic verification of ultrasonographic diagnosis of meniscal pathology in dogs. Vet Surg 2005;34:318–323.

O'Connor PJ, Grainger AJ. Ultrasound imaging of joint disease. In: *Practical Musculoskeletal Ultrasound*, McNally EG (ed), first edition. Philadelphia: Elsevier, 2005, pp. 245–262.

Reed AL, Payne JT, Constantinescu GM. Ultrasonography anatomy of the normal canine stifle. Vet Radiol Ultrasound 1995;36:315–321.

Reef VB, Sertich PL, Turner RM. Musculoskeletal ultrasonography. In: *Equine Diagnostic Ultrasound*, Reef VB, Sertich PL, Turner RM (eds). Philadelphia: WB Saunders, 1998, pp. 39–186.

Samii VF, Long CD. Musculoskeletal system. In: Small Animal Diagnostic Ultrasound, Nyland TG, Mattoon JS (eds), second edition. Philadelphia: WB Saunders, 2002, pp. 267–284.

Seong Y, Eom K, Lee H, et al. Ultrasonographic evaluation of cranial cruciate ligament rupture via dynamic intra-articular saline injection. Vet Radiol Ultrasound 2005;46:80–82.

Soler M, Murciano J, Latorre R, et al. Utrasonographic, computed tomographic and magnetic resonance imaging anatomy of the normal canine stifle joint. Vet J 2007;174:351–361.

Thieman KM, Tomlinson JL, Fox DB, et al. Effect of meniscal release on rate of subsequent meniscal tears and owner-assessed outcome in dogs with cruciate disease treated with tibial plateau leveling osteotomy. Vet Surg 2006;35:705–710.

Vasseur PB, Arnoczky SP. Collateral ligaments of the canine stifle joint: Anatomic and functional analysis. Am J Vet Res 1981;42:1133–1137.

20 Computed Tomography of the Stifle

Ingrid Gielen, Jimmy Saunders, Bernadette Van Ryssen, and Henri van Bree

Introduction

In dogs, the stifle is a frequently injured joint. Ligamentous and meniscal damages are frequent injuries and are associated with secondary degenerative changes (Vasseur 1993; Johnson et al. 1994). Diagnosis of stifle joint disorders is generally based on a history of lameness, physical examination, and radiography. For decades radiography has been the most often used medical imaging technique to diagnose stifle disorders, and has been proven to be very useful during clinical workup. In contrast to radiography, where there is a summation of the overlying structures, cross-sectional imaging, such as computed tomography (CT), allows identification of the internal joint structures without superimposition. CT has been proven to be extremely sensitive in demonstrating calcified or bony structures and also allows demonstration of the soft tissues (Figure 20.1) with selection of appropriate windows (Soler et al. 2007). Also the use of computed tomographic arthrography (CTA) has been described (Samii 2004) and although the results for identifying simulated meniscal injury are encouraging (Tivers &

Advances in the Canine Cranial Cruciate Ligament, Edited by Peter Muir, © 2010 ACVS Foundation, This Work is a co-publication between the American College of Veterinary Surgeons Foundation and Wiley-Blackwell.

Corr 2008), a recent clinical study in dogs reported that CTA had limited value in the detection of naturally occurring meniscal injuries (Samii et al. 2009). Although gross meniscal lesions can be evaluated (Figure 20.2), the problem we experienced with CTA is that in inflamed stifle joints the injected contrast medium is very rapidly absorbed and diluted, making an accurate interpretation of possible lesions difficult and in some cases even impossible. Research on the use of dimeric contrast agents (van Bree et al. 1992) and a mixture of epinephrine with conventional contrast agents (van Bree 1989; Vande Berg et al. 2002) in order to slow down resorption is needed in future work.

We examined the use and diagnostic value of CT in a retrospective study in a cohort of 50 clinical patients with stifle disorders. Inclusion criteria were a complete medical file including results of the clinical examination, radiographic examination, CT findings, and results of an arthroscopic examination or artrotomy. The final diagnosis was confirmed either with artrotomy or arthroscopy.

Technique

The CT images were performed with either a conventional axial CT scanner (Pace, GE Medical

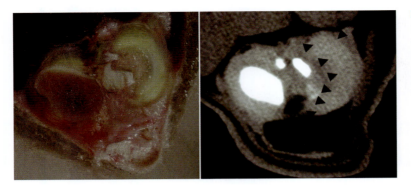

Figure 20.1 Anatomical specimen of a normal medial meniscus and associated CT image displayed in a soft tissue window (WW 400, WL 65). Although the silhouette of the medial meniscus (arrow heads) is visible, the exact delineation cannot be evaluated.

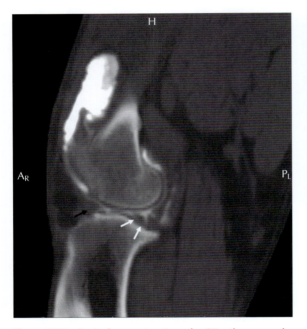

Figure 20.2 Sagittal reconstruction of a CT arthrogram of a dog after partial medial meniscectomy. We can see that the cranial pole is missing (black arrow) and the caudal pole seems to be crushed (white arrows).

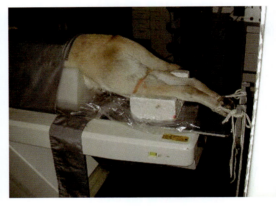

Figure 20.3 Positioning of a dog for stifle CT scanning: ventral recumbency with both stifles extended and scanned simultaneously.

Systems, Milwaukee, WI), or a single slice helical scanner (Prospeed, GE Medical Systems, Milwaukee, WI). Under general anesthesia, the dogs were scanned in ventral recumbency with both stifles extended and scanned simultaneously. Care should be taken to position them symmetrically (Figure 20.3).

Transverse scans were made parallel to the joint space using a bone algorithm and a standard algorithm. The slice thickness varied between 1 mm in the joint space and 2 mm at the level of the distal femur and proximal tibia (Figure 20.4).

Afterwards sagittal and dorsal reconstructions were made. The images were displayed and read in both a bone window (WW 3500; WL 500) and a soft tissue window (WW 400; WL 65). In case of soft tissue involvement intravenous contrast application was used at a dose of 2 ml/kg body weight.

Results

The final diagnosis in these 50 dogs was 22 osteochondritis dessicans (OCD), 13 cruciate ligament problems (5 avulsion fractures, 4 cranial cranial cruciate ligament [CrCL] ruptures, 1 caudal cruciate ligament rupture [CaCL], 5 stable partial

CrCL ruptures, 3 complete CrCL ruptures), 4 m. extensor digitorum longus problems (3 avulsions of the muscle origin), 1 m. popliteus avulsion, 7 neoplasia, and 3 patella luxations.

- Using CT, arthritic changes could be detected in an earlier stage than with conventional radiography, and they looked more severe (Figure 20.5).
- OCD lesions have typical features being radiolucencies surrounded by a sclerotic rim. More lesions could be detected by the use of CT. More intra-articular fragments could be seen as well (Figure 20.6).
- CT was very useful for the detection of avulsion fractures of the CrCL (Figure 20.7).
- CT was useful for the detection of avulsion fractures of the CaCL (Figure 20.8).
- CT was useful for the detection of avulsion of the origin of the m. extensor digitorum longus (Figure 20.9).
- and the m. popliteus (Figure 20.10).
- The depth of the fossa patellaris could be evaluated (Figure 20.11).

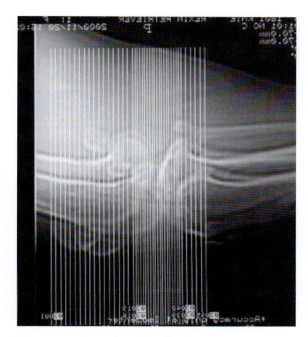

Figure 20.4 Scout view of a stifle CT scan: transverse scans are made parallel to the joint space. The slice thickness varies between 1 mm in the joint space and 2 mm at the level of the distal femur and proximal tibia.

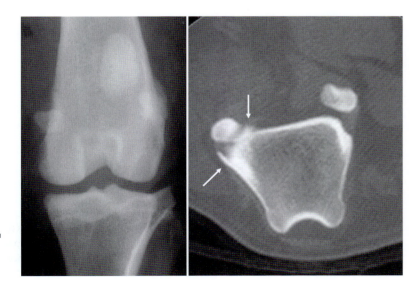

Figure 20.5 Radiograph and corresponding CT image of the distal part of the femur showing new bone formation and subchondral sclerosis in the area of the medial fabella (white arrows). These lesions are hardly visible on the radiograph.

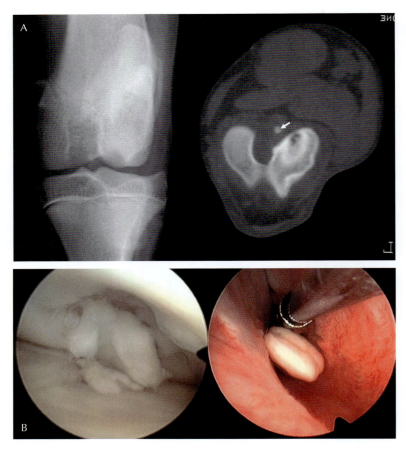

Figure 20.6 (A) Radiograph and corresponding CT image of the distal femur showing an obvious OCD lesion in the lateral femoral condyle not visible on the radiograph. A small fragment can be seen as well (white arrow). (B) The corresponding arthroscopic pictures of the OCD lesion and the floating fragment.

- The extension of neoplastic processes could be better evaluated with CT than with conventional radiography (Figure 20.12).
- CT was not very useful in evaluating the integrity of the cruciate ligaments and menisci.

Discussion

CT appeared to be useful in every case where superimposition of the bony structures had to be avoided. From the results of this study it was clear that CT was useful in detecting avulsions of the different intra-articular structures including both the CrCL and the CaCL, the m. extensor digitorum longus, and the m. popliteus. In these avulsion fractures, detection of a small bone fragment with CT imaging was superior to other imaging techniques. A stress radiographic technique, based on the clinical tibial compression test, has been introduced in an attempt to improve the diagnostic accuracy of clinical evaluation of craniocaudal instability. It is a valuable asset in the diagnosis of

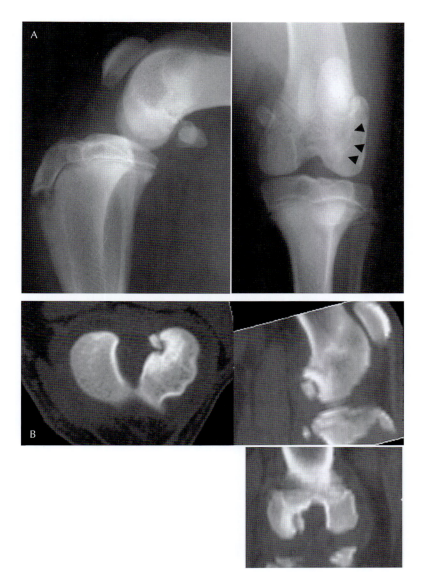

Figure 20.7 (A) Radiographs of a 5-month-old golden retriever with an avulsion of the cranial cruciate ligament (CrCL). On the caudocranial view subchondral sclerosis in the area of the medial part of the lateral femoral condyle can be appreciated (black arrow heads). (B) Corresponding transverse CT image, and sagittal and dorsal reconstructed images showing clearly the avulsed proximal attachment of the CrCL at the medial part of the lateral condyle with associated subchondral sclerosis.

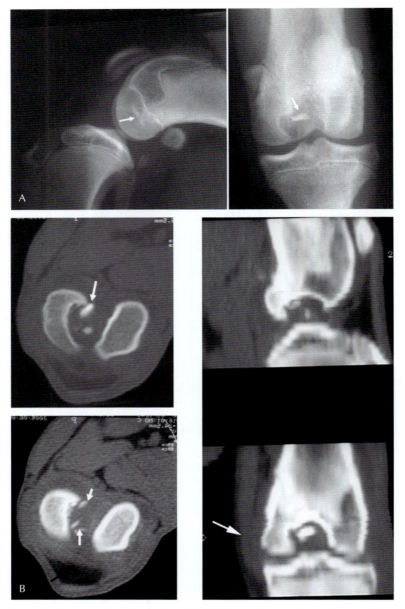

Figure 20.8 (A) Radiographs of a 6-month-old American Staffordshire with an avulsion of the caudal cruciate ligament (CaCL). On the mediolateral and caudocranial views, a fragment is visible (white arrow). On the caudocranial view an associated radiolucency in the medial area of the distal medial femoral condyle can also be appreciated. (B) Corresponding transverse, sagittal, and dorsal reconstructed CT images showing multiple fragments (white arrows) in the area of the proximal attachment of the CaCL in the medial area of the medial condyle. A prominent distension of the joint capsule is present (white arrow in the dorsal reconstructed CT images).

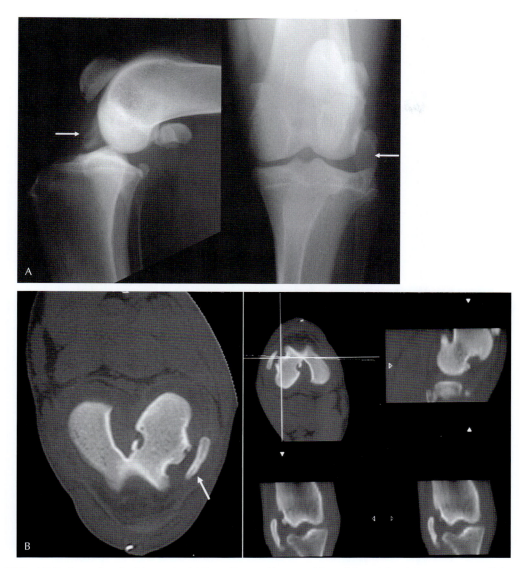

Figure 20.9 (A) Radiographs of a 14 month-old Great Dane with an avulsion of the origin of the m. extensor digitorum longus. On the medio-lateral and caudo-cranial views, a radiodense shadow (white arrow) can be identified in the lateral part of the stifle, of which the origin is unclear. (B) Corresponding transverse, sagittal, and dorsal reconstructed CT images showing this dense shadow originating from the origin of the m. extensor digitorum longus.

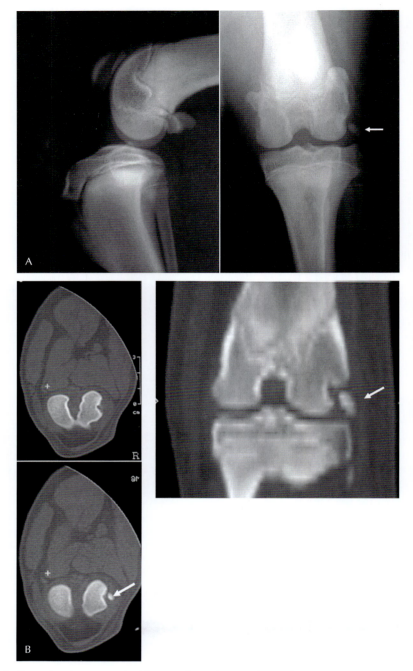

Figure 20.10 (A) Radiographs of an 8-month-old Rottweiler with an avulsion of the origin of the popliteus muscle. On the caudocranial view a rounded opacity (white arrow) can be identified in the lateral part of the stifle. Its origin is unclear from these radiographs. (B) Corresponding transverse and dorsal reconstructed CT images showing this opacity originating from the origin of the popliteus muscle (white arrow).

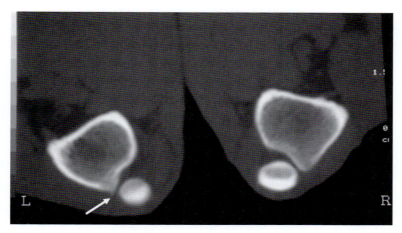

Figure 20.11 Transverse CT images of the left and right stifles of a 13 month-old Chesapeake Bay retriever with bilateral lateral patellar luxation. The patellar groove appears to be shallow and shows bony reaction in the area of the left lateral trochlear ridge of the femur (arrow).

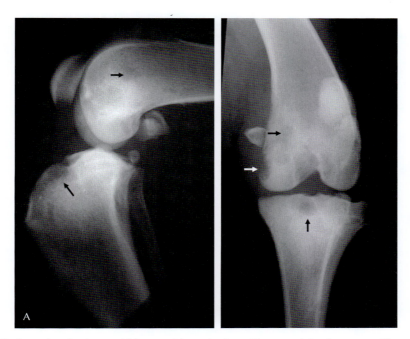

Figure 20.12 (A) Radiographs of a 6-year-old Bernese Mountain dog with a synovial cell sarcoma. The radiographs show several radiolucencies in the subchondral bone (arrows). (B) Transverse images of the distal femur and proximal tibia clearly demonstrate the osteolysis caused by the tumor (arrows). One transverse image in a soft tissue window after intravenous contrast administration shows enhancement of the severely swollen synovia (black arrow heads). These CT images better show the extent and severity of the neoplastic process. (C) Sagittal and dorsal reconstructed images giving a clear overview of the extent of the tumor.

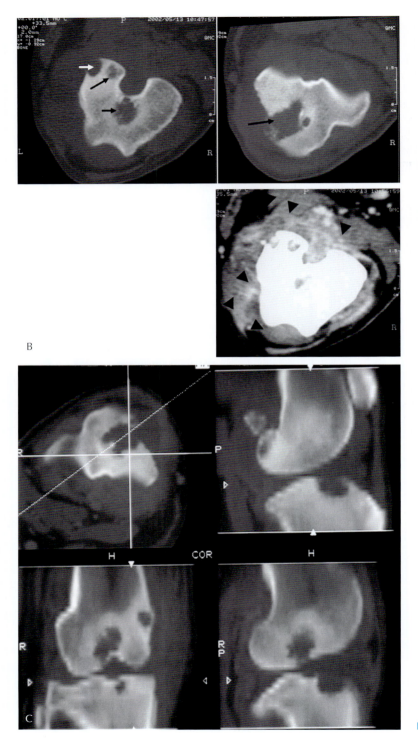

Figure 20.12 *Continued*

canine stifle instability because of CrCL tearing. It is a useful technique in proving (or disproving) a tentative diagnosis of CrCL damage, especially when there is a lack of cranial drawer sign on clinical examination. Tibial compression radiography is able to detect complete or partial tears of the CrCL (de Rooster et al. 1998; de Rooster & van Bree 1999). However, plain CT images were not very useful in evaluating the integrity of the cruciate ligaments and the menisci. In some of the patients with stifle problems we could detect a fragment or calcified structure on the radiographs without knowing its origin. CT helped us to clarify where the fragment originated from. From this study it appeared that especially in the diagnosis of CrCL avulsions in young dogs, CT was very useful and could confirm a working diagnosis. CrCL avulsion is considered rare and is suggested to be a disease primarily in skeletally immature dogs. In these animals the ligamentous attachment to the bone is stronger than the immature bone itself, allowing avulsion to occur under a force insufficient to cause ligament rupture. The diagnosis is of clinical importance as the avulsed fragment may be reattached if large enough and consequently the function of the CrCL could be restored in these young dogs.

References

de Rooster H, van Bree H. Use of compression stress radiography for the detection of partial tears of the canine cranial cruciate ligament. J Small Anim Pract 1999;40:573–576.

de Rooster H, Van Ryssen B, van Bree H. Diagnosis of cranial cruciate ligament injuries in dogs by tibial compression radiography. Vet Rec 1998;142:366–368.

Johnson JA, Austin C, Breur GJ. Incidence of canine appendicular musculoskeletal disorders in 16 veterinary teaching hospitals from 1980 through 1989. Vet Comp Orthop Traumatol 1994;7:56–69.

Samii VF DJ. Computed tomographic arthrography of the normal canine stifle. Vet Radiol Ultrasound 2004;45:402–406.

Samii V DJ, Pozzi A, Drost WT, et al. Computed tomographic arthrography of the stifle for detection of cranial and caudal cruciate ligament and meniscal tears in dogs. Vet Radiol Ultrasound 2009;50:144–150.

Soler M, Murciano J, Latorre R, Belda E, Rodrıguez MJ, Agut A. Ultrasonographic, computed tomographic and magnetic resonance imaging anatomy of the normal canine stifle joint. Vet J Journal 2007;174:351–361.

Tivers MS, Mahoney P, Corr SA. Canine stifle positive contrast computed tomography arthrography for assessment of caudal horn meniscal injury: A cadaver study. Vet Surg 2008;37:269–277.

van Bree H. Epinephrine enhanced positive contrast shoulder arthrography in the dog. J Vet Med A Physiol Pathol Clin Med 1989;36:687–691.

van Bree H, Van Ryssen B, Tshamala M, Maenhout T. Comparison of the nonionic contrast agents, iopromide and iotrolan, for positive-contrast arthrography of the scapulohumeral joint in dogs. Am J Vet Res 1992;53:1622–1626.

Vande Berg BC, Lecouvet FE, Poilvache P, Maldague B, Malghem J. Spiral CT arthrography of the knee: Technique and value in the assessment of internal derangement of the knee. Euro Radiol 2002;12:1800–1810.

Vasseur P. Stifle joint. In: *Textbook of Small Animal Surgery*, Slatter D, (ed), second edition. Philadelphia: WB Saunders, 1993, pp. 1817–1865.

21 Magnetic Resonance Imaging of the Stifle

Peter V. Scrivani

Introduction and image acquisition

Joints limit motion between bones to a particular range and dissipate stress during use (Dyce et al. 2002). The ability to perform these functions is based on the type of joint (synovial, cartilaginous, fibrous), bone conformation, and supporting soft tissues (Dyce et al. 2002). Loss of function, therefore, is manifested as excessive motion, restricted motion, or pain. In dogs the most common cause of joint dysfunction is osteoarthritis, which is a chronic degenerative disease of the articular cartilage and underlying bone because of a combination of genetic and environmental factors. Other common arthropathies are a result of inflammatory, traumatic, or neoplastic causes. Relative to this information and to the stifle joint in particular, the aims of magnetic resonance imaging (MRI) are early diagnosis of osteoarthritis and more specific diagnosis of the arthropathy, and to guide therapy decisions, to offer more detailed prognosis, and to assess response to treatment. MRI should be performed when achieving one of these goals to improve patient care. The beneficial impact of

Advances in the Canine Cranial Cruciate Ligament,
Edited by Peter Muir, © 2010 ACVS Foundation, This Work is a co-publication between the American College of Veterinary Surgeons Foundation and Wiley-Blackwell.

musculoskeletal MRI in humans is undisputed. In veterinary medicine, however, there is minimal evidence yet available that MRI actually improves patient care relative to the cost of the examination and additional anesthesia time. Competing diagnostic modalities, such as radiography, ultrasonography, or arthroscopy, offer benefits such as guiding therapy without the need for anesthesia or the ability to treat the underlying problem during the same procedure. MRI is promising and might have advantages in early detection of lesions in the subchondral bone, articular cartilage or menisci, or for establishing the cause of lameness that has not been diagnosed by conventional methods.

MRI recognition of joint lesions is based on alterations of signal intensity (SI) and morphologic changes (Rubin 2005). For subtle lesions, detecting these changes depends on acquiring images with high contrast and spatial resolution (Rubin 2005). It is difficult to make exact recommendations for optimal image acquisition because of different scanners (e.g., low-field, high-field), various manufacturer names for sequences, individual preferences, minimal evidence of efficacy of one protocol versus another, various breed conformations, and coils and algorithms that are optimized for humans. As a basic protocol the joint should be examined using a local coil—preferably one that surrounds the joint, and the joint should be located in the magnetic isocenter. The degree of joint flexion may be dictated by coil configurations. Obtain T2-weighted fast spin echo sequences in the transverse, sagittal, and dorsal planes using a long TR (3500–6000 msec) and moderate TE (28–38 msec), small field-of-view centered on the area of interest, and a large matrix size (e.g., 512 in frequency direction and 384 in phase direction). Additionally for the stifle obtain a proton density fast spin echo sequence with a shorter TE and short echo train length in the sagittal plane and a fat-suppressed T2-weighted sequence (e.g., short-tau inversion recovery or STIR) in the dorsal plane. For larger joints use a slice thickness of 3–4 mm; for smaller joints use 1–2 mm. Very thin slices (1 mm) may require a T2-weighted 3-dimensional (3D) gradient recall echo sequence. Additional sequences or planes may be of use in certain conditions. Intravenous or intra-articular contrast medium is not used routinely. Image orientation is accomplished by obtaining scout images in three planes. The dorsal plane is aligned parallel to the patellar tendon on the sagittal scout and parallel to the caudal aspect of the femoral condyles on the transverse scout. The transverse plane is made parallel to the distal aspect of the femoral condyles on the dorsal scout and perpendicular to the patellar tendon on the sagittal scout. The sagittal plane is made such that slices bisect the patellar tendon and intercondylar fossa (femur) on the transverse scout and parallel to the patellar tendon on the dorsal scout (Winegardner et al. 2007). High-quality images depend on the patient being still, which often requires anesthesia. Implants or metallic objects may reduce image quality (Banfield & Morrison 2000). High-field scanners provide superior signal-to-noise ratio but are not always available.

Synovial structures

Evaluation of synovial joints is one of the most important reasons for hospital visits relating to gait abnormality or lameness. Synovial joints consist of a fibrous joint capsule, synovial membrane, fluid-filled joint space, and articular cartilage (Dyce et al. 2002). The combination of the joint capsule and synovial membrane is seen as a low SI structure on MR images (Rubin 2005). The synovial membrane is usually too small to differentiate as a separate structure; it also lines joint recesses, bursas, and tendon sheaths. The normal synovial membrane does not enhance (or minimally) after intravenous contrast-medium administration (Rubin 2005). An inflamed synovial membrane is thick and may be nodular or mass-like, especially when chronic (Rubin 2005). When there is active inflammation the synovial membrane rapidly enhances with intravenous contrast-medium administration (Rubin 2005). Therefore intravenous contrast-medium administration might be helpful when an inflammatory arthropathy (e.g., immune-mediated, infectious) is suspected. Joint effusion (Figure 21.1) that is a result of increased synovial fluid production has similar signal characteristics as normal joint fluid. Joint fluid that contains proteinaceous debris or blood products has a different and variable SI (Rubin 2005). This different appearance may be referred to as "clean"

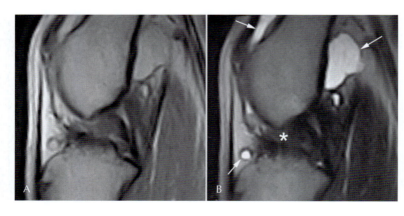

Figure 21.1 Sagittal (A) proton density MR image and Sagittal (B) SE T2-weighted MR image of a 2-year-old, neutered female, Mastiff with a complete tear of the cranial cruciate ligament. There is increased fluid within the stifle joint. Compare the SI of the "clean" (arrows) and "dirty" synovial fluid (asterisk) on the two images.

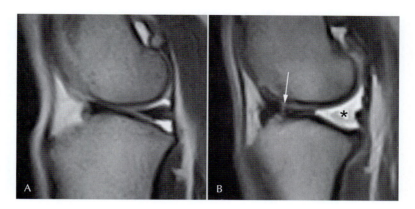

Figure 21.2 Sagittal (A) SE T2-weighted MR image of a 2.5-year-old, neutered female, Saint Bernard and (B) Sagittal SE T2-weighted MR image of a 2.5-year-old, neutered female, Rottweiler. Compare the normal appearance of the medial meniscus (A) to the abnormal (B). A full thickness tear is present in the cranial part of the medial meniscus (arrow) and the caudal portion is absent (*).

or "dirty" fluid. The appearance of normal articular cartilage reflects its chemical composition and 3D histological organization (Rubin 2005). For example articular cartilage has a low T2 SI that progressively increases from deep to superficial. Cartilage abnormalities appear as defects in the smooth articular surface, which may extend to the subchondral bone plate. Traumatic articular lesions are often sharply demarcated (Rubin 2005).

Meniscus

Within the stifle joint, there are lateral and medial menisci, which are crescent-shaped fibrocartilaginous structures that partially divide the joint cavity and provide structural integrity during movement (Dyce et al. 2002). Each meniscus has unnamed cranial-tibial and caudal-tibial ligaments. The lateral meniscus also has an attachment to the femur (meniscofemoral ligament). The transverse ligament connects the cranial-tibial ligaments of the two menisci. The normal MRI appearance of the meniscus is triangular or bow tie-shaped (sagittal and dorsal planes) and is of uniform low SI, although some exceptions regarding SI exist (Martig et al. 2006). Meniscal tears are common in dogs secondary to cranial cruciate ligament (CrCL) rupture and the medial meniscus is affected more commonly (Blond et al. 2008). The MRI appearance of a meniscal tear is a primarily linear intrameniscal area of high SI that extends definitively to one or both articular surfaces, or abnormal meniscal shape (Figure 21.2; Rubin 2005; Blond et al. 2008).

A grading system for describing meniscal injuries during MRI has been proposed in dogs: 0 (normal) to 4 (Martig et al. 2006). False-positive results for meniscal tears however are reported and may be a result of misinterpretation of the appearance of normal structures adjacent to the meniscus or artifact (Baird et al. 1998; Hashemi et al. 2004). A truncation artifact appears as alternating bright and dark bands at high-contrast interfaces such as the meniscus and synovial fluid (Figure 21.3; Hashemi et al. 2004). It is a result of an inability to approximate exactly a step-like change in the signal intensity because of a limited number of samples or sampling time, and it usually occurs in the phase direction (Hashemi et al. 2004). It may be remedied by increasing the sample time to reduce the ripples or decrease the pixel size by increasing the number of phase encodes or decreasing the field of view (Hashemi et al. 2004).

Tendons, ligaments, and muscles

Tendons, ligaments, and muscles of the stifle joint (Table 21.1; Figures 21.4–21.9), along with bone conformation, restrict movement primarily to a craniocaudal plane with minimal rotation and translation. Tendons and ligaments normally appear as homogeneous low SI sharply margined linear structures; on cross-section they are round, oval, or flat (Rubin 2005; Soler et al. 2007). Higher SI may be seen normally if muscle is interspersed with the fibers or if the orientation of the fibers approaches 55° relative to the magnetic field

138 Clinical Features

Table 21.1 Key for Figures 21.4 to 21.9

Anatomic structures

1. Femur
2. Patella
3. Tibia
4. Fibula
5. Lateral collateral ligament
6. Medial collateral ligament
7. Meniscofemoral ligament
8. Cranial cruciate ligament
9. Caudal cruciate ligament
10. Transverse ligament
11. Quadriceps muscle
    a. Vastus lateralis muscle
    b. Vastus intermedius muscle
    c. Rectus femoris muscle
    d. Vastus medialis muscle
    e. Quadriceps tendon
    f. Patellar tendon
12. Infrapatellar fat pad
13. Sartorious muscle
    a. Cranial
    b. Caudal
14. Biceps femoris muscle
15. Abductor cruralis caudalis muscle
16. Semitendinous muscle
17. Semimembranosus muscle
18. Gracilis muscle
19. Adductor muscle
20. Aponeurosis of pectineus muscle
21. Long digital extensor muscle
    a. Tendon
22. Extensor hallucis longus muscle
23. Fibularis longus muscle (*formerly peroneus longus*)
24. Lateral digital extensor muscle
25. Flexor hallucis longus muscle
26. Popliteus muscle
    a. Tendon
    b. Sesamoid bone
27. Cranial tibial muscle
28. Caudal tibial muscle
29. Long digital flexor muscle
30. Gastrocnemius muscle
    a. Fabella (sesamoid bone)
    b. Lateral head
    c. Medial head
31. Superficial digital flexor muscle

(magic-angle artifact; Spriet & McKnight 2009). During tendon degeneration or ligament sprain the structure may have increased SI, altered size (usually increased), irregular margins, or abnormal shape (Rubin 2005). With an acute tendon or ligament tear total discontinuity may be detected (Rubin 2005). With chronic ligament tear there may be complete absence of the ligament or a low SI scar that does not have the normal morphology of the ligament (Figure 21.10; Rubin 2005).

Bone

Cortical bone has a uniform low SI on all sequences. The normal periosteum is not visible (Rubin 2005). New bone formation (periosteal, osteophytes, enthesophytes) has an intermediate to low SI and is differentiated by location on the bone (Rubin 2005; D'Anjou et al. 2008). The SI of yellow and red bone marrow is similar to fat (high T1 and T2 SI); red marrow has a slightly lower T1 SI (Rubin 2005; Armbrust et al. 2008). In dogs the SI of the marrow in the femoral condyles on STIR images varies with age. At 4 months the SI relative to fat is inhomogeneous and is intermediate to low: 8–16 months, it is uniformly low SI (Armbrust et al. 2008). On STIR images high SI lesions may be detected in the bone marrow and may be a result of trauma (blunt or repetitive), hyperemia, ischemia, infarction, inflammation, or neoplasia (Rubin 2005).

In dogs with CrCL rupture it is common to detect varying degrees of increased SI on STIR images that are deep to the proximal and distal attachments of the CrCL (Figure 21.11; Baird et al. 1998; Martig et al. 2007; Winegardner et al. 2007). Whereas these lesions develop after surgical resection of CrCL they also have been observed in dogs with a partial CrCL tear or an intact CrCL (Winegardner et al. 2007). This observation suggests that multiple pathogeneses are possible and questions whether the surgical model of osteoarthrosis is the best representation of CrCL rupture in dogs. Additionally the location of the high SI lesions is different than in people with anterior cruciate ligament rupture, further suggesting a different or multiple pathogeneses. One possibility is a "stress reaction" especially if muscle strength is not developed sufficiently to absorb the load because of inconsistent exercise. A stress fracture is distinguished from other stress injuries by detecting a visible fracture line, periosteal reaction, or both (Rubin 2005).

Figure 21.3 Sagittal (A) SE T2-weighted MR image of a 2-year-old, intact male, Great Dane and (B) Dorsal SE T1-weighted MR image of a 2.5-year-old, neutered female, Rottweiler. Note the linear, high SI band within the meniscus (arrows) that are parallel to the interface between meniscus and synovial fluid that does not extend to the articular surface.

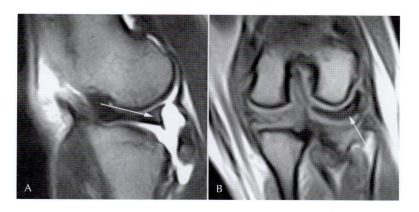

Figure 21.4 Sagittal (A) proton density MR image of a 2-year-old, neutered female, Chesapeake Bay retriever and (B) dorsal SE T1-weighted MR image of a 2.5-year-old, neutered female, Saint Bernard. The cranial aspect of the joint capsule and synovium (black arrow) is seen immediately caudal to the infrapatellar fat pad.

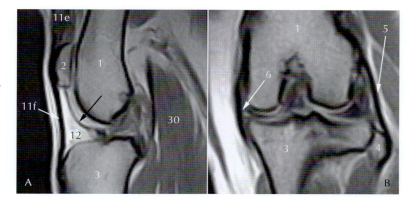

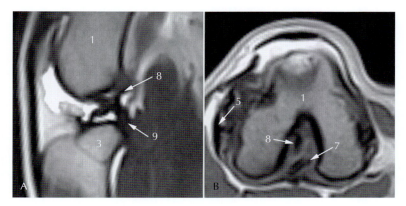

Figure 21.5 Sagittal (A) SE T2-weighted MR image of a 10-year-old, neutered female, Labrador retriever and (B) transverse SE T1-weighted MR image of a 2.5-year-old, neutered female, Saint Bernard. The proximal attachment of the cranial cruciate ligament is on the medial aspect of the lateral femoral condyle. The proximal attachments of the caudal cruciate and meniscofemoral ligaments are on the lateral aspect of the medial femoral condyle. The distal attachments of the cruciate ligaments are on the tibia. The distal attachment of the meniscofemoral ligament is on the lateral meniscus.

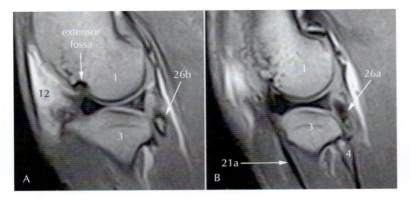

Figure 21.6 Sagittal SE T1-weighted MR images of a 2.5-year-old, neutered female, Great Dane depicting some normal anatomic structures.

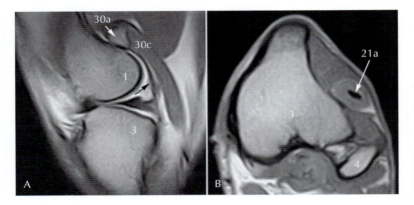

Figure 21.7 Sagittal (A) proton density MR image and (B) transverse SE T1-weighted MR image of a 2-year-old, male, Great Dane depicting some normal anatomic structures. The caudal aspect of the joint capsule and synovium (black arrow) is seen between the joint space and gastrocnemius muscle.

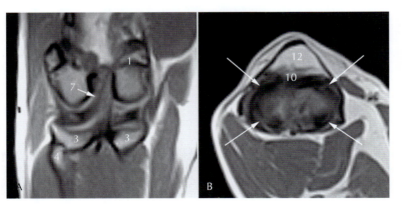

Figure 21.8 Dorsal (A) and transverse (B) SE T1-weighted MR image (TR860/TE26) MR images of a 2-year-old, neutered female, Chesapeake Bay retriever depicting some normal anatomic structures. The transverse scan is obtained through both menisci: the menisci (arrows) appear as apposing crescents with heterogeneous low SI because of slice thickness artifacts.

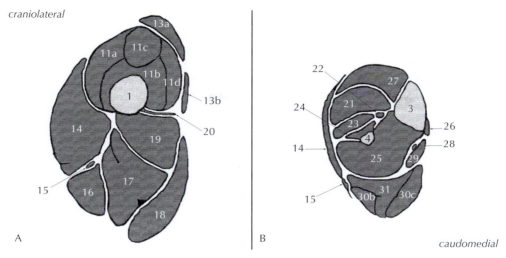

Figure 21.9 Schematic transverse section through the thigh (A) and crus (B) depicting the anatomic relationship of muscles and bones. The positional relationship of the supporting musculature is important when assessing joints. Reproduced from *Miller's Anatomy of the Dog*, with permission from Elsevier.

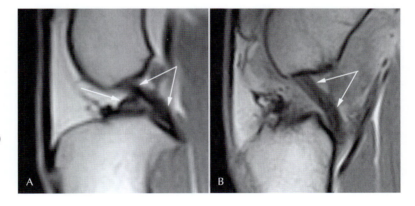

Figure 21.10 Sagittal (A) SE T1-weighted MR image of a 9-year-old, intact female, mixed-breed dog and sagittal (B) SE T1-weighted MR image of a 2.5-year-old, neutered female, Great Dane. Note the normal caudal cruciate ligament (CaCL, double arrow) and cranial cruciate ligament (CrCL, single arrow) (A). In the other dog (B), the CaCL (double arrow) is visible and the CrCL is completely torn.

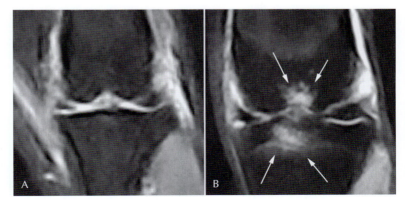

Figure 21.11 Dorsal GE_STIR MR image of a 2-year-old, neutered female, Chesapeake Bay retriever (A) and a 2-year-old, intact male, Great Dane (B). Compare the normal appearance (A) to the high SI lesions (arrows) at the proximal and distal attachments of the cranial cruciate ligament (B).

141

Conclusion

Musculoskeletal MRI is an emerging technique in veterinary medicine. Consequently there is minimal evidence to show that MRI is better than other types of examinations justified for cost and risk. Continued research, however, has the potential to show improved patient care through early lesion detection in areas inaccessible by other methods, which may establish the cause of a lameness that is undiagnosed by conventional methods, and lead to earlier, novel, or more specific treatments.

References

Armbrust LJ, Ostmeyer M, McMurphy R. Magnetic resonance imaging of bone marrow in the pelvis and femur of young dogs. Vet Radiol Ultrasound 2008;49: 432–437.

Baird DK, Hathcock JT, Kincaid SA, et al. Low-field magnetic resonance imaging of early subchondral cyst-like lesions in induced cranial cruciate ligament deficient dogs. Vet Radiol Ultrasound 1998;39:167–173.

Banfield CM, Morrison WB. Magnetic resonance arthrography of the canine stifle joint: Technique and applications in eleven military dogs. Vet Radiol Ultrasound 2000;41:200–213.

Blond L, Thrall DE, Roe SC, et al. Diagnostic accuracy of magnetic resonance imaging for meniscal tears in dogs affected with naturally occurring cranial cruciate ligament rupture. Vet Radiol Ultrasound 2008;49: 425–431.

D'Anjou MA, Moreau M, Troncy E, et al. Osteophytosis, subchondral bone sclerosis, joint effusion and soft tissue thickening in canine experimental stifle osteoarthritis: Comparison between 1.5T magnetic resonance imaging and computed radiography. Vet Surg 2008; 37:166–177.

Dyce KM, Sack WO, Wensing CJG. *Textbook of Veterinary Anatomy*, third edition. Philadelphia: WB Saunders, 2002.

Hashemi RH, Bradley WG, Lisanti CJ. *MRI The Basics*, second edition. Philadelphia: Lippincott Williams & Wilkins, 2004.

Martig S, Konar M, Schmökel HG, et al. Low-field MRI and arthroscopy of meniscal lesions in ten dogs with experimentally induced cranial cruciate ligament insufficiency. Vet Radiol Ultrasound 2006;47:515–522.

Martig S, Boisclair J, Konar M, et al. MRI characteristics and histology of bone marrow lesions in dogs with experimentally induced osteoarthritis. Vet Radiol Ultrasound 2007;48:105–112.

Rubin DA. Magnetic resonance imaging: practical considerations. In: *Bone and Joint Imaging*, Resnick D, Kransdorf MJ (eds), third edition. Philadelphia: Elsevier Saunders, 2005, pp. 118-132.

Soler M, Murciano J, Latorre R, et al. Ultrasonographic, computed tomographic and magnetic resonance imaging anatomy of the normal canine stifle joint. Vet J 2007;174:351–361.

Spriet M, McKnight A. Characterization of the magic angle effect in the equine deep digital flexor tendon using a low-field magnetic resonance system. Vet Radiol Ultrasound 2009;50:32–36.

Winegardner KR, Scrivani PV, Krotscheck U, Todhunter RJ. Magnetic resonance imaging of subarticular bone marrow lesions in dogs with stifle lameness. Vet Radiol Ultrasound 2007;48:312–317.

Section IV

Surgical Treatment

Introduction

A large number of different surgical procedures have been described for treatment of stifle instability in the dog, and decision making regarding surgical treatment remains controversial. Currently, widely used surgical procedures are aimed at treatment of stifle instability, not at reconstruction or repair of the ruptured cranial cruciate ligament (CrCL). Stabilization is accomplished either by osteotomy of the tibia or by extracapsular stabilization. Historically, by extrapolation from surgical treatment of human patients with anterior cruciate ligament rupture, intra-articular stabilization procedures have also been popular. Although initial results in experimental dogs were promising, use of intra-articular grafting procedures has become less popular over time. Recent longitudinal studies of surgical treatment have challenged the widely held belief that stifle instability is always the primary reason for lameness in affected dogs.

This section provides a detailed discussion of current surgical procedures used for treatment of dogs affected with CrCL rupture.

22 Arthroscopy versus Arthrotomy for Surgical Treatment

Brian S. Beale and Don A. Hulse

Introduction

Arthroscopy has revolutionized the treatment of joint disease in human beings and animals. Arthroscopic-assisted surgical techniques reduce postoperative pain and shorten the length of hospital stay and the time required for return to function (Whitney 2003; Hoelzler et al. 2004; Pozzi et al. 2008; Ertelt & Fehr 2009). At present, arthroscopy in animals is used primarily by veterinary surgeons having advanced training, usually working out of specialty practices or in a university hospital. General practitioners who routinely perform joint surgery have been slow to adopt arthroscopy due to the learning curve involved. Traditional arthrotomy gives a level of comfort to the surgeon at the consequence of sacrificing the benefits of arthroscopy. Consideration should be given to implementing arthroscopy at the time of arthrotomy to enhance joint examination, improve surgical treatment, and assist in arthroscopic training. The arthroscopic procedure is simplified when using arthroscopy at the time of arthrotomy. Many conditions affecting the joints are best viewed arthroscopically, including osteochondritis dessicans (OCD) of the shoulder and elbow, ligamentous and tendinous injuries of the shoulder, fragmented medial coronoid process, partial tears of the cranial cruciate ligament (CrCL), and meniscal tears (Whitney 2003; Hoelzler et al. 2004; Pozzi et al. 2008; Ertelt & Fehr 2009). Arthroscopic and minimally invasive arthrotomy has been reported to be an effective method of treating CrCL ruptures and meniscal injury (Whitney 2003; Ertelt & Fehr 2009).

Arthrotomy of the stifle

Arthrotomy of the stifle can be performed in a traditional open or a minimally-invasive manner (Hoelzler et al. 2004; Piermattei & Johnson 2004; Pozzi et al. 2008; Ertelt & Fehr 2009). Traditional arthrotomy can be performed by a medial or lateral parapatellar approach depending on the surgeon's preference (Piermattei & Johnson 2004). Some surgeons prefer a medial parapatellar approach because they claim to have an improved view and better access to the medial meniscus, but other surgeons claim the same using a lateral arthrotomy. A lateral arthrotomy may be best if a lateral extracapsular prosthetic CrCL is to be placed due to the need to have exposure to the caudolateral aspect of the joint (Figure 22.1A). A

Advances in the Canine Cranial Cruciate Ligament,
Edited by Peter Muir, © 2010 ACVS Foundation, This Work is a co-publication between the American College of Veterinary Surgeons Foundation and Wiley-Blackwell.

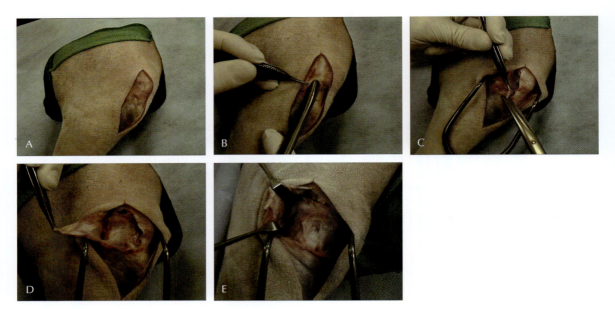

Figure 22.1 (A) A lateral parapatellar incision is most commonly used to approach the stifle joint for extracapsular treatment of cranial cruciate ligament tears. (B) The deep fascia is incised in a longitudinal direction cranial to the biceps femoris muscle. The fascial incision is continued distally along the lateral edge of the patellar tendon. (C) The deep fascia is incised and elevated from Gerdy's tubercle at the lateral aspect of the proximal tibia. (D) The incision is continued caudally in a transverse manner, exposing the lateral aspect of the stifle. (E) Retraction of the fascia allows adequate access to the lateral fabella, the caudal joint capsule, lateral collateral ligament, fibular head, long digital extensor tendon, extensor groove, and the cranial joint capsule.

medial arthrotomy may be most convenient if a tibial plateau leveling osteotomy or a tibial tuberosity advancement are to be performed due to the need to have medial exposure to the tibial diaphysis.

Traditional arthrotomy should be performed meticulously. The skin is initially incised, followed by subcutaneous tissue, deep fascia, and joint capsule. Each tissue layer should be identified and incised separately. If a lateral parapatellar approach is used, the deep fascia is incised at the cranial border of the biceps femoris muscle (Figure 22.1B). The fascial incision is continued distally 5–10 mm lateral to the edge of the straight patellar tendon. The deep fascia should be elevated from the joint capsule and its bony attachment to Gerdy's tubercle at the craniolateral aspect of the proximal tibia (Figure 22.1C). This allows optimal exposure to the caudal aspect of the stifle and closure of the joint capsule and deep fascia in separate layers. The fascia and attached biceps muscle is retracted caudally, giving good exposure to the lateral fabella, lateral condyle of the femur, fibular head, caudal joint capsule, long digital extensor tendon, extensor groove, and cranial joint capsule (Figure 22.1D,E). This approach is particularly useful when placing an extracapsular prosthetic CrCL. The joint capsule is incised longitudinally just lateral to the patellar tendon along its entire length. The patella is luxated medially. The proximal aspect of the femoropatellar joint and medial and lateral gutters along the femoral condyles are evaluated for trochlear groove depth, cartilage integrity, periarticular osteophytes, and degree of synovitis. The stifle is flexed and a Gelpi retractor is used to retract the joint capsule. A Senn retractor is used to retract the patellar fat pad distally, allowing a good view of the intercondylar notch, CrCL, and caudal cruciate ligament (CaCL). Torn fibers of the CrCL are typically resected by most surgeons. Removal of torn fibers allows an improved view of the weight-bearing surfaces of the femoral condyle and tibial plateau and the menisci. A portion of the fat pad can also be resected if needed to improve examination of the joint. An improved view of the menisci is obtained by placing the tip of a narrow, sturdy Hohmann retractor on the caudal aspect of the tibial plateau. The blade of the retractor is levered against the trochlear groove of the femoral condyle, resulting in a separation of the joint surfaces and improved access to the menisci. The menisci should be examined, probed, and treated as indicated while maintaining retraction. A stifle distractor can also be used in the intercondylar notch to enhance view of the menisci (Böttcher et al. 2009; Gemmill & Farrell 2009).

Increased morbidity occurs with arthrotomy due to the need for a more aggressive surgical approach. The initial skin incision must be longer and subsequent tissues beneath the skin, including subcutaneous tissue, deep fascia, muscle, and joint capsule, must be incised. Incised tissues cause pain due to initiation of inflammatory pathways and stimulation of sensory innervation. The surgeon should strive to minimize trauma to the regional soft tissues of the stifle to reduce the activation of pain stimuli. Smaller arthrotomy incisions and meticulous surgical technique are recommended. Joint tissues should be prevented from dessication by frequent lavage. Dessication of soft tissue and articular cartilage is deleterious, leading to increased tissue damage and patient morbidty.

Minimally invasive arthrotomy can be used to assess the joint in an effort to reduce postoperative morbidity. The arthrotomy can be made just medial or lateral to the patellar tendon, extending from the distal pole of the patella to the proximal tibia. A small Gelpi retractor is used to retract the joint capsule (Figure 22.2A). Resection of the fat pad provides an improved view of the joint. Luxation of the patella is not necessary to explore the joint. The CrCL is inspected and torn remnants are removed. Care should be taken during fat pad and CrCL resection to avoid severing the cranial meniscotibial ligaments and the transverse meniscal ligament. A Hohmann retractor or stifle distractor can be inserted to separate the joint surfaces of the femur and tibia, providing a better view of the menisci (Figures 22.2B–D and 22.3). The Hohmann retractor should be narrow but have adequate stiffness (thickness) to prevent bending. The tip of the Hohmann should have minimal cur-

vature. Critics of using a minimally invasive arthrotomy cite a reduced ability to view and gain access to the menisci, increasing the chance of leaving a meniscal tear behind at the time of surgery. In addition, partial meniscectomy performed through a minimally invasive arthrotomy may be difficult due to the inability to accurately assess the torn meniscus while attempting to resect the damaged portion of the meniscus. Iatrogenic cartilage damage may also occur due to inadvertent trauma to the joint surfaces while resecting meniscal tissue. The view obtained through the small window of the minimally invasive arthrotomy may also be inadequate to allow adequate examination of partial tears of the CrCL.

Arthroscopy of the stifle

Arthroscopy of the canine and feline stifle is rapidly becoming the method of choice for joint exploration and is performed as previously described (Whitney 2003). Arthroscopic management of CrCL rupture reduces short-term postoperative morbidity compared to traditional arthrotomy technique (Hoelzler et al. 2004). The advantages of arthroscopy include magnification, greater access to anatomic regions of the joint, evaluation of the joint structures in a fluid medium, and reduced intraoperative and postoperative morbidity.

A magnified view of anatomic structures of the stifle allows more accurate diagnosis and precise treatment of pathological conditions (Figure 22.4). Arthroscopic evaluation of the stifle allows more thorough evaluation of the patella, trochlear groove, femoral condyles, tibial plateau, CrCL, CaCL, and menisci. Arthroscopy of the stifle is commonly used to evaluate and treat CrCL tears, meniscal tears, osteochondrosis, osteochondral fragments, intraarticular foreign bodies, and septic arthritis. Arthroscopy provides a means of evaluating and treating intra-articular structures within the stifle with extreme precision and minimal morbidity.

The CrCL can be assessed for partial or complete tears before making an arthrotomy. Complete tears of the ligament are easy to see by arthrotomy or arthroscopy. Partial tears, on the other hand, are often not visible to the naked eye

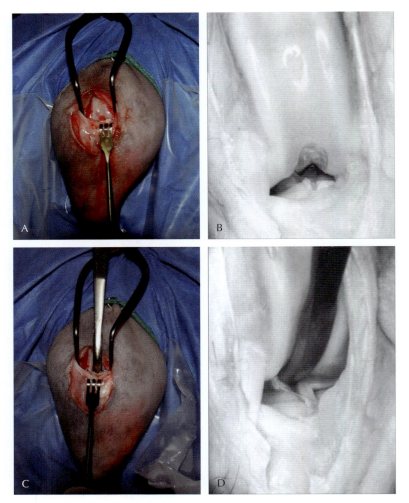

Figure 22.2 (A) A minimally invasive arthrotomy has been used to explore the stifle. The joint capsule is retracted using a small Gelpi retractor. The fat pad and cranial joint capsule are retracted distally using a Senn retractor. (B,C) Examination of caudal parts of the menisci can be difficult using an arthrotomy. A Hohmann retractor can be used to improve the view of the menisci. The tip of the retractor is inserted just caudal to or on the caudal edge of the proximal tibia. The body of the retractor is levered against the trochear groove of the femoral condyle. This action separates the joint surfaces, giving a better view of the joint. An assistant is required when using this procedure. (D) Distraction using the Hohmann retractor provides a good view for inspection of the menisci and adequate access for partial meniscectomy or meniscal release.

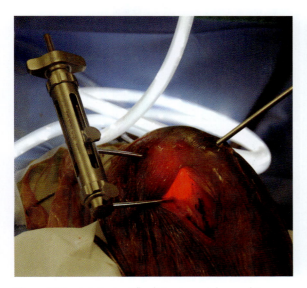

Figure 22.3 A Leipzig stifle distractor can be used to separate the space between the femoral condyle and tibial plateau, giving an improved view of, and better access to, the menisci. The distractor is attached to the medial femoral condyle and proximal tibia using threaded fixator pins. Distraction is achieved using the turnbuckle device on the distractor. An assistant is not required when using this device.

(Figure 22.5). Arthroscopic examination of the CrCL gives the surgeon the ability to identify and document partial tears of the ligament before progression of osteoarthritis (OA) and complete tearing of the ligament. Surgical intervention in the early stages of cruciate rupture may help reduce the severity of future OA, preserve the integrity of the remaining fibers of the ligament, and thereby decrease the potential of postliminary meniscal tears.

Examination of menisci is also improved due to the ability to position the arthroscope directly adjacent to the meniscus in both the cranial and the caudal joint compartment. Arthroscopy is superior to arthrotomy for diagnosis of meniscal injuries (Pozzi et al. 2008). A Hohmann retractor can be placed through a separate lateral portal in the intercondylar notch and levered against the femoral condyle to separate the joint surfaces and give better access to the menisci if needed. A stifle distractor has also recently been described to improve the arthroscopic view and surgical access for meniscectomy (Böttcher et al. 2009; Gemmill &

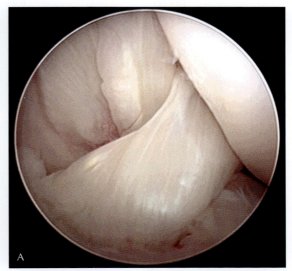

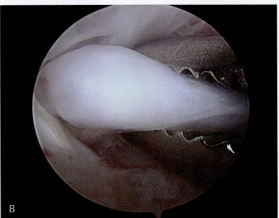

Figure 22.4 The cranial and caudal cruciate ligaments are more accurately assessed when viewed with an arthroscope due to magnification and evaluation in a fluid medium (A). The flow of fluid improves the appearance because the tissues do not dessicate and hemorrhage is flushed away. A bucket-handle tear of the medial meniscus is better viewed and more precisely removed using arthroscopy (B).

Farrell 2009; Figure 22.6). Bucket-handle tears of the medial meniscus are the most common type of tear found at the time of treatment of CrCL rupture. Only a small portion of these tears are actually displaced cranially at the time of surgical intervention. Arthroscopic evaluation of the meniscus allows the surgeon to better evaluate the integrity of the meniscus due to the magnified

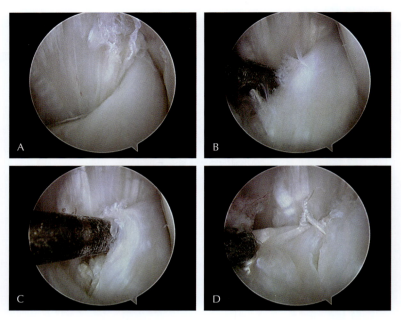

Figure 22.5 (A) The cranial cruciate ligament (CrCL) of this dog initially appears normal. (B–D) A partial tear of the cranial medial band of the CrCL was found when the insertion of the ligament was carefully probed. This CrCL partial tear would be difficult to see using traditional arthrotomy.

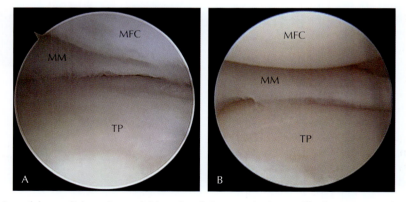

Figure 22.6 The view of the medial meniscus of this patient is improved using a stifle distractor. (A) The view of, and access to, the menisicus is inadequate initially. (B) With the use of a stifle distractor, meniscal evaluation and access for partial meniscectomy are improved. MFC: medial femoral condyle; MM: medial meniscus; TP: tibial plateau.

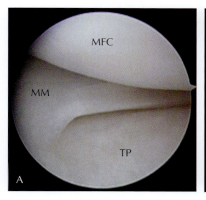 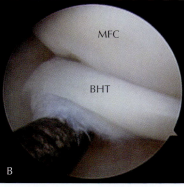 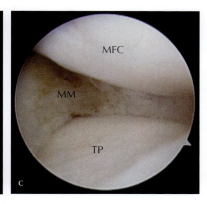

Figure 22.7 Meniscal tears can be difficult to see during routine arthrotomy. (A) This patient appeared to have a normal meniscus on initial arthroscopic inspection. (B) Careful probing of the medial meniscus revealed a bucket-handle tear. (C) A partial meniscectomy was performed, leaving the remaining healthy portion of the meniscus intact. MFC: medial femoral condyle; MM: medial meniscus; TP: tibial plateau; BHT: bucket-handle tear of medial meniscus.

view. The femoral surface of the caudal horn of the medial meniscus may appear to have wearing of the fibers or a change in the character of the surface of the meniscus. These changes may be impossible to see without magnification and often are associated with nondisplaced tears of the medial meniscus. Small radial and axial tears of the menisci often become evident only after magnification. The meniscus should be carefully probed on the tibial and femoral surface to assess for latent tears (Figure 22.7). Pozzi et al. (2008) found an increase in the ability to detect meniscal tears when the meniscus was probed using arthroscopic examination. Partial meniscectomy can be performed more accurately when assessed arthroscopically. Meniscectomy performed with the naked eye often leads to iatrogenic cartilage damage or inadequate removal of damaged meniscal tissue. Arthroscopic-assisted meniscectomy through an arthrotomy incision (see Arthroscopic-assisted arthrotomy) also gives a magnified view of the meniscus, which helps prevent inadvertent damage to the cartilage during instrumentation and allows the surgeon to assess the meniscus repeatedly to ensure complete removal of damaged portions of the meniscus.

Medial meniscal release is a commonly performed procedure designed to lessen the chance of postliminary meniscal tears after treatment of CrCL tears. Meniscal release can be performed under arthroscopic guidance by transection of the caudal meniscotibial ligament or by percutaneously incising transversely across the medial meniscus, just caudal to its attachment to the medial collateral ligament (Whitney 2003; Figure 22.8).

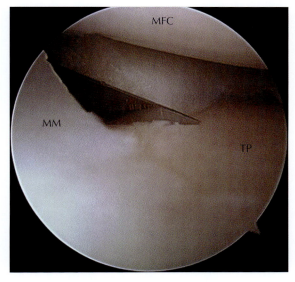

Figure 22.8 A mid-body medial meniscal release was performed using a #11 scalpel blade through a percutaneous stab incision made in the caudal medial aspect of the stifle joint. Meniscal release can be accurately performed and assessed using arthroscopy. MFC: medial femoral condyle; MM: medial meniscus; TP: tibial plateau.

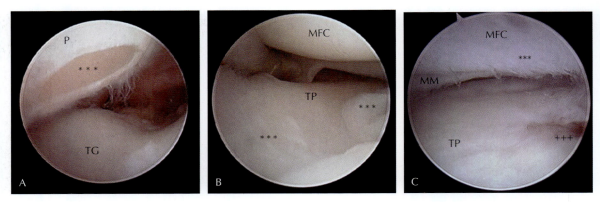

Figure 22.9 Arthroscopy improves the ability of the surgeon to assess the condition of articular cartilage. (A) A small focal area of full-thickness erosion of the patellar cartilage (***) is seen on the underside of the patella (P) adjacent to the trochlear groove (TG) in this patient with medial patellar luxation. (B) Chondromalacia (***) of the articular cartilage of the tibial plateau (TP) can be seen in this patient with a cranial cruciate ligament tear. (C) Fine fibrillation (***) of the articular cartilage of the medial femoral condyle (MFC) and fibrillation and erosion (+++) of the cartilage of the TP can be seen in this patient with a cranial cruciate ligament tear. Changes to cartilage as seen in (B) and (C) are typically only visible with magnification.

Magnification of intraarticular structures allows for more accurate identification of pathological change to articular cartilage. Early osteoarthritic changes to articular cartilage, not visible to the naked eye, are clearly seen arthroscopically (Figure 22.9). Fine and coarse fibrillation, superficial erosions, and neovascularization of the cartilage are readily evaluated and documented (Figure 22.9). Evidence of damage to the articular cartilage may help the surgeon devise a plan to treat or protect the cartilage in the future with adjunctive medications, nutritional supplements, or activity recommendations.

Arthroscopic-assisted arthrotomy

Arthroscopy is easier to perform when used at the time of arthrotomy. An arthroscope can be introduced into the arthrotomy incision to dramatically enhance the view of the patella, trochlear groove, femoral condyle, tibial plateau, CrCL, CaCL, and the menisci. Advantages of using an arthroscope through an arthrotomy compared with the traditional arthroscopic technique include the ability to use the arthrotomy incision for all three portals (egress, arthroscope, and instrument portals), a dramatic shortening of the arthroscopy learning curve, and a decreased chance of developing fluid extravasation in the soft tissues of the stifle. Other important advantages of arthroscopic-assisted arthrotomy compared with traditional arthrotomy include decreased pain, earlier return to function, improved viewing of intra-articular structures, and more precise and accurate treatment. Smaller arthrotomy incisions can be made when arthroscopy is used at the same time, thus capturing some of the benefits gained from the use of arthroscopy. The arthroscope can be quickly and easily moved in and out of the joint as needed. The surgeon's orientation of the arthroscope and anatomic target is improved. The arthroscope can be positioned in the desired location by gross observation, while the anatomic structure of interest can be assessed more completely using the magnification and enhanced viewing field provided by the arthroscope. Instruments used to treat the primary condition can be inserted adjacent to the arthroscope through the same arthrotomy incision. Triangulation, an arthroscopic skill that is difficult to learn, is no longer a problem because surgical instruments can be applied to the target tissue under gross observation. The arthroscope is then positioned next to the instrument to allow a magnified view while treatment of the damaged tissue is performed. Over time, the surgeon will improve their arthroscopic skills to the point where arthrotomy may no longer be needed. Extravasation of fluids into the subcutaneous tissues, a common problem with arthroscopy leading to poor viewing of intra-articular structures, is unlikely due to the ease of fluid egress from the arthrotomy incision.

A small arthrotomy is initially performed when using arthroscopic-assisted arthrotomy (Figure 22.10A). When first trying this procedure, the recommended arthrotomy should be made just medial or lateral to the patellar tendon, extending from the distal pole of the patella to the proximal tibia. As the surgeon gains experience, the length of the arthrotomy incision can be decreased. A small Gelpi retractor is used to retract the joint capsule (Figure 22.10B). Resection or retraction of the fat pad allows improved viewing. Luxation of the patella is not necessary to explore the joint. The proximal joint pouch and medial and lateral gutters can be examined by directing the arthroscope proximally (Figure 22.10C). Synovitis and osteophytes can be seen, assessed, and documented with images obtained using the arthroscopic camera. The synovium can be evaluated for hyperplasia, hyperemia, and fibrosis (Figure 22.11A). Synovial biopsies can be obtained using arthroscopic assistance to ensure that optimal tissue samples are obtained. Arthroscopic-assisted arthrotomy gives the surgeon the ability to fully assess and document the size and impact of osteophytes present in the joint (Figure 22.11B,C). The CrCL is inspected and torn remnants are removed (Figure 22.12A). Care should be taken during fat pad and CrCL resection to avoid severing the cranial meniscotibial ligaments and the transverse meniscal ligament. A Hohmann retractor or stifle distractor can be inserted to separate the joint surfaces of the femur and tibia, providing a better view of the menisci (Figure 22.12B,C). The joint is explored and precisely treated using the magnified view of the arthroscope. The arthroscope can be stabilized by resting the surgeon's hand against the patient or a folded sterile towel positioned on the patient to avoid a shaky image and inadvertently withdrawing the arthroscope from the joint (Figure 22.13). The surgeon can also steady the image and prevent inadvertent pulling of the

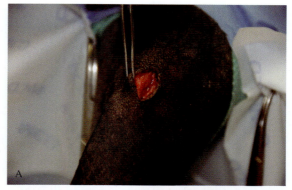

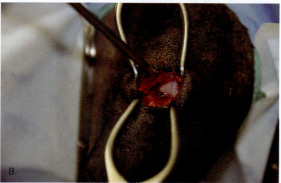

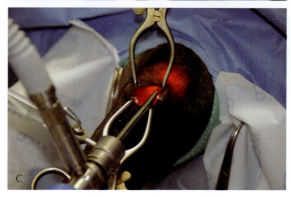

Figure 22.10 (A) Arthroscopic-assisted arthrotomy can be used to evaluate the stifle with similar advantages of arthroscopy but with the ease of arthrotomy. The arthrotomy incision is typically small as seen in this patient, but any size arthrotomy incision can be used with arthroscopic assistance. (B) Gelpi retractors can be used to retract the joint capsule and improve exposure to the joint. (C) The arthroscope is positioned in the proximal aspect of the joint to assess the patella, trochlear groove, synovial membrane, and the medial and lateral gutters for osteophytes. Fluid enters the joint through the arthroscope cannula and drains from the arthrotomy incision.

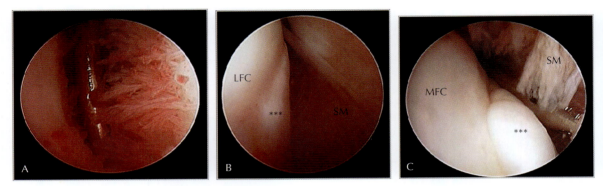

Figure 22.11 Arthroscopic-assisted arthrotomy facilitates assessment of intra-articular pathology at the time of arthrotomy (A). The synovium can be evaluated for hyperplasia, hyperemia, and fibrosis. Synovial biopsies can be obtained using arthroscopic assistance to ensure optimal tissue samples are obtained. (B) Small osteophytes (***) along the attachment of the joint capsule to the lateral femoral condyle (LFC) can be seen in this patient having an early cranial cruciate ligament (CrCL) tear. Minimal inflammation of the synovial membrane (SM) is seen. (C) Moderate sized osteophytes are present along the medial femoral condyle (MFC) in this patient with a chronic CrCL tear. The synovial membrane appears hyperplastic in the area of the ostophytes.

arthroscope out of the joint by grasping the shaft of the arthroscope near the arthrotomy incision. (Figure 22.13). Fluids are administered through the arthroscope cannula, similar to routine arthroscopy. The rate of fluid administration should be lowered due to the decreased resistance of the arthrotomy incision compared with traditional arthroscopy portals. Fluid egress occurs freely and fluid collection should be performed. Fluid egress can be captured using a drainage pouch with suction attachment or floor drain, or by simply placing towels or absorbent towels on the floor (Figure 22.13). A water-impervious drape should be used to avoid contamination of the surgical site (Figure 22.13). The tip of the arthroscope should be placed near the target tissue to provide the best view. Bubbles will often obscure the view if the tip of the arthroscope is drawn too far away from the tissue (Figure 22.14A). Surgical instruments are used with a combination of gross and arthroscopic observation. The instrument is initially positioned with gross observation, but manipulation of the instrument is best viewed arthroscopically to ensure precise treatment of the damaged tissue. Arthroscopic treatment also helps to prevent iatrogenic injury to the articular cartilage. A scrubbed assistant can be used to hold a grasper or probe during resection of the CrCL remnants or partial meniscectomy (Figure 22.14B). The surgeon typically holds the arthroscope and the cutting instrument or shaver. The meniscus should be carefully probed to assess for meniscal tears (Figure 22.15). Bucket-handle tears should be removed by partial meniscectomy. Arthroscopic-assisted arthrotomy allows the surgeon to perform a partial meniscectomy with great precision (Figure 22.16). After treatment, the affected tissue should be reevaluated using the arthroscope to ensure complete treatment. This is particularly important when performing a partial meniscectomy when treating a bucket-handle tear of the medial meniscus. It is common to find a second or third bucket-handle tear after removal of the first (Figure 22.17). The meniscus should be probed under arthroscopic viewing to ensure that additional damaged meniscal tissue is not left behind. Medial mensical release can also be performed more accurately using arthroscopic guidance (Figure 22.18).

Patient morbidity

Postoperative pain

Pain after surgery of the stifle can be substantial. Disruption of tissues leads to pain. Pain is generated locally by cellular mechanisms and activation of pain receptors. The perception of pain is

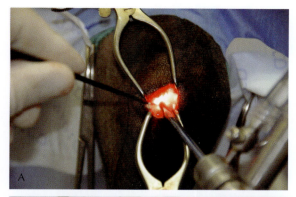

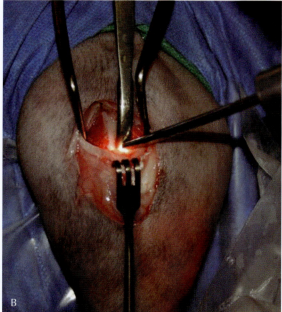

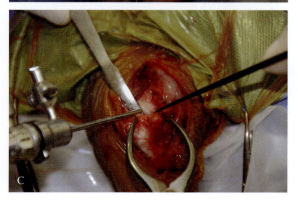

dependent on the transmission of impulses through the peripheral and central neural pathways. The source of pain may include skin, subcutaneous tissues, muscle, ligaments, tendons, synovial membrane, and subchondral bone. Inflammatory mediators within the synovial fluid also cause pain. Surgical pain can be decreased by appropriate preemptive analgesia and adjunctive nonsteroidal anti-inflammatory drug (NSAID) therapy, by reducing the number and extent of tissues incised, and by meticulous handling of tissues. Arthroscopic-assisted surgery is minimally invasive, sparing soft tissues around the joint, thereby reducing painful stimuli. Persistent synovitis has been identified after arthrotomy or arthroscopy during the initial 8-week postoperative period. The presence of persistent inflammation in the joint postoperatively may warrant a longer duration of NSAID after surgery. Persistent synovitis may increase patient morbidity and slow rehabilitation postoperatively. Anecdotal clinical improvement has been seen by the author if NSAID therapy is continued for 2–8 weeks after surgical treatment of CrCL tears.

Return to function

Early return to function is desirable to reduce muscle atrophy and preserve joint motion after surgery. Limb disuse quickly leads to muscle atrophy. The loss of muscle mass results in increased force on the joint, which may predispose to OA and additional injury to ligamentous structures. Pain, tissue swelling, activity restriction, and bandaging contribute to postoperative loss of joint range-of-motion. Early range-of-motion exercise is advantageous due to the tendency for joints

Figure 22.12 Arthroscopic-assisted arthrotomy. (A) The cranial cruciate ligament is inspected with a probe. Diagnosis of partial tears of the CrCL is facilitated because of the magnified view supplied by the arthroscope. (B) A Hohmann retractor has been inserted into the mini-arthrotomy adjacent to the arthroscope, allowing an improved view of the menisci. (C) The menisci are probed while viewed with an arthroscope. The magnified view and ability to position the scope into an optimal position next to the meniscus increases the surgeon's accuracy in finding meniscal tears.

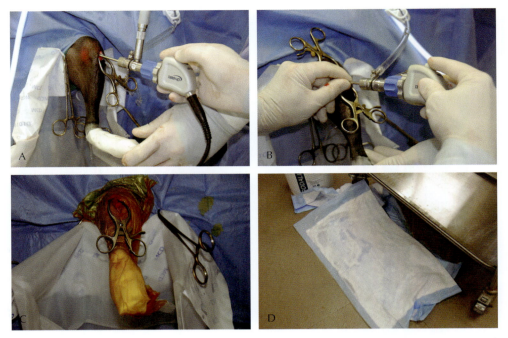

Figure 22.13 During arthroscopic-assisted arthrotomy, the arthroscope can be stabilized by resting the surgeon's hand against the patient or a sterile towel positioned on the patient to avoid a shaky image and inadvertently withdrawing the arthroscope from the joint (A). (B) The surgeon can steady the image and prevent inadvertent pulling of the arthroscope out of the joint by grasping the shaft of the scope near the arthrotomy incision. (C) Fluid egress occurs freely, and fluid collection should be performed. A water-impervious drape is used on patients having arthroscopic-assisted arthrotomy to avoid contamination of the surgical site. The drape used in this patient is an antimicrobial surgical incise drape with an iodophor-impregnated adhesive, designed to provide a sterile surface all the way to the wound edge and continuous antimicrobial activity throughout the procedure. Fluid egress can be captured using a drainage pouch with a suction attachment. (D) Fluids falling to the floor can be collected with a suction floor drain or by simply placing absorbent towels on the floor.

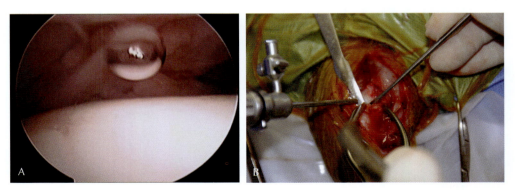

Figure 22.14 (A) The tip of the arthroscope should be placed near the target tissue to provide the best view. Bubbles will often obscure the view if the tip of the scope is drawn too far away from the tissue. (B) A scrubbed assistant can be used to hold a retractor, a grasper, or a probe during resection of the CrCL remnants or partial meniscectomy. The surgeon typically holds the scope and the cutting instrument or shaver.

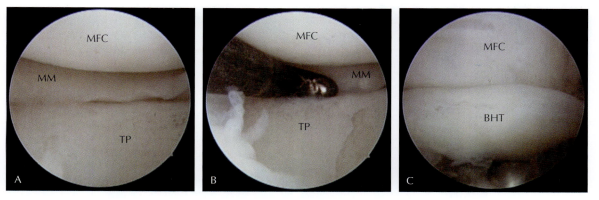

Figure 22.15 The meniscus should be carefully probed to assess for meniscal tears. This meniscus of this patient was examined using an arthroscopic-assisted arthrotomy technique. (A) The meniscus appears normal. (B) A probe is introduced to palpate and assess the meniscal integrity. (C) A bucket-handle tear of the medial meniscus is found and displaced cranially using the probe. MFC: medial femoral condyle; MM: medial meniscus; TP: tibial plateau; BHT: bucket-handle tear.

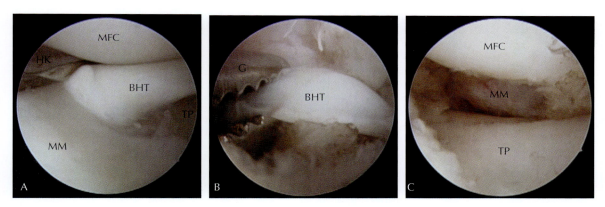

Figure 22.16 Bucket-handle tears should be removed by partial meniscectomy. Arthroscopic-assisted arthrotomy allows the surgeon to perform a partial meniscectomy with great precision. (A) A hook knife is used to cut the abaxial attachment to the bucket-handle tear of the medial meniscus. (B) The torn portion of the meniscus is grasped and tension is applied before cutting the axial attachment of the torn fragment. (C) Appearance of the periphery of the medial meniscus and articular surfaces following partial meniscectomy. MFC: medial femoral condyle; MM: medial meniscus; TP: tibial plateau; BHT: bucket-handle tear; HK: hook knife, G: grasper.

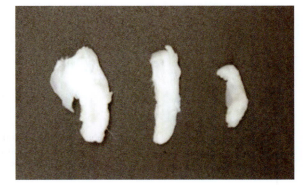

Figure 22.17 It is particularly important to reassess the meniscus with a probe after performing a partial meniscectomy to treat a bucket-handle tear of the medial meniscus. It is relatively common to find a second or even a third bucket-handle tear after removal of the first. This patient had a triple bucket-handle tear of the medial meniscus.

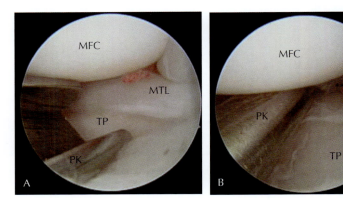

Figure 22.18 Medial mensical release can also be performed more accurately using arthroscopic guidance. (A) A meniscal release was performed by cutting the medial meniscotibial ligament using a meniscal push knife. (B) The caudal horn of the medial ligament has displaced caudally after cutting the ligament. Note the gap (***) at the site of transection of the meniscotibial ligament. MFC: medial femoral condyle; MTL: medial meniscotibial ligament; TP: tibial plateau; PK: push knife.

to become stiff after surgery. Periarticular fibrosis may lead to irreversible loss of range of motion and long-term morbidity and should be avoided. A formal rehabilitation program should be initiated during the early postoperative period to preserve muscle mass and joint range-of-motion. Consultation with a trained rehabilitation therapist is recommended. Therapists can develop a custom in-hospital and home rehabilitation program to reduce patient morbidity, speed up recovery, and improve the maximum functional outcome. Arthroscopic-assisted techniques also help to preserve joint range of motion due to its effect on decreasing postoperative pain and swelling.

References

Böttcher P, Winkels P, Oechtering G. A novel pin distraction device for arthroscopic assessment of the medial meniscus in dogs. Vet Surg 2009;38:595–600.

Ertelt J, Fehr M. Cranial cruciate ligament repair in dogs with and without meniscal lesions treated by different minimally-invasive methods. Vet Comp Orthop Traumatol 2009;22:21–26.

Gemmill TJ, Farrell M. Evaluation of a joint distractor to facilitate arthroscopy of the canine stifle. Vet Surg 2009;38:588–594.

Hoelzler MG, Millis DM, Francis DA, et al. Results of arthroscopic versus open arthrotomy for surgical management of cranial cruciate ligament deficiency in dogs. Vet Surg 2004;33:146–155.

Piermattei DL, Johnson KA. *An Atlas of Surgical Approaches to the Bones and Joints of the Dog and Cat.* Philadelphia: WB Saunders, 2004, pp. 338–351.

Pozzi A, Hildreth BE, Rajala-Schulz PJ. Comparison of arthroscopy and arthrotomy for diagnosis of medial meniscal pathology: An ex vivo study. Vet Surg 2008;37:749–755.

Whitney WO. Arthroscopically assisted surgery of the stifle joint. In: *Small Animal Arthroscopy*, Beale BS, Hulse DA, Schulz KS, Whitney WO (eds). Philadelphia: WB Saunders, 2003, pp. 117–157.

23 Joint Lavage

Peter Muir

Introduction

Pharmacologic treatment of arthritis often includes systemic or intra-articular administration of various types of drugs, particularly anti-inflammatory drugs. Common intra-articular therapies used for the treatment of arthritis include corticosteroids and hyaluronic acid (Jüni et al. 2007; Habib 2009). However, these treatments may be associated with adverse effects. Relief from arthritic pain after joint lavage has been noted by arthrosopists since 1934 (Burman et al. 1934). Subsequently, it has been suggested that large-volume lavage or irrigation of joints may facilitate removal of cartilage degradation products, inflammatory cells, pro-inflammatory cytokines, and matrix-degrading enzymes. However, this remains a provocative question that has been little considered in canine orthopaedic surgery.

Clinical studies

To address the question of joint lavage efficacy, a number of clinical trials have been conducted in human patients, principally studying knee osteoarthritis. Results of these trials have been conflicting. It has been suggested that the benefit of joint lavage is due to a placebo effect (Bradley et al. 2002). In at least one well-controlled trial, when arthroscopic debridement was compared with arthroscopic lavage or placebo surgery, no significant differences between groups were detected (Moseley et al. 2002). However, knee arthritis patients undergoing arthroscopic lavage have experienced persistent pain relief for up to 24 weeks in other trials (Ravaud et al. 1999). Comparison of arthroscopic lavage with lavage plus intra-articular corticosteroids suggested that little additional benefit is gained from use of corticosteroids; benefits from intra-articular corticosteroids appear short-lived in the range of 2–4 weeks (Ravaud et al. 1999; Smith et al. 2003). In at least one study, no interaction between steroid injection and joint lavage was found (Ravaud et al. 1999), suggesting that joint lavage may have a different mechanism of action from injection of corticosteroids. Effects of these two treatments have also been found to be additive (Ravaud et al. 1999).

Mechanism for relief of joint pain

Little experimental data are available to provide insight into the mechanism by which joint lavage

Advances in the Canine Cranial Cruciate Ligament,
Edited by Peter Muir, © 2010 ACVS Foundation, This Work is a co-publication between the American College of Veterinary Surgeons Foundation and Wiley-Blackwell.

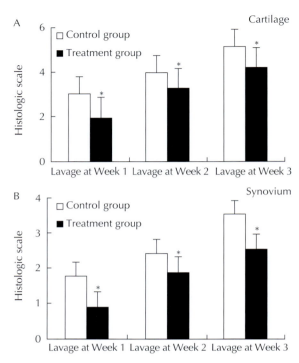

Figure 23.1 Histologic grading of cartilage from femoral condyles and synovium of osteoarthritis in a rabbit model ($n = 10$/group). Bilateral meniscectomy was performed with unilateral lavage, with the contralateral joint acting as a control. Treatment was joint lavage with saline, with euthanasia performed 1 week later. (A) Histologic grading of cartilage. (B) Histologic grading of synovium. Joint lavage was performed at 1 week, 2 weeks, and 3 weeks after meniscectomy. *$p < 0.05$ versus control group, which received no lavage treatment. Reproduced from Fu et al. (2009), with permission from Wiley-Blackwell.

Table 23.1 Influence of joint lavage on inflammatory markers in synovial fluid in a rabbit meniscectomy model

	Weeks after meniscectomy before joint lavage		
	1 week	2 weeks	3 weeks
IL-1β (pg/mL)			
Control ($n = 10$)	81.35 ± 2.41	67.39 ± 2.95	53.86 ± 3.79
Saline lavage ($n = 10$)	35.79 ± 3.50*	39.85 ± 4.78*	29.94 ± 3.99*
TNF-α (pg/mL)			
Control ($n = 10$)	599.36 ± 25.40	761.97 ± 17.28	446.32 ± 26.83
Saline lavage ($n = 10$)	313.02 ± 24.61*	459.15 ± 18.15*	309.88 ± 27.69*

Note: Euthanasia was performed 1 week after lavage. IL-1β concentrations were determined by ELISA. Reproduced from Fu et al. (2009), with permission from Wiley-Blackwell.
*$p < 0.05$ versus control group.

might induce relief from joint pain. However, in a recent experimental study using a rabbit meniscectomy model, joint lavage was found to significantly reduce joint degeneration at 1–3 weeks after induction of joint instability (Fu et al. 2009). Synovial inflammation and degradation of articular cartilage were both significantly reduced (Figure 23.1 and Table 23.1; Fu et al. 2009). Joint lavage treatment also led to reduced expression of the pro-inflammatory cytokines interleukin-1 beta (IL-1β) and tumor necrosis factor alpha (TNF-α) in synovial fluid (Fu et al. 2009).

Conclusion

Collectively, these clinical trial and experimental findings suggest that joint lavage may have efficacy in the treatment of arthritis, particularly through reduction of joint inflammation. In conclusion, when designing clinical trials using arthroscopy for treatment of dogs with stifle arthritis and cranial cruciate ligament rupture, the possibility that a significant treatment effect from arthroscopic lavage may exist should be considered in the experimental design of the trial project. Further work is needed to more comprehensively understand the mechanistic effects of joint lavage on arthritic canine joints, particularly as the beneficial effect of joint lavage appears much more durable, when compared to intra-articular corticosteroid treatment.

References

Bradley JD, Heilman DK, Katz BP, et al. Tidal irrigation as treatment for knee osteoarthritis. A sham-controlled, randomized, double-blinded evaluation. Arthritis Rheum 2002;46:100–108.

Burman MS, Finkelstein H, Mayer L. Arthroscopy of the knee joint. J Bone Joint Surg Am 1934;16:255–268.

Fu X, Lin L, Zhang J, Yu C. Assessment of the efficacy of joint lavage in rabbits with osteoarthritis of the knee. J Orthop Res 2009;27:91–96.

Habib GS. Systemic effects of intra-articular corticosteroids. Clin Rheumatol 2009;28:749–756.

Jüni P, Reichenbach S, Trelle S, et al. Efficacy and safety of intraarticular hylan or hyaluronic acids for osteoarthritis of the knee. Arthritis Rheum 2007;56:3610–3619.

Moseley JB, O'Malley K, Petersen NJ, et al. A controlled trial of arthroscopic surgery for osteoarthritis of the knee. N Eng J Med 2002;347:81–88.

Ravaud P, Moulinier L, Giraudeau B, et al. Effects of joint lavage and steroid injection in patients with osteoarthritis of the knee. Arthritis Rheum 1999;42:475–482.

Smith MD, Wetherall M, Darby T, et al. A randomized placebo-controlled trial of arthroscopic lavage versus lavage plus intra-articular corticosteroids in the management of symptomatic osteoarthritis of the knee. Rheumatology 2003;42:1477–1485.

24 Extracapsular Stabilization

James L. Cook

Introduction

Extracapsular stabilization (ES) is a time-tested option for the correction of joint instability as part of comprehensive management for cranial cruciate ligament (CrCL) rupture in dogs. ES procedures have been used for this purpose since the 1960s and have consistently produced good outcomes with respect to safety and efficacy. The basic concept for ES involves the use of a biologic or synthetic material with femoral and tibial fixation points to provide passive resistance to cranial tibial translation, internal rotation, and/or hyperextension in the stifle joint such that sufficient periarticular fibrosis can be produced for long-term stability and function. The potential advantages of ES over other joint instability corrective procedures include the safety profile, potential for addressing abnormal internal rotation, relative technical ease, and a small requirement for surgical equipment with low associated costs. The potential disadvantages primarily relate to the fact that all materials stretch or break at some point after implantation, which may result in failure of

instability correction, and resultant dysfunction. Many surgeons have suggested that outcomes after ES are inferior to those seen after osteotomies of various types. However, every prospective, head-to-head, cohort study published in the peer-reviewed literature to date has shown no differences in outcomes for ES and the osteotomies evaluated based on kinetics, kinematics, client-based and veterinarian-based subjective assessments, radiographic progression of osteoarthritis, or muscle mass measures (Conzemius et al. 2005; Lazar et al. 2005; Millis et al. 2008; Au et al. 2009; Cook et al. 2010; Evans, unpublished data). In addition, head-to-head comparison data have shown significantly better stifle range-of-motion measurements for ES compared with osteotomies and, most importantly, a better safety profile for ES (Millis et al. 2008; Cook et al. 2010; Evans, unpublished data).

Surgical approach and fixation points

While the basic mechanistic concept is consistent among ES procedures, the variations in technique are expansive. In the author's opinion, the stabilization procedure should be performed only after comprehensive assessment and treatment of intra-articular pathology via arthrotomy or arthroscopy. For subsequent ES, the surgical approach can be performed via medial or lateral skin inci-

---

Advances in the Canine Cranial Cruciate Ligament, Edited by Peter Muir, © 2010 ACVS Foundation, This Work is a co-publication between the American College of Veterinary Surgeons Foundation and Wiley-Blackwell.

sions and medial or lateral parapatellar arthrotomies (Payne & Constantinescu 1993). Because of the mobility of the skin over the stifle joint in dogs, access to relevant structures for ES can be readily achieved via either approach for all of the various ES techniques. For all of the ES procedures, fixation points for the stabilizing tissue or materials should be placed in anatomic locations that are as isometric as possible. This will optimize re-establishment of joint kinematics (counteraction of instability in all planes with maintenance of range of motion) while minimizing wear on the stabilizing tissue or material. In theory, use of isometric fixation points in ES procedures will allow for greater joint stability for a longer duration such that function of periarticular connective tissue is superior to that for non-isometric techniques. The most isometric points on the lateral aspect of the canine stifle have been described (Hyman et al. 2001; Roe et al. 2008). For application of these points to ES procedures using consistent anatomic landmarks, the tibial fixation point should be centered in or near the muscular groove of the tibia (taking care to protect the long digital extensor tendon) and should be placed as proximal as possible without entering the joint. The femoral fixation point is in the lateral femoral condyle, distal to its articulation with the lateral fabella and as caudal as safely possible (Figure 24.1). Use of the lateral fabella as a fixation point is also considered acceptable for addressing optimal isometry. Accurate identification and use of these points is absolutely critical to success for patients treated by ES procedures.

Stabilization methods

For the purposes of this chapter, the various ES techniques will be divided into the following basic categories: *Biologic* or *synthetic* and *medial* or *lateral* (Table 24.1). The majority of current ES procedures use synthetic implants placed on the lateral side of the stifle, but all of the major techniques will be briefly addressed.

Biological stabilization

Currently used biologic techniques involve the transfer or transposition of local tissues for stifle

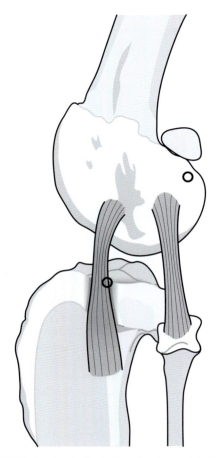

Figure 24.1 Anatomic illustration showing points that are most isometric on the lateral aspect of the canine stifle. Copyright © Samantha J. Elmhurst at www.livingart.org.uk.

joint stabilization. Fascial strips, the sartorius muscle, and the popliteal tendon have been used in biologic ES procedures, but currently the most commonly used techniques for biologic ES are fibular head transposition (FHT; Smith & Torg 1985) and fascial/biceps tendon advancement/ imbrication procedures (Childers 1966; McCurnin et al. 1971; Pearson et al. 1971). Fascial/biceps tendon advancement/imbrication procedures were the first reported means for ES for CrCL rupture and continue to be used to this day. Currently, these techniques are typically combined with another ES procedure with the intent of augmenting the initial stabilization and encouraging more optimal periarticular fibrosis. When used alone, fascial/biceps tendon advancement/imbri-

Table 24.1 Categorization and outcomes reported for common ES procedures in dogs

Procedure	Biologic or Synthetic	Location	Success rate (%)	Complication rate (%)
Fascial imbrication	Biologic	Lateral	NA	NA
FHT	Biologic	Lateral	64–90	17–50
LFTS	Synthetic	Lateral	90–95	17–25
MRIT	Synthetic	Medial and Lateral	90–95	17–25
LSA	Synthetic	Lateral	~91	≥21
TR	Synthetic	Lateral	91.6–95.6	9.1–12.5

NA: not available; FHT: fibular head transposition; LFTS: lateral fabellotibial suture; MRIT: modified retinacular imbrication technique; LSA: lateral suture anchor(s); TR: TightRope.

cation procedures have been successful in improving function as shown by anecdotal evidence and subjective assessments in small numbers of clinical patients (Childers 1966; McCurnin et al. 1971; Pearson et al. 1971; Aiken et al. 1992). To the author's knowledge, these techniques have not been directly compared with others for treatment of CrCL rupture in dogs.

FHT is designed to help stabilize the CrCL-deficient stifle by reorienting the lateral collateral ligament (LCL) such that it helps to counteract cranial tibial translocation and internal rotation. After FHT in experimental dogs, elongation and remodeling of the LCL occur such that stifle instability recurs, secondary meniscal pathology is seen, and osteoarthritis progresses (Dupuis et al. 1994a,b). However, clinical studies have shown efficacy in 64%–90% of patients with some reporting superiority (Smith & Torg 1985) and others, inferiority (Chauvet et al. 1996) of FHT in direct comparison with other CrCL stabilization procedures. Complication rates range from 17% to 50% for FHT and complications reported include fibular fracture, subsequent meniscal tears, instability, pain, and infection (Smith and Torg 1985; Mullen & Matthiesen. 1989; Dupuis et al. 1994b; Chauvet et al. 1996).

Stabilization using synthetic implants

ES procedures based on the use of synthetic implants typically use laterally placed devices while some also include a medially placed device.

The most common procedures from this category currently performed include the lateral fabellotibial suture (LFTS), medial and lateral modified retinacular imbrication technique (MRIT), lateral suture anchor techniques (LSA), and the lateral TightRope CrCL (TR; Arthrex, Naples, FL) procedure (Figure 24.2). The LFTS and MRIT procedures use sutures of various materials passed around the fabellae for the femoral fixation point and through a tunnel drilled in the metaphysis for the tibial fixation point. Both techniques employ an LFTS, and the MRIT adds a medial fabellotibial suture. A tremendous amount of *in vitro* and clinical research has been performed evaluating the various materials used for these two procedures. The major factors considered include strength, stiffness, creep, knot/fastener security, and biocompatibility of the materials. In general, multifilament braided materials (e.g., polyester, polybutester, kevlar, fiberwire) typically have superior material properties (load-to-failure, stiffness, creep, knot security), while monofilament (e.g., fishing line, leader line, polypropylene, nylon) materials allow for crimp fastening and are associated with less susceptibility for infection, tissue reaction, and sinus formation. The assumption is that all of these materials break or significantly elongate over time, but that if stifle stability is maintained for a sufficient period after surgery (~6–8 weeks), then adequate periarticular fibrosis will occur to maintain long-term functional stability. Interestingly, to the author's knowledge, the material properties of the fabella and its attachments to the femur have never been critically

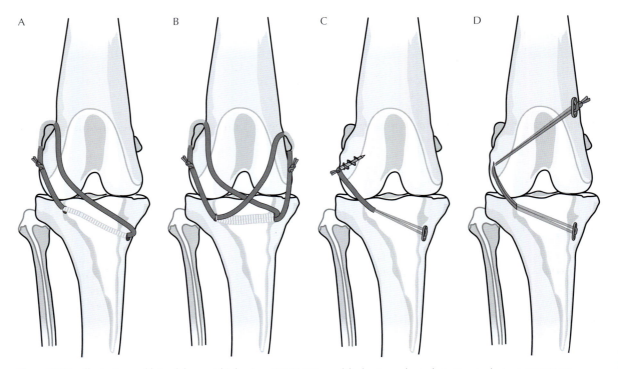

Figure 24.2 Illustrations of lateral femorotibial suture (LFTS) (A), modified retinacular imbrication technique (MRIT) (B), lateral suture anchor technique (LSA) (C), and TightRope (TR) (D) methods for extracapsular stabilization in the dog. Copyright © Samantha J. Elmhurst at www.livingart.org.uk.

evaluated with respect to ES procedures using this attachment site. Clinically, results for LFTS and MRIT for up to 6 years after surgery have been consistently good, with success rates in the range of 90%–95% (Chauvet et al. 1996; Innes et al. 2000; Conzemius et al. 2005; Millis et al. 2008; Au et al. 2009). Based on assessment of kinetics, kinematics, and/or radiographic progression of osteoarthritis, these techniques have been reported to be superior to FHT and intracaspular stabilization procedures and not statistically or clinically different from tibial plateau leveling osteotomy (TPLO; Chauvet et al. 1996; Conzemius et al. 2005; Millis et al 2008; Au et al. 2009). Complications with LFTS and MRIT can be expected in 17%–25% of cases and include infection, tissue reaction, sinus formation, subsequent meniscal tears, peroneal nerve damage, pain and instability (DeAngelis & Lau 1970; Dulisch 1981; Chauvet et al. 1996; Casale & McCarthy 2009). The majority of these complications are thought to be related to premature failure of the stabilizing materials, which may be the result of inferior mechanical properties, nonisometric placement, or material and/or fixation failure.

In an attempt to use a femoral fixation point that may be more isometric and a fixation method that may prove stronger and less susceptible to creep, lateral ES procedures using next-generation synthetic materials and bone anchors or tunnels have been developed. The LSA technique for ES uses a bone anchor of various types placed in the femur at the location described above as most isometric and a bone tunnel or another anchor in the most isometric tibial location. Suture material used may be determined separately for some anchors or anchors with preloaded sutures may be used as well. Currently, the only published study evaluating the clinical use of an LSA procedure used a subcortical femoral anchor and double tibial bone tunnel technique with a coated, braided polyester suture (Guénégo et al. 2007). These authors reported a 91% success rate using this technique despite the fact that 21% of the anchors had pulled out of the femoral condyle at mean follow-up of 18 months. This relatively high anchor failure rate was likely related to the fixation strength of the anchor as well as the non-isometric placement of femoral and/or tibial fixation points. Newer LSA techniques using transcortical femoral anchors in conjunction with isometrically placed tibial tunnel(s) or transcortical anchors and newer generation synthetic implants have been developed, and anecdotal data suggest excellent outcomes with very low complication rates (Hulse & Beale, Arthrex, Naples, FL, unpublished data).

The TR technique is an ES procedure that uses femoral and tibial bone tunnels placed at isometric locations using guide wires and drilling with a cannulated bit. The material used for stabilization is a synthetic braided tape (Fibertape, Arthrex), which is passed through the tunnels and secured on the medial aspects of femur and tibia using a toggle and button. *In vitro*, TR had superior mechanical properties for creep, stiffness, yield load, and load-at-failure when compared to LFTS using monofilament suture with crimps and braided suture with knots (Cook et al. 2010). Clinically, TR was compared with TPLO in a prospective head-to-head study (Cook et al. 2010). In that study, TR resulted in 6-month outcomes that were not different from TPLO in terms of client-evaluated level of function and radiographic progression of osteoarthritis. TR was associated with shorter anesthesia and surgery times as well as lower complication rates. Anecdotal multicenter data compiled on safety and efficacy of TR in 1,215 cases treated at 31 centers and evaluated at 3 months to 3 years postoperatively showed a 94.1% success rate. Complications requiring further treatment were reported to occur in 9.8% of cases (Cook, Arthrex, Naples, FL unpublished data).

Postoperative management for patients treated with ES procedures will vary based on the technique used, the patient, and surgeon preference. In general, the author recommends soft-padded bandaging for 24–72 hours postoperatively, careful attention to incision care and healing, restriction of activity to strictly controlled walking for 8 weeks after surgery, and strength-building rehabilitation from 8 weeks after surgery until full return to function. Rehabilitation during the postoperative period is discussed in Chapter 36.

Conclusion

ES is an effective method for surgical treatment of CrCL rupture in dogs. Comprehensive assessment and treatment of all joint pathology, isometric fixation points, and postoperative management that allows for adequate periarticular fibrosis and strength building are considered factors critical to successful outcomes. These procedures have been associated with the highest safety profile and outcomes that are equal to or better than all other techniques for surgical treatment of CrCL rupture in dogs.

Disclosure

The author receives direct financial benefit associated with sales of one of the products/techniques described in this chapter (TightRope CCL, Arthrex, Naples, FL).

References

Aiken SW, Bauer MS, Toombs JP. Extra-articular fascial strip repair of the cranial cruciate deficient stifle: Technique and results in seven dogs. Vet Comp Orthop Traumatol 1992;5:145–150.

Au KK, Gordon-Evans WJ, Johnson AL, et al. Comparison of short and long term function and radiographic osteoarthrosis in dogs with naturally occurring cranial cruciate ligament injury receiving postoperative physical therapy and tibial plateau leveling osteotomy or lateral fabellar suture. *Proceedings of the Veterinary Orthopedic Society Annual Conference.* Steamboat Springs, CO, 2009, p. 14.

Casale SA, McCarthy RJ. Complications associated with lateral fabellotibial suture surgery for cranial cruciate ligament injury in dogs: 363 cases (1997–2005). J Am Vet Med Assoc 2009;234:229–235.

Chauvet AE, Johnson AL, Pijanowski GJ, et al. Evaluation of fibular head transposition, lateral fabellar suture, and conservative treatment of cranial cruciate ligament rupture in large dogs: A retrospective study. J Am Anim Hosp Assoc 1996;32:247–255.

Childers HE. New methods for cruciate ligament repair: II. Repair by suture technique. Mod Vet Pract 1966; 47:59–60.

Conzemius MG, Evans RB, Besancon MF, et al. Effect of surgical technique on limb function after surgery for rupture of the cranial cruciate ligament in dogs. J Am Vet Med Assoc 2005;226:232–236.

Cook JL, Luther JK, Beetem J, et al. Clinical comparison of a novel extracapsular stabilization procedure and tibial plateau leveling osteotomy for treatment of cranial cruciate ligament deficiency in dogs. Vet Surg 2010;39:315–323.

Dulisch ML. Suture reaction following extra-articular stabilization in the dog. Part II: A prospective study of 66 stifles. J Am Anim Hosp Assoc 1981;17:572–574.

DeAngelis M, Lau RE. A lateral retinacular imbrication technique for the surgical correction of anterior cruciate ligament rupture in the dog. J Am Vet Med Assoc 1970;57:79–84.

Dupuis J, Harari J, Papageorges M, et al. Evaluation of fibular head transposition for repair of experimental cranial cruciate ligament injury in dogs. Vet Surg 1994a;23:1–12.

Dupuis J, Harari J, Blackketter DM, Gallina AM. Evaluation of the lateral collateral ligament after fibular head transposition in dogs. Vet Surg 1994b;23:456–465.

Guénégo L, Zahra A, Madelénat A, et al. Cranial cruciate ligament rupture in large and giant dogs. A retrospective evaluation of a modified lateral extracapsular stabilization. Vet Comp Orthop Traumatol 2007;20:43–50.

Hyman W, Hulse D, Saunders B, et al. Strain analysis of femoral and tibial anchorage sites for extracapsular reconstruction of the cranial cruciate deficient stifle joint. *Proceedings of the Veterinary Orthopedic Society Annual Conference.* Chateau Lake Louise, CA, 2001, p. 32.

Innes JF, Bacon D, Lynch C, Pollard A. Long-term outcome of surgery for dogs with cranial cruciate ligament deficiency. Vet Rec 2000;147:325–328.

Lazar TP, Berry CR, de Haan JJ, et al. Long-term radiographic comparison of tibial plateau leveling osteotomy versus extracapsular stabilization for cranial cruciate ligament rupture in the dog. Vet Surg 2005;34:133–141.

McCurnin DM, Pearson PT, Wass WM. Clinical and pathologic evaluation of ruptured cranial cruciate ligament repair in the dog. Am J Vet Res 1971;32:1517–1524.

Millis DL, Durant A, Headrick J, Weigel JP. Long term kinetic and kinematic comparison of cruciate-deficient dogs treated with tibial plateau leveling osteotomy or modified retinacular imbrications technique. *Proceedings of the Veterinary Orthopedic Society Annual Conference.* Big Sky, MT, 2008, p. 12.

Mullen HS, Matthiesen DT. Complications of transposition of the fibular head for stabilization of the cranial cruciate-deficient stifle in dogs: 80 cases (1982–1986). J Am Vet Med Assoc 1989;195:1267–1271.

Payne JT, Constantinescu GM. Stifle joint anatomy and surgical approaches in the dog. Vet Clin North Am Small Anim Pract 1993;23:691–701.

Pearson PT, McCurnin DM, Carter JD, Hoskins JD. Lembert suture technique to surgically correct ruptured cruciate ligaments. J Am Anim Hosp Assoc 1971;7:1–13.

Roe SC, Kue J, Gemma J. Isometry of potential suture attachment sites for the cranial cruciate ligament deficient canine stifle. Vet Comp Orthop Traumatol 2008;21:215–220.

Smith GK, Torg JS. Fibular head transposition for repair of cruciate-deficient stifle in the dog. J Am Vet Med Assoc 1985;187:375–383.

25 Tibial Plateau Leveling Osteotomy

Milan Milovancev and Susan L. Schaefer

Introduction

Tibial plateau leveling osteotomy (TPLO) was first described by Slocum and Slocum (1993) to address stifle instability due to cranial cruciate ligament (CrCL) rupture. By decreasing the natural caudodistal orientation of the tibial plateau, TPLO limits the shear force generated by compression of stifle during weight-bearing, thereby abating cranial tibial thrust (Reif et al. 2002). The dynamic stability imparted to the CrCL-deficient stifle via TPLO is achieved by performing a radial osteotomy of the proximal tibia and rotating the proximal segment to decrease the tibial plateau angle (TPA; Figure 25.1).

Preoperative determination of the patient's TPA allows calculation of the magnitude of rotation necessary to achieve a desired postoperative TPA. The minimum amount of rotation required to neutralize cranial tibial thrust results in a postoperative TPA of $6.5° \pm 0.9°$. Further rotation increases strain on the caudal cruciate ligament (CaCL); rotating from $6.5°$ to $0°$ increases CaCL strain by $37.7\% \pm 17.4\%$ (Warzee et al. 2001). It

is important to note that the TPLO procedure itself only addresses dynamic stifle instability; therefore, inspection of intra-articular structures with appropriate treatment of meniscal injuries or other abnormalities must accompany the procedure. An excellent review of the proposed mechanism of action for TPLO is available (Boudrieau 2009).

TPLO technique

The magnitude of rotation planned preoperatively generally correlates well with realized postoperative TPA result (Windolf et al. 2008). However, achieving an accurate TPA measurement and executing the osteotomy and tibial rotation in such a manner as to accurately achieve the desired postoperative TPA without inadvertently creating angular or rotational limb deformities involves a complex interplay of factors. Intra- and interobserver variability in TPA assessment has the potential to influence preoperative planning and subsequent postoperative TPA. Interobserver variability in TPA measurement has been shown to be relatively small (standard deviation of $0.8°$) but statistically significant, whereas intraobserver variability and between groups of observers was not statistically significant (Caylor et al. 2001; Fettig et al. 2003). Limb position has been shown to influ-

---

Advances in the Canine Cranial Cruciate Ligament,
Edited by Peter Muir, © 2010 ACVS Foundation, This Work is a co-publication between the American College of Veterinary Surgeons Foundation and Wiley-Blackwell.

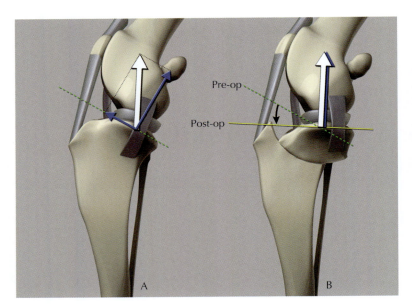

Figure 25.1 Schematic drawing depicting the reduction in tibial plateau angle following a tibial plateau leveling osteotomy and the subsequent change in individual tibiofemoral forces. (A) The tibiofemoral forces are broken down into a perpendicular and a parallel force relative to the tibial plateau (blue arrows). The force parallel to the tibial plateau represents tibial femoral shear. (B) With rotation of the tibial plateau. Note the elimination of tibial femoral shear. The resultant compressive force remains unchanged and is represented by the white arrow in both (A) and (B). Reproduced from Boudrieau (2009), with permission from Wiley-Blackwell.

ence radiographic TPA measurement: cranial and proximal positioning of the limb relative to the X-ray beam results in overestimation, whereas caudal and distal positioning results in underestimation of the TPA (Reif et al. 2004). An emphasis on osteotomy reduction at the expense of medial cortex alignment minimizes angular and rotational deformities due to TPLO (Wheeler et al. 2003). Distal positioning of the osteotomy (versus centering on the proximal tibial long axis point dividing the intercondylar tubercles) results in a postoperative TPA greater than is expected. In addition, undesired craniodistal translation of the tibial plateau and tibial long axis shift are also noted (Kowaleski et al. 2005).

Recently, the necessity of jig use during TPLO has been questioned by some authors. One study found no significant differences in postsurgical TPA, tibial crest thickness, varus–valgus malalignment, or tibial torsion between TPLOs performed with or without a jig (Bell & Ness 2007). The same author found that use of a jig resulted in a more distally positioned osteotomy. Another group found no significant difference in postsurgical TPA, fragment reduction, or proximodistal osteotomy orientation when a jig was not used, as long as the limb was held in 10°–15° of internal rotation and parallel to horizontal while performing a vertically oriented osteotomy (Schmerbach et al. 2007).

TPLO reportedly eliminates the wedge effect of the medial meniscus, which may protect it from postoperative injury (Pozzi et al. 2006). Hence, the necessity of medial meniscal release during TPLO has been debated and appears to be related to the quality of intraoperative meniscal evaluation. A subsequent meniscal tear is 3.8 times more likely to occur when meniscal evaluation is performed via arthrotomy and no meniscal release is performed, as compared with either meniscal evaluation via arthroscopy with no release or meniscal evaluation via arthrotomy with a release performed (Thieman et al. 2006). Importantly, although TPLO eliminates dynamic craniocaudal stifle instability and may impart protection to the medial meniscus, it fails to restore normal femorotibial contact mechanics. Postoperative femorotibial contact areas are significantly smaller than normal, with higher peak contact pressures (Kim et al. 2009).

Patient selection

Appropriate case selection is important to the success of TPLO. TPLO results in increased strain

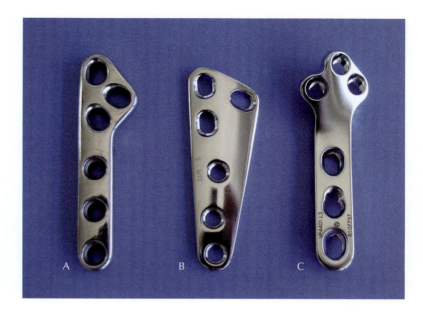

Figure 25.2 Example of three commercial manufacturer's tibial plateau leveling osteotomy plates: (A) Slocum 3.5 mm, (B) Securos 3.5 mm, (C) Synthes 3.5 mm. Plates (A) and (B) required contouring and utilize conventional screws. Plate (C) is a pre-bent locking plate.

on the CaCL ligament; therefore, patients with a compromised CaCL are not candidates for the procedure (Warzee et al. 2001). Patient size in itself is not a concern as long as appropriately sized implants are chosen for the procedure. Patients as small as a cat (Hoots & Petersen 2005) and as large as an alpaca (Ray et al. 2004) have been successfully treated with TPLO. TPLO in patients with concurrent patellar luxation allows for limited correction of tibial torsional deformity. Anecdotally, TPLO has been advocated in cases with a lack of cranial drawer where partial rupture of the CrCL is suspected as a means to decrease the biomechanical strain on the CrCL and theoretically protect it from further damage. To the authors' knowledge, this claim has not been systematically evaluated in any peer-reviewed publication.

TPLO implant selection

A wide range of orthopaedic implant manufacturers produce commercially available TPLO implants in various sizes. Both locking and non-locking implants are available (Figure 25.2). A biomechanical comparison between three different commercial manufacturer's TPLO plates has been performed in an axially loaded gap model: Synthes TPLO plate (Synthes Vet, West Chester, PA)/tibia constructs were found to be significantly stiffer than Slocum TPLO plate (Slocum Enterprises, Inc., Eugene, OR)/tibia constructs, which were found to be not significantly different from Securos TPLO plate (Securos, Fiskdale, MA)/tibia constructs (Kloc et al. 2009). Notably, the Synthes TPLO implant used in the above study was a locking bone plate, whereas the Slocum and Securos implants were conventional (non-locking) bone plates.

Concerns related to the use of the original Slocum TPLO plate center around plate corrosion *in vivo* with subsequent generation of chemical species that have the potential to cause disease, presence of plate magnetism, and findings showing the plate to be a cast stainless steel implant (Boudrieau et al. 2006; Charles & Ness 2006). Furthermore, Slocum TPLO implant-associated sarcoma has been reported (Boudrieau et al. 2005). To the authors' knowledge, no metallurgical analysis of alternative TPLO implants has been reported by an independent, unbiased party.

Use of locking bone screws causes significantly less translational movement of the proximal tibial segment toward the bone plate compared with use of conventional bone screws in an identical plate.

However, no significant difference exists between locking and conventional screw constructs in mean stiffness or cycles to failure under load sharing conditions (Leitner et al. 2008).

Complications after TPLO

The overall postoperative complication rate of TPLO has been reported to vary from 18% to 28% (Pacchiana et al. 2003; Priddy et al. 2003; Stauffer et al. 2006). Higher complication rates have been found in dogs undergoing simultaneous bilateral TPLO (Priddy et al. 2003). Notably, most complications can be resolved without surgical intervention (Pacchiana et al. 2003). Examples of complications include hemorrhage, incision site issues, patellar tendon enlargement, fractures involving the fibula or tibia, subsequent meniscal injury, and implant failures.

Dogs with preoperative TPA of ≥35° have a higher incidence of postoperative complications, with loss of postoperative TPA (colloquial term "rockback") during the convalescent period being the most common; addition of ancillary implants to TPLO significantly reduces the incidence of this problem (Duerr et al. 2008). Combination of TPLO with a cranial closing wedge ostectomy has been suggested as one possible means of addressing excessive TPA (Talaat et al. 2006). Small losses of postoperative TPA (approximately 1.5°) during the convalescent period have been documented in the face of apparently stable implant fixation, and by itself do not appear to have any deleterious effects on clinical outcome (Hurley et al. 2007; Moeller et al. 2006).

Radiographic evidence of patellar tendon enlargement is a common finding after TPLO with up to 80% of clinical cases showing evidence of moderate to severe thickening 2 months postoperatively (Carey et al. 2005; Figure 25.3). Despite these findings, only 7% of the dogs in this study showed clinical signs of patellar tendinosis, with most dogs improving with medical management.

Dogs that were cranial tibial thrust negative immediately after surgery occasionally become thrust-positive after surgery. Affected dogs often have poor limb function and pivot shift on ambulation. Pivot shift is created by a combination of

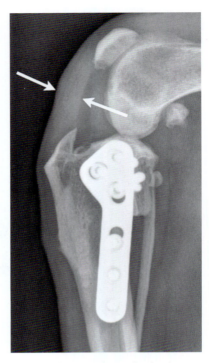

Figure 25.3 Lateral view radiograph of a dog 8 weeks after tibial plateau leveling osteotomy demonstrating marked thickening of the patellar tendon (white arrows).

cranial translation of the tibia with internal rotation of the stifle. The mechanism for this complication is unclear and is more commonly identified in heavily muscled dogs with genu varum conformation. Most cases improve with aggressive physical therapy; however, a lateral fabellar imbrication suture or a femoral corrective osteotomy may be required in severe cases.

Fractures of the fibula or tibia are potentially more serious complications that may be encountered during or after the TPLO procedure (Figure 25.4). Fibular fractures occurred in 5.4% of cases in a series of 168 TPLO procedures, with identified risk factors including increased body weight, greater preoperative TPA, greater change in TPA, and TPLO performed without the use of a jig (Tuttle & Manley 2009). Risk factors for tibial tuberosity fracture after TPLO include simultaneous bilateral TPLO, thinner postoperative mean thickness of the tibial tuberosity, and an increase in TPA during convalescence (Kergosien et al. 2004; Bergh et al. 2008).

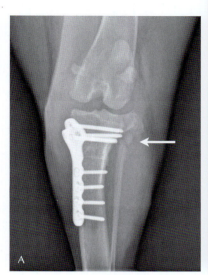 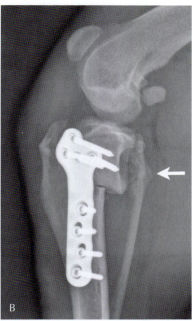

Figure 25.4 Cranial–caudal (A) and lateral (B) radiographic views of a dog 10 weeks after tibial plateau leveling osteotomy showing a short oblique proximal fibular fracture (white arrows).

Utilization of a structured postoperative physiotherapy program has been shown to result in greater stifle range of motion (ROM) for dogs undergoing TPLO at 3 and 6 weeks postoperatively as compared with standard home-exercise-restricted dogs (Monk et al. 2006). This suggests the importance of postoperative physiotherapy, as loss of ≥10° ROM has been associated with significantly higher subjective clinical lameness scores than dogs with <10° ROM loss. Loss of extension is also correlated with osteoarthritis in the cranial femorotibial joint (Jandi & Shulman 2007). Although progression of osteoarthritis after TPLO occurs (Boyd et al. 2007; Hurley et al. 2007), in general, presence of stifle osteoarthritis correlates poorly with clinical function (Gordon et al. 2003).

Outcome after TPLO

Despite these potential complications, outcome after TPLO has generally been reported as favorable as assessed by subjective and, less frequently, objective means. Most studies have employed subjective clinical assessments such as lameness scoring, radiographic osteophyte scoring, and client questionnaires (Kergosien et al. 2004; Stauffer et al. 2006; Thieman et al. 2006; Boyd et al. 2007). Objective evaluation of limb use after TPLO via force plate and kinematic analysis has corroborated a good outcome after TPLO with improvement of ground reaction forces comparable to lateral fabellotibial suture stabilization (Conzemius et al. 2005; Millis et al. 2008). Although *in vitro* work (Warzee et al. 2001) has demonstrated that a postoperative TPA of 6.5 ± 0.9 neutralizes cranial tibial thrust, a recent study of 32 client-owned Labrador retrievers with naturally occurring CrCL rupture undergoing TPLO evaluated via force plate analysis preoperatively and ≥4 months postoperatively found no relationship between postoperative TPA (range 0°–14°) and postoperative ground reaction forces (Robinson et al. 2006). Client satisfaction with postoperative outcomes of TPLO is reported as very good in multiple studies, even though such subjective assessments often do not correlate with incidence of postoperative complications or objective measures of limb function (Priddy et al. 2003; Talaat et al. 2006; Thieman et al. 2006; Boyd et al. 2007; Waxman et al. 2008).

Conclusion

Overall, TPLO is a viable surgical technique providing dynamic stability in the CrCL-deficient stifle.

References

Bell JC, Ness MG. Does use of a jig influence the precision of tibial plateau leveling osteotomy surgery? Vet Surg 2007;36:228–233.

Bergh MS, Rajala-Schultz P, Johnson KA. Risk factors for tibial tuberosity fracture after tibial plateau leveling osteotomy in dogs. Vet Surg 2008;37:374–382.

Boudrieau RJ. Tibial plateau leveling osteotomy or tibial tuberosity advancement? Vet Surg 2009;38:1–22.

Boudrieau RJ, McCarthy RJ, Sisson RD, Jr. Sarcoma of the proximal portion of the tibia in a dog 5.5 years after tibial plateau leveling osteotomy. J Am Vet Med Assoc 2005;227:1613–1617.

Boudrieau RJ, McCarthy RJ, Sprecher CM, et al. Material properties of and tissue reaction to the Slocum TPLO plate. Am J Vet Res 2006;67:1258–1265.

Boyd DJ, Miller CW, Etue SM, Monteith G. Radiographic and functional evaluation of dogs at least 1 year after tibial plateau leveling osteotomy. Can Vet J 2007;48:392–396.

Carey K, Aiken SW, DiResta GR, et al. Radiographic and clinical changes of the patellar tendon after tibial plateau leveling osteotomy 94 cases (2000–2003). Vet Comp Orthop Traumatol 2005;18:235–242.

Caylor KB, Zumpano CA, Evans LM, Moore RW. Intra- and interobserver measurement variability of tibial plateau slope from lateral radiographs in dogs. J Am Anim Hosp Assoc 2001;37:263–268.

Charles AE, Ness MG. Crevice corrosion of implants recovered after tibial plateau leveling osteotomy in dogs. Vet Surg 2006;35:438–444.

Conzemius MG, Evans RB, Besancon MF, et al. Effect of surgical technique on limb function after surgery for rupture of the cranial cruciate ligament in dogs. J Am Vet Med Assoc 2005;226:232–236.

Duerr FM, Duncan CG, Savicky RS, et al. Comparison of surgical treatment options for cranial cruciate ligament disease in large-breed dogs with excessive tibial plateau angle. Vet Surg 2008;37:49–62.

Fettig AA, Rand WM, Sato AF, et al. Observer variability of tibial plateau slope measurement in 40 dogs with cranial cruciate ligament-deficient stifle joints. Vet Surg 2003;32:471–478.

Gordon WJ, Conzemius MG, Riedesel E, et al. The relationship between limb function and radiographic osteoarthrosis in dogs with stifle osteoarthrosis. Vet Surg 2003;32:451–454.

Hoots EA, Petersen SW. Tibial plateau leveling osteotomy and cranial closing wedge ostectomy in a cat with cranial cruciate ligament rupture. J Am Anim Hosp Assoc 2005;41:395–399.

Hurley CR, Hammer DL, Shott S. Progression of radiographic evidence of osteoarthritis following tibial plateau leveling osteotomy in dogs with cranial cruciate ligament rupture: 295 cases (2001–2005). J Am Vet Med Assoc 2007;230:1674–1679.

Jandi AS, Shulman AJ. Incidence of motion loss of the stifle joint in dogs with naturally occurring cranial cruciate ligament rupture surgically treated with tibial plateau leveling osteotomy: Longitudinal clinical study of 412 cases. Vet Surg 2007;36:114–121.

Kergosien DH, Barnhart MD, Kees CE, et al. Radiographic and clinical changes of the tibial tuberosity after tibial plateau leveling osteotomy. Vet Surg 2004;33:468–474.

Kim SE, Pozzi A, Banks SA, et al. Effect of tibial plateau leveling osteotomy on femorotibial contact mechanics and stifle kinematics. Vet Surg 2009;38:23–32.

Kloc PA, Kowaleski MP, Litsky AS, et al. Biomechanical comparison of two alternative tibial plateau leveling osteotomy plates with the original standard in an axially loaded gap model: An in vitro study. Vet Surg 2009;38:40–48.

Kowaleski MP, Apelt D, Mattoon JS, Litsky AS. The effect of tibial plateau leveling osteotomy position on cranial tibial subluxation: An *in vitro* study. Vet Surg 2005;34:332–326.

Leitner M, Pearce SG, Windolf M, et al. Comparison of locking and conventional screws for maintenance of tibial plateau positioning and biomechanical stability after locking tibial plateau leveling osteotomy plate fixation. Vet Surg 2008;37:357–365.

Millis D, Durant A, Headrick J, et al. Long term kinetic and kinematic comparison of cruciate-deficient dogs treated with tibial plateau leveling osteotomy or modified retinacular imbrications technique. Vet Surg 2008;37:E23.

Moeller EM, Cross AR, Rapoff AJ. Change in tibial plateau angle after tibial plateau leveling osteotomy in dogs. Vet Surg 2006;35:460–464.

Monk ML, Preston CA, McGowan CM. Effects of early intensive postoperative physiotherapy on limb function after tibial plateau leveling osteotomy in dogs with deficiency of the cranial cruciate ligament. Am J Vet Res 2006;67:529–536.

Pacchiana PD, Morris E, Gillings SL, et al. Surgical and postoperative complications associated with tibial plateau leveling osteotomy in dogs with cranial cruciate ligament rupture: 397 cases (1998–2001). J Am Vet Med Assoc 2003;222:184–193.

Pozzi A, Kowaleski MP, Apelt D, et al. Effect of medial meniscal release on tibial translation after tibial plateau leveling osteotomy. Vet Surg 2006;35:486–494.

Priddy NH, Tomlinson JL, Dodam JR, Hornbostel JE. Complications with and owner assessment of the outcome of tibial plateau leveling osteotomy for treatment of cranial cruciate ligament rupture in dogs: 193 cases (1997–2001). J Am Vet Med Assoc 2003;222:1726–1732.

Ray WM, Gustafson SB, Huber MJ. Tibial plateau leveling osteotomy in a llama with a ruptured cranial cruciate ligament. J Am Vet Med Assoc 2004;225:1739–1742.

Reif U, Hulse DA, Hauptman JG. Effect of tibial plateau leveling on stability of the canine cranial cruciate-deficient stifle joint: An in vitro study. Vet Surg 2002;31:147–154.

Reif U, Dejardin LM, Probst CW, et al. Influence of limb positioning and measurement method on the magnitude of the tibial plateau angle. Vet Surg 2004;33:368–375.

Robinson DA, Mason DR, Evans R, Conzemius MG. The effect of tibial plateau angle on ground reaction forces 4–17 months after tibial plateau leveling osteotomy in Labrador retrievers. Vet Surg 2006;35:294–299.

Schmerbach KI, Boeltzig CK, Reif U, et al. In vitro comparison of tibial plateau leveling osteotomy with and without use of a tibial plateau leveling jig. Vet Surg 2007;36:156–163.

Slocum B, Slocum TD. Tibial plateau leveling osteotomy for repair of cranial cruciate ligament rupture in the canine. Vet Clin North Am Small Anim Pract 1993;23:777–795.

Stauffer KD, Tuttle TA, Elkins AD, et al. Complications associated with 696 tibial plateau leveling osteotomies (2001–2003). J Am Anim Hosp Assoc 2006;42:44–50.

Talaat MB, Kowaleski MP, Boudrieau RJ. Combination tibial plateau leveling osteotomy and cranial closing wedge osteotomy of the tibia for the treatment of cranial cruciate ligament-deficient stifles with excessive tibial plateau angle. Vet Surg 2006;35:729–739.

Thieman KM, Tomlinson JL, Fox DB, et al. Effect of meniscal release on rate of subsequent meniscal tears and owner-assessed outcome in dogs with cruciate disease treated with tibial plateau leveling osteotomy. Vet Surg 2006;35:705–710.

Tuttle TA, Manley PA. Risk factors associated with fibular fracture after tibial plateau leveling osteotomy. Vet Surg 2009;38:355–360.

Warzee CC, Dejardin LM, Arnoczky SP, Perry RL. Effect of tibial plateau leveling on cranial and caudal tibial thrusts in canine cranial cruciate deficient stifles. Vet Surg 2001;30:278–286.

Waxman AS, Robinson DA, Evans RB, et al. Relationship between objective and subjective assessment of limb function in normal dogs with an experimentally induced lameness. Vet Surg 2008;37:241–246.

Wheeler JL, Cross AR, Gingrich W. In vitro effects of osteotomy angle and osteotomy reduction on tibial angulation and rotation during the tibial plateau-leveling osteotomy procedure. Vet Surg 2003;32:371–377.

Windolf M, Leitner M, Schwieger K, et al. Accuracy of fragment positioning after TPLO and effect on biomechanical stability. Vet Surg 2008;37:366–373.

26 Tibial Tuberosity Advancement

Randy J. Boudrieau

Introduction

Advancement of the tibial tuberosity was first described by Maquet, where the premise of the procedure was that an increase in the efficiency of the quadriceps mechanism would subsequently decrease retropatellar pressure, thus alleviating pain associated with the patellofemoral joint in humans (Maquet 1976). Other possible effects on the biomechanics of the tibiofemoral joint included evidence that a variable tibiofemoral shear force was present in the knee joint, which was either anteriorly or posteriorly directed depending on the angle of knee joint extension or flexion (and patellar tendon angle [PTA]), respectively (Nisell 1985), and that the magnitude and direction of the tibiofemoral shear force were determined by the PTA (Nisell et al. 1986; Figure 26.1). An increase in translational knee joint instability has been demonstrated by a number of biomechanical studies in humans as a result of variations in tibial plateau slope (TPS; Giffin et al. 2004), axial loading (Li et al. 1998), and knee flexion angle (Nisell et al. 1989). A recent three-dimensional (3-D) nonlinear

finite element model of the human knee evaluating the Maquet procedure found it to be effective in decreasing the femorotibial contact forces in stifle joint extension in addition to decreasing retropatellar pressure (Shirazi-Adl & Mesfar 2007). Similarly, changes in tibiofemoral shear forces were observed depending on the knee flexion angle, which placed more or less stress on the anterior and posterior cruciate ligaments depending on the amount of tibial tuberosity advancement (Shirazi-Adl & Mesfar 2007). A relationship between tibial tuberosity advancement, knee joint flexion/extension, tibiofemoral shear force, retropatellar pressure (including femorotibial contact forces), and patellar tendon force has been suggested and supported by a variety of experimental studies (Maquet 1976; Nakamura et al. 1985; Nisell 1985; Nisell et al. 1986; Nisell et al. 1989; Li et al. 1998; Giffin et al. 2004; Shirazi-Adl & Mesfar 2007).

Stifle biomechanics

Based on the data published by Maquet and Nisell, Montavon and Tepic proposed that a similar situation existed in the dog, and that tibial tuberosity advancement (TTA) would neutralize cranial tibiofemoral shear force in a cranial cruciate ligament (CrCL)-deficient stifle joint in the dog (Maquet

---

Advances in the Canine Cranial Cruciate Ligament,
Edited by Peter Muir, © 2010 ACVS Foundation, This Work is a co-publication between the American College of Veterinary Surgeons Foundation and Wiley-Blackwell.

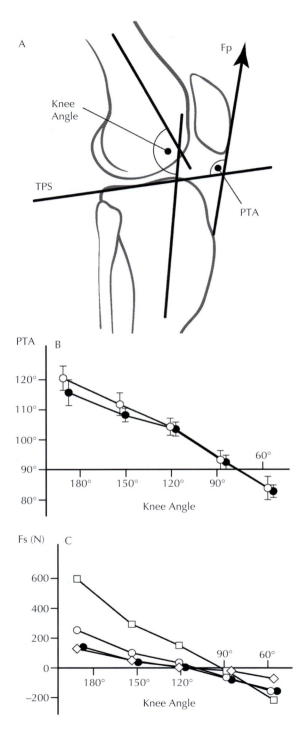

1976; Nisell et al. 1986; Montavon et al. 2002; Tepic et al. 2002). A PTA of 90° was suggested as the crossover point at 135° of stifle joint extension, thus the TTA technique was developed to achieve this PTA (Figure 26.2). These assumptions have since been validated in four experimental models (Apelt et al. 2007; Miller et al. 2007; Kipfer et al. 2008; Hoffmann et al. 2009). These models were used to evaluate cranial tibiofemoral shear force either indirectly with cranial tibial subluxation (Apelt et al. 2007; Miller et al. 2007; Kipfer et al. 2008) or directly with cranial tibial thrust under varying loading conditions (Hoffmann et al. 2009) (Figure 26.3).

A 3-D nonlinear joint finite element model reconstruction, which was based on a cadaver knee joint of a human, was used to evaluate the reduction in retropatellar pressure and patellar tendon force. The analysis confirmed not only a decrease in patellofemoral contact forces after TTA, but also femorotibial contact forces with stifle joint extension (Shirazi-Adl & Mesfar 2007). A decrease in retropatellar pressure after TTA has recently been demonstrated experimentally in the dog (Hoffmann et al. 2009). Theoretically, this diminished force can protect the articular cartilage of both the patella and the femur from subsequent damage. Femorotibial contact pressure and loca-

Figure 26.1 (A) Anatomic landmarks of the radiographic and morphologic studies of the knee. The patellar tendon force (Fp) is shown, which is approximately of the same magnitude and direction as that of the tibiofemoral compressive force, and results in a variable amount of tibiofemoral shear force depending on the knee flexion angle and tibial plateau slope (TPS), both of which influence the patellar tendon angle (PTA). (B) The relationship between the PTA (y-axis) and knee flexion angle (x-axis); note that the PTA = 90° at a knee flexion angle of ~100°; the 95% confidence intervals of the means are shown for men (filled circles) and women (open circles). (C) Tibiofemoral shear force (Fs; y-axis) during isometric knee extension at various knee flexion angles (x-axis) for men (filled circle) and women (unfilled symbols). During knee extension, application of posteriorly directed external forces of 100 N (squares and circles) and 50 N (diamonds) against the anterior tibia at 0.4, 0.2, and 0.2 m distal to the tibial plateau, respectively. Positive values (Fs) indicate that the tibia tends to slide anteriorly in relationship to the femur (anterior tibiofemoral shear). Reproduced and modified from Nisell (1985), published by Taylor & Francis.

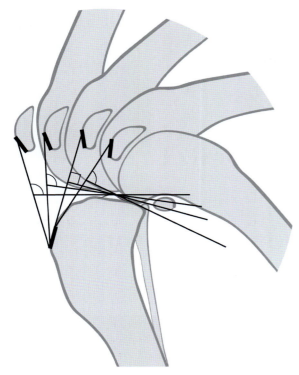

Figure 26.2 Schematic representation of stifle joint flexion with respect to PTA. In full extension, the PTA is >90°, and in full flexion the PTA is <90°. There is a point at which the PTA is 90°, which is termed the "crossover" point (see Figure 26.1C, Fs = 0.0). At this point, there is neither cranial nor caudal tibiofemoral shear force present. The premise of the tibial tuberosity advancement (TTA), according to Tepic, is to alter the geometry of the proximal tibia such that the PTA is maintained at ≤90° throughout the stifle joint range-of-motion during weight-bearing; the TTA will change the PTA and move the crossover point such that Fs = 0.0 N when PTA = 90° when the stifle joint is in full extension. Further stifle joint flexion ensures that Fs always is ≤0.0 N and PTA ≤90°. The PTA is thus maintained at ≤90° throughout the stifle joint range-of-motion during weight-bearing. Compare with Figure 26.5. Reproduced from Boudrieau (2009), with permission from Wiley-Blackwell.

tion have been evaluated *in vitro* using an experimental model of a CrCL-deficient stifle joint, which demonstrated an ~40% decrease in contact area with an associated 100% increase in peak pressure; furthermore, the positioning of the peak pressure was found to shift caudally (Kim et al. 2009). The TTA appeared to restore the normal femorotibial contact and pressure (Kim et al. 2009), which may spare the meniscus from risk of trauma after TTA (Figure 26.4). The work of Kim et al. (2009) also suggested that because TTA did not change the geometry of the joint, and the pressure distributions essentially remained unchanged, there may be less development of osteoarthritis over time. All of these findings could support clinical studies that implied an absence of problems with the patellar tendon and the joint surfaces after TTA (Hoffmann et al. 2006; Lafaver et al. 2007; Stein & Schmoekel 2008; Kim et al. 2009).

As the resultant PTA is crucial to the determination of the amount of TTA, there has been a suggestion that the PTA is more accurately determined by the method of the common tangent (PTA^{CT}) (Dennler et al. 2006; Schwandt et al. 2006; Boudrieau 2009) as opposed to the method using the tibial plateau angle (PTA^{TPA}) (Boudrieau 2009; Hoffmann et al. 2009). The former method has been proposed to be clinically more accurate as it takes into account the anatomic relationship between the femoral condyles and tibial plateau, as opposed to a static relationship of the tibial plateau with the patellar tendon (Boudrieau 2009; Figure 26.5). Based on these suppositions, this method has been recommended for clinical use (2007 Veterinary Symposium—The Surgical Summit; Pre-Symposium Laboratories: TTA Laboratory; Chicago, IL). Support for this concept has been demonstrated experimentally whereby less variability was observed with PTA^{CT} versus PTA^{TPA} when compared to the target PTA of 90° (Hoffmann et al. 2009).

TTA case selection

Several factors specific to the anatomic configuration of the limb should be considered before selection of this surgical technique (Boudrieau 2009).

Low versus high patellar tendon insertion point

The tibial tuberosity may be at greater risk for possible fracture with the TTA in cases with a low

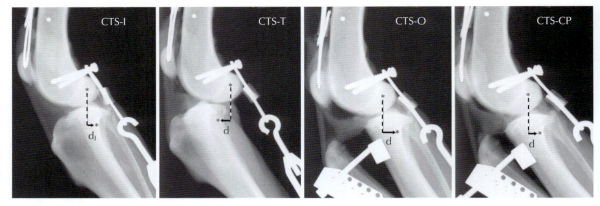

Figure 26.3 Lateral radiographic images of cranial tibial subluxation (CTS) in a loaded stifle joint within an experimental limb press model: before cranial cruciate ligament (CrCL) transection (CTS-I), after CrCL transection (CTS-T), post-tibial tuberosity advancement after maximal tibial tuberosity advancement (CTS-O), and at critical point tibial tuberosity advancement (CTS-CP) (The critical point for the tibial tuberosity advancement distance in this model was defined as the position one revolution before stifle joint instability occurred). The CTS was defined as "d" in each figure: CTS-T/CTS-O/CTS-CP = d–d_I, where d_I (arrow) is the horizontal distance between the tibial marker (*) and the vertical passing through the femoral marker (dotted line) in the intact CrCL (the intact CrCL was the reference position), and d is the same horizontal distance (arrows) for each respective position (CTS-T, CTS-O, and CTS-CP). In this specimen, CTS-T was positive, CTS-O was negative, and CTS-CP was slightly negative. Reproduced from Apelt et al. (2007), with permission from Wiley-Blackwell.

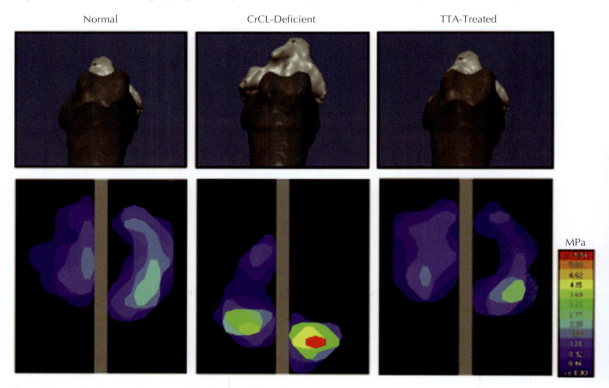

Figure 26.4 Axial view of bone models depicting three-dimensional poses of normal, cranial cruciate ligament-deficient (CrCL-deficient), and tibial tuberosity advancement (TTA-treated stifles), with corresponding contact maps representative of each testing condition. The tibia (light gray) is cranially displaced and internally rotated relative to the femur (dark gray) after CrCL transection; femorotibial pose of normal and TTA-treated stifles are similar. CrCL transection resulted in caudal shift, reduced area, and increased pressure of femorotibial contact; TTA contact patterns are similar to normal. Left: lateral; top: cranial. Reproduced from Kim et al. (2009), with permission from Wiley-Blackwell.

Tibial Tuberosity Advancement

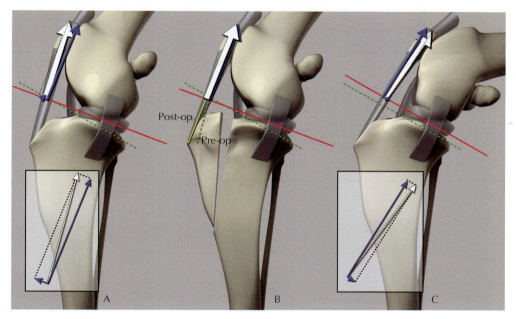

Figure 26.5 Schematic representation of the tibiofemoral forces in the stifle joint, according to Tepic, before (A) and after (B) tibial tuberosity advancement (TTA). The resultant compressive force (large white arrows) across the stifle joint is parallel to the patellar tendon. Using the common tangent at the tibiofemoral contact point as the baseline (solid red line), whereby the femur can move along this surface if the cranial cruciate ligament (CrCL) is deficient, the resultant force can be broken down into its two orthogonal components (small blue arrows), one perpendicular and one parallel to the tibial plateau. The latter represents the tibiofemoral shear force. If the angle of the tibial tuberosity is advanced cranially until the patellar tendon angle (PTA) is reduced to 90°, the tibiofemoral shear force vector becomes zero, and the joint compressive force and resultant force become one and the same. Notice that the cranial tibiofemoral shear force is smaller than that depicted with the PTA using the tibial plateau slope (TPS), which is indicated by the green dotted line. Notice that the common tangent and TPS are similar in stifle joint flexion (C). Insets clarify the force vectors depicted on the schematic bone models. Compare with Figure 26.2. Reproduced from Boudrieau (2009), with permission from Wiley-Blackwell.

patellar tendon insertion point, as a smaller plate is applied to the tibial crest and the usual position of the interspersed cage is above the most proximal position of the plate with little bone present for support (interestingly, this conformation may be better suited for a tibial plateau leveling osteotomy (TPLO) as there is increased buttress support of the tibial tuberosity with greater amounts of tibial plateau rotation). In dogs with a high insertion point, the TTA is preferable, as a larger TTA plate can be applied to the tibial crest, and the interspersed cage that is placed within the gap remains buttressed with adequate bone. Finally, the larger plate better disperses all the forces to the tibial crest (Figure 26.6). There are, however, no experimental or clinical studies reported that support these assumptions.

Excessive tibial plateau angle

Cases where there is excessive tibial plateau angle are not conducive to TTA. The target PTA is 90°, but achieving this angle in such cases would likely require advancement beyond that obtained with the currently available implants (the maximal cage width for the osteotomy gap is 15 mm). Perhaps more importantly, there is a conformational deformity of the joint with excessive tibial plateau angle that places it in a relative angle of hyperextension despite the limb itself not being in the extended position (Figure 26.7). The TTA does not address this malformation. The maximal tibial plateau angle to perform a TTA has yet to be determined. No data have been published regarding the range of tibial plateau angles in dogs with

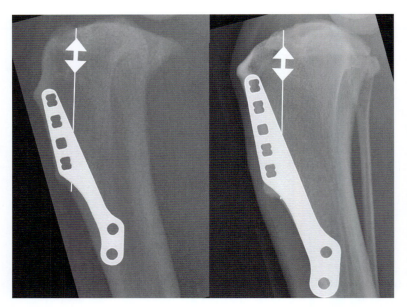

Figure 26.6 Lateral radiographs of the stifle joint demonstrating the variation between the insertion points of the patellar tendon into the tibial tuberosity. (A) Tibial tuberosity with a low insertion point, and (B) tibial tuberosity with a high insertion point. A smaller plate must be applied when a shorter tibial tuberosity distance is available. The result is an increase in the forces at each tine of the fork; additionally, the overall plate length is shortened, potentially creating a stress riser at the distal end of the osteotomy and the screws placed to secure the distal end of the plate (recall that the tuberosity shifts proximally with advancement in order to maintain patellar position). Furthermore, cage position (double-headed arrow) provides greater buttress support of the tuberosity, and also buttresses the proximal attachment of the plate when a high insertion point is present.

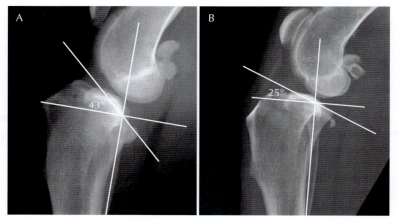

Figure 26.7 Lateral stifle joint radiographs demonstrating differences in the anatomic shape of the proximal tibia such that the tibial plateau angle (TPA) is either considered excessive (A) at 43° or within normal limits (B) at 25°. This conformational deformity of the stifle joint angle in part (A) places the joint in a relatively hyperextended position (compare with part (B)). Advancing the tibial tuberosity does not correct this hyperextension as the TPA remains unaltered. Reproduced from Boudrieau (2009), with permission from Wiley-Blackwell.

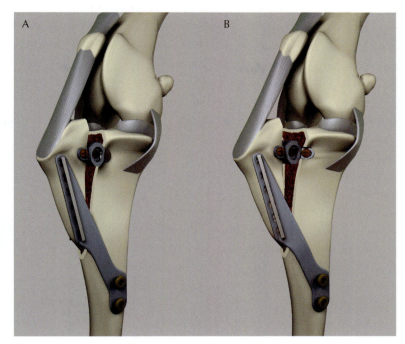

Figure 26.8 Craniomedial view of the proximal tibia after tibial tuberosity transposition (TTA) performed routinely (A) and after simultaneous lateral transposition (B) with the advancement (for a medial patellar luxation). Notice that the caudal cage ear has been recessed slightly into the caudal (tibial) bone fragment (this is done by bending this ear at ~45° without removing a large amount of bone); the plate also is contoured such that it meets the tuberosity more laterally. (Alternatively, or additionally, the cranial cage ear may be elevated off of the bone (tuberosity) by placing 1–2 small metal washers under this ear).

TTA, although it has been reported that successful procedures have been performed in dogs with a TPS of ~30° and anecdotally proposed that angles >30° probably are not well suited for a TTA (2007 Veterinary Symposium—The Surgical Summit; Pre-Symposium Laboratories: TTA Laboratory, Chicago, IL).

Angular and torsional limb deformities

Angular and torsional limb deformities may be treated with TTA; however, a separate osteotomy is required for correction of any tibial varus, valgus, or torsion. The disadvantage of performing a separate osteotomy is that the medial side of the bone already has a plate positioned for the TTA in the proximal one-third of the medial tibial surface, which will interfere with subsequent additional medial plate fixation. Although a standard plate could be applied over the thin TTA plate, this is far from ideal and generally not recommended. Therefore, a TTA generally is not recommended under these circumstances.

Patellar luxation

Patellar luxation requiring tibial tuberosity transposition may be very well suited for a TTA, as any desired transposition may be simultaneously performed with the advancement. In this instance, the TTA plate is slightly overbent to conform to the new laterally (or medially) transposed tibial crest. The alteration in the surgical technique occurs with cage application. For example, in a medial patellar luxation, where the tibial crest is moved laterally, either the caudal "ear" of the cage is recessed into the proximal tibia, or the cranial "ear" of the cage is elevated above the surface of the tibial tuberosity by interposing some washers, or both (Figure 26.8). Ancillary fixation generally is unnecessary. This technique has been briefly described (2007 Veterinary Symposium—The Sur-

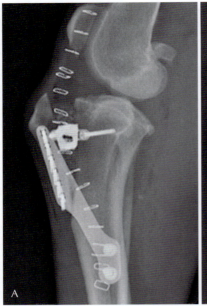
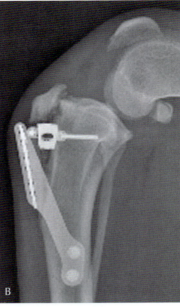

Figure 26.9 Mediolateral radiographs of a 2.5-year-old, male neutered Labrador retriever. (A) Immediately postoperatively a 9-mm cage is observed 1.2 cm distally within the osteotomy gap along the tibia (with 2.3 cm of tibial tuberosity proximal to the cage). The granular material observed within and below the cage is the allograft of corticocancellous chips. (B) At 8 weeks postoperatively, the tibial tuberosity has fractured just above the cage. Reproduced from Burns and Boudrieau (2008), with permission from Schattauer.

gical Summit; Pre-Symposium Laboratories: TTA Laboratory, Chicago, IL; Boudrieau 2005), and an abstract has been presented on a series of cases (Fitzpatrick et al. 2007).

Patient size

TTA has been performed in dogs as small as 5 kg and as large as 92 kg (Hoffmann et al. 2006; Lafaver et al. 2007). Size limitation is dependent on the availability of appropriately sized implants (two- to eight-hole plates, and 3- to 15-mm cage widths—Kyon, Zürich, Switzerland). The implants are produced in a variety of sizes such that they can be used in almost any sized dog. In some instances, in the very large breeds of dogs, a limitation of the TTA may be the large distance (>15 mm) of TTA that is required (not necessarily the heavier dogs, but rather the taller dogs, e.g., Great Danes) (Burns & Boudrieau 2008). The widest cage currently available to support the osteotomy gap is 15-mm, which only became available in early 2009 (before this time a 12-mm cage was the widest available). While the cage can be moved further distally to increase the width of the gap, this must be done judiciously, as the tibial tuberosity above the cage may become prone to fracture because of a large stress riser created above the cage, which could result in fracture of the tuberosity at that level (Burns & Boudrieau 2008; Figure 26.9). One alternative described has been to buttress the tibial tuberosity above the cage with a block of cancellous bone allograft; however, adding this graft adds a considerable additional expense to the procedure (Burns & Boudrieau 2008).

Outcome and complications

The TTA has been in general use for <6 years; as such, it can be considered a relatively new procedure. There are anecdotal reports of good to excellent results, and some early clinical results published (Hoffmann et al. 2006; Lafaver et al. 2007; Stein et al. 2008). These early clinical results are the experiences of a number of surgeons and, as such, are influenced by the respective learning curves for these individuals. These three studies

(249 total cases) report an overall complication rate of 20.0%–59.0% in CrCL-deficient stifle joints stabilized using the TTA (Hoffmann et al. 2006; Lafaver et al. 2007; Stein et al. 2008). A number of minor complications were reported in these studies, including postoperative swelling and bruising, which accounted for 19.3%–21.0% of these complications (Hoffmann et al. 2006; Lafaver et al. 2007). The major complications accounted for 12.3%–38.0% (Hoffmann et al. 2006; Lafaver et al. 2007; Stein et al. 2008). A reoperation rate of 11.3%–14.0% was reported (Lafaver et al. 2007; Stein et al. 2008). Combining the data, these complications, in order of frequency, were as follows: meniscal tears (7.6%, or 16.5% of the intact menisci), infection (4.0%), medial patellar luxation (0.4%), tibial fractures (0.08%), and catastrophic implant failure (0.08%; Hoffmann et al. 2006; Lafaver et al. 2007; Stein et al. 2008). The primary discrepancies between these reports were the fre-

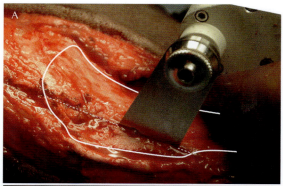

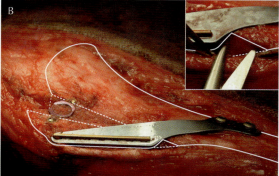

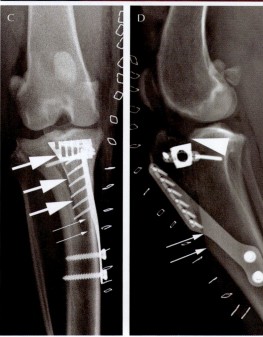

Figure 26.10 Intraoperative photographs (A,B) and postoperative radiographs (C,D) illustrating key points in appropriate surgical technique (in both (A) and (B), the dog is in dorsal recumbency and the right pelvic limb is rotated to align the tibia parallel to the floor [for orientation, both photographs show the outline of the medial tibial surface]). (A) An osteotomy is performed parallel to the frontal plane extending from the distal extent of the tibial crest to a point immediately cranial to the medial meniscus (and cranial to the long digital extensor tendon). (B) Completed appearance of the tibial tuberosity advancement, a seven-hole plate and a 12-mm cage have been applied; the fracture gap has been filled with a corticocancellous autograft. Inset: notice the slight proximal displacement of the tibial crest to ensure a center of rotation of the patellar tendon's attachment to the tibial tuberosity based at the patella. Craniocaudal (C) and lateral (D) postoperative radiographs of a completed tibial tuberosity advancement immediately postoperatively. The slight proximal shift of the tibial crest can be seen (small arrows, compare with (B)). Notice that the plate is parallel to the cranial tibial margin of the tibial crest. The lateral border of the osteotomized tibial crest can also be seen; notice that the lateral margin of the cage follows the contour of the bone at this level (large arrows). The cage is placed 2–3 mm below the proximal extent of the tibia (arrowhead). Also notice that the caudal extent of the osteotomy at the level of the tibial joint surface: immediately cranial to the medial meniscus (this position is also cranial to the long digital extensor tendon laterally). Reproduced from Lafaver et al. (2007), with permission from Wiley-Blackwell.

quency of meniscal tears (16%–21.7%; Lafaver et al. 2007; Stein et al. 2008) and technical failures (22%; Hoffmann et al. 2006).

Radiographic healing was reported to be partially complete by ~7–8 weeks postoperatively and fully complete as early as 8–10 weeks postoperatively in one report (Hoffmann et al. 2006), bridging bone at one site in >94% of the cases (Stein et al. 2008), and at a mean of 9.4 weeks postoperatively in the other report (Lafaver et al. 2007). Overall function (outcome and lameness) of the dogs postoperatively was reported to be good to excellent in >90% of the dogs (Hoffmann et al. 2006; Lafaver et al. 2007; Stein et al. 2008).

In all studies, two major points are discussed: early technical errors with the procedure and meniscal injury (Hoffmann et al. 2006; Lafaver et al. 2007; Stein et al. 2008). Elimination of technical errors, which were associated with the early learning curve in performing this surgical procedure, would have significantly reduced the number of major complications; attention to the technical details of the procedure is paramount (Figure 26.10). The issue with the meniscus is more confounding, as there is much controversy as to the best method of approach: meniscal release or no meniscal release. The TTA was originally performed without a meniscal release, but it appears that the majority of complications occurring postoperatively in two of the studies were because of meniscal tears, either those that may have been missed at the time of the original surgery or those that subsequently occurred (Lafaver et al. 2007; Stein et al. 2008). A suggestion was made that meniscal release may eliminate this issue (Lafaver et al. 2007). Furthermore, it was reported that dogs with/without meniscal debridement (meniscal tears or not) were not different based on clinical outcome (Stein et al. 2008). Therefore, it was suggested a meniscal release might be appropriate as minimal morbidity could be expected; however, this supposition needs to be further evaluated with long-term follow-up (Stein et al. 2008).

Given the limited information in TTA biomechanics, debate remains as to whether or not to perform a medial meniscal release. It appears there are two opposing opinions regarding the necessity of meniscal release at this time with TTA. Further discussion of meniscal release is presented in Chapters 31 and 32.

Conclusion

Currently, there is no documented evidence (published scientific reports) of any superiority to any one of the surgical techniques in the dog for stifle stabilization in dogs with CrCL rupture over the long term, and the specific technique chosen primarily depends on individual surgeon preference (Leighton 1999). However, there has been much anecdotal evidence that there may be a quicker recovery (return to full function) in a shorter period with the TTA (similar to and perhaps also quicker than the TPLO). The rapid return to function is one of the primary reasons that this technique is more frequently performed. In addition, there is anecdotal evidence from owners (again not scientific data) that dogs with this technique (and also the TPLO) do better, interpreted as returning to work (hunting, field trials), than dogs with either the extra-articular, for example, lateral suture/imbrication, and intra-articular techniques, for example, over-the-top. These supposed benefits of the TTA over the other surgical techniques need to be documented long term.

References

Apelt D, Kowaleski M, Boudrieau RJ. Effect of tibial tuberosity advancement on cranial tibial subluxation in canine cranial cruciate-deficient stifle joints: An in vitro experimental study. Vet Surg 2007;36:170–177.

Boudrieau RJ. Tibial tuberosity advancement (TTA): Clinical results. *Proceedings of the ACVS Veterinary Symposium.* San Diego, CA, 2005, pp. 443–445.

Boudrieau RJ. Tibial plateau leveling osteotomy or tibial tuberosity advancement? Vet Surg 2009;38:1–22.

Burns CG, Boudrieau RJ. Modified tibial tuberosity advancement procedure with tibial tuberosity advancement in excess of 12 mm in four large breed dogs with cranial cruciate ligament-deficient joints. Vet Comp Orthop Traumatol 2008;21:250–255.

Dennler R, Kipfer NM, Tepic S, et al. Inclination of the patellar ligament in relation to flexion angle in stifle joints of dogs without degenerative joint disease. Am J Vet Res 2006;67:1849–1854.

Fitzpatrick N, Yeadon R, Kowaleski M. Tibial tuberosity transposition-advancement for treatment of medial patellar luxation and concomitant cranial cruciate ligament disease in the dog. *Proceedings of the 34th Annual Conference of the Veterinary Orthopedic Society.* Sun Valley, ID, 2007, p. 67.

Giffin JR, Vogrin TM, Zantop T, et al. Effects of increasing tibial slope on the biomechanics of the knee. Am J Sports Med 2004;32:376–382.

Hoffmann DE, Miller JM, Ober CP, et al. Tibial tuberosity advancement in 65 canine stifles. Vet Comp Orthop Traumatol 2006;19:219–227.

Hoffmann DE, Kowaleski MP, Johnson KA, et al. *In vitro* biomechanical evaluation of the canine CrCL deficient stifle with varying angles of stifle joint flexion and axial loads after TTA. *Proceedings of the 18th Annual Scientific Meeting of the European College of Veterinary Surgeons*. Nantes, France, 2009, pp. 557–559.

Kim SE, Pozzi A, Banks SA, et al. Effect of tibial tuberosity advancement on femorotibial contact mechanics and stifle kinematics. Vet Surg 2009;38:33–39.

Kipfer NM, Damur DM, Guerrero T, et al. Effect of tibial tuberosity advancement on femorotibial shear in cranial cruciate-deficient stifles: An *in vitro* study. Vet Comp Orthop Traumatol 2008;21:385–390.

Lafaver S, Miller NA, Stubbs WP, et al. Tibial tuberosity advancement for stabilization of the canine cranial cruciate ligament-deficient stifle joint: Surgical technique, early results and complication in 101 dogs. Vet Surg 2007;36:573–586.

Leighton RL. Letter to the Editor. Preferred method of repair of cranial cruciate ligament rupture in dogs: A survey of ACVS diplomates specializing in canine orthopedics. Vet Surg 1999;28:194.

Li G, Rudy TW, Allen C, et al. Effect of combined axial compressive and anterior tibial loads on in situ forces in the anterior cruciate ligament: A porcine model. J Orthop Res 1998;16:122–127.

Maquet P. Tibial tuberosity advancement. Clin Orthop Rel Res 1976;115:225–230.

Miller JM, Shires PK, Lanz OI, et al. Effect of 9 mm tibial tuberosity advancement on cranial tibial translation in the canine cranial cruciate ligament-deficient stifle. Vet Surg 2007;36:335–340.

Montavon PM, Damur DM, Tepic S. Advancement of the tibial tuberosity for the treatment of cranial cruciate deficient canine stifle. *Proceedings of the 1st World Orthopaedic Veterinary Congress*. Munich, Germany, 2002, p. 152.

Nakamura N, Ellis M, Seedhom BB. Advancement of the tibial tuberosity: A biomechanical study. J Bone Joint Surg Br 1985;67:255–260.

Nisell R. Mechanics of the knee. A study of joint and muscle load with clinical applications. Acta Orthop Scand Supp 1985;56:3–42.

Nisell R, Németh G, Ohlsén H. Joint forces in the extension of the knee: Analysis of a mechanical model. Acta Orthop Scand 1986;57:41–46.

Nisell R, Ericson MO, Németh G, Ekholm J. Tibiofemoral joint forces during isokinetic knee extension. Am J Sports Med 1989;17:49–54.

Schwandt CS, Bohorquez-Vanelli A, Tepic S, et al. Angle between the patellar ligament and the tibial plateau in dogs with partial rupture of the cranial cruciate ligament. Am J Vet Res 2006;67:1855–1860.

Shirazi-Adl A, Mesfar W. Effect of tibial tubercle elevation on biomechanics of the entire knee joint under muscle loads. Clin Biomech 2007;22:344–351.

Stein S, Schmoekel H. Short-term and eight to 12 months results of a tibial tuberosity advancement as treatment of canine cranial cruciate ligament damage. J Small Anim Pract 2008;49:398–404.

Tepic S, Damur D, Montavon PM. Biomechanics of the stifle joint. *Proceedings of the 1st World Orthopaedic Veterinary Congress*. Munich, Germany, 2002, pp. 189–190.

27 Intra-articular Stabilization

Paul A. Manley

Introduction

The idea of surgical treatment of a torn cruciate ligament has intrigued surgeons for nearly a century. Numerous reports in the human and veterinary literature have detailed techniques to either primarily repair or replace the torn cranial cruciate ligament (CrCL). This chapter will focus on three distinct areas of intra-articular stabilization and will present historic and current information on techniques, results of clinical and experimental work, and future considerations. First, intra-articular primary ligament repair will be discussed, then intra-articular ligament replacement, and finally intra-articular augmentation and repair.

Intra-articular repair

Healing of injured ligaments that are extra-articular occurs as for most connective tissue with formation and organization of a hematoma at the site of injury, recruitment of inflammatory cells to remove necrotic tissue, recruitment of fibroblasts and stem cells to reorganize the granulation tissue into fibrous tissue, and finally maturation of the scar and realignment of collagen fibers to provide strength and durability of the repaired tissue (Bray et al. 1996; Fu et al. 1999).

A major factor that complicates healing of the CrCL is its biological environment. Unlike extra-articular ligaments, the CrCL is intra-articular and completely ensheathed by a fold of synovial membrane rendering it extrasynovial. This synovial sheath is richly endowed with vessels that play a part in the nutritional support of the ligament (Arnoczky & Marshall 1981). Small gaps in the synovial covering may allow joint fluid access to the ligament and may serve as a secondary pathway for nutritional support (Kobayashi et al. 2006). Any injury to the CrCL also injures the synovial sheath and its vessels, resulting in hemorrhage, but the blood dissipates throughout the joint and does not stay at the site of injury to form an organized hematoma. The constant flow of the synovial fluid and the presence of inflammatory mediators and circulating inflammatory proteins prevent the formation of a hematoma necessary for normal ligament repair (Fu et al. 1999; Murray et al. 2006). Experimentally in dogs, acute transections of the CrCL have demonstrated some ability to heal if the ends of the ligaments were surgically apposed and the stifle was immobilized, but the mechanical strength of the liga-

Advances in the Canine Cranial Cruciate Ligament, Edited by Peter Muir, © 2010 ACVS Foundation, This Work is a co-publication between the American College of Veterinary Surgeons Foundation and Wiley-Blackwell.

ment did not reach that of control ligaments, even after 10 weeks of immobilization (O'Donoghue et al. 1966).

Additional factors complicating healing of the CrCL are the constant mechanical load applied to the ligament during healing, the long time required for healing of any ligament tissue, and the inability to protect the healing process for a sufficient time to allow maturation of the healing scar (O'Donoghue et al 1966). A central defect model of CrCL injury was developed to evaluate healing of the ligament without destabilizing it. In this model, a small (3.5 mm) incision was made in the central portion of the canine CrCL leaving the peripheral bands of the ligament intact to provide intrinsic stability (Spindler et al. 2006). The ligament showed minimal capacity to heal until a collagen–platelet-rich plasma scaffold was placed into the defect. This allowed formation and organization of a fibrin clot, and at 6 weeks there was histologic evidence of ligament healing (Murray et al. 2006).

Failure of the CrCL to heal is based on its unique extrasynovial and intra-articular environment, failure of a fibrin clot formation, premature loss of the fibrin clot, and the mechanical stresses on the ligament that are difficult to neutralize (Murray et al. 2007). Future studies regarding the capacity of CrCL injuries to be primarily repaired will have to address these issues.

Intra-articular ligament replacement

The CrCL is a not just a simple longitudinal band, but rather a ligament consisting of twisting bundles of collagen arranged into two physiologic components (Arnoczky 1983). The craniomedial portion forms a band that twists almost 90° from its attachment on the femur to its attachment on the tibia and remains tight in both flexion and extension, whereas the caudolateral portion forms the bulk of the ligament, but is only tight when the stifle is in extension (Arnoczky & Marshall 1977). Additionally, the CrCL has a broad fan-like attachment to the medial aspect of the lateral femoral condyle and another broad attachment on the craniomedial intercondylar area of the tibia (Arnoczky 1983; de Rooster et al. 2006). The anatomic configuration of the CrCL and its fan-like attachments to bone make it challenging to replicate with any type of intra-articular graft. Many biologic and prosthetic grafts have been described, but premature failure of the graft has often been attributed more to the failure to recreate the mechanical environment than to the inherent strength of the graft.

Autografts

As early as 1917, Hey Groves utilized an iliotibial band to replace a torn anterior cruciate ligament in a human patient. It was not until 1952 that Paatsama reported the use of fascia lata as a replacement for the CrCL in dogs (Figure 27.1; Knecht 1976; Burnett & Fowler 1985). Paatsama's technique was a modification of the 1917 Hey Groves technique in which a lateral fascial strip was harvested from the lateral thigh of a dog and passed through tunnels drilled in the femur and tibia to replicate the position of the original CrCL. The free end of the strip was either tightened and sutured to the patellar tendon or passed through a hole in the tibial tuberosity to the lateral side of the tibia and sutured to the fascia (Knecht 1976). Modifications of the fascia lata technique were reported by Singleton in 1957, Titemeyer and Brinker in 1958, Rudy in 1974, and Hulse in 1980 (Knecht 1976; Hulse et al. 1980).

Other tissue autografts have been reported in dogs including skin, the tendon of the peroneus longus, the flexor digitalis pedis longus, the long digital extensor, the central and medial aspect of the patellar tendon, and a semitendinosus–gracilis combination (Chiroff 1975; Knecht 1976; Arnoczky et al. 1979a; Lopez et al. 2003). The patellar tendon autograft was first reported in dogs by Dueland in 1966 and was modified from the bone–patellar tendon–bone graft utilized in human patients and reported by Campbell in 1936 (Dueland 1966; Burnett & Fowler 1985). Dueland utilized the central third of the patellar tendon with a wedge of patella (Figure 27.2). The proximal end of the graft with the bone wedge was passed through a tunnel in the femur proximally and sutured to the gastrocnemius. Modifications of the patellar tendon graft were reported by Arnoczky in 1979 where the graft was created from the medial one-third of the patellar tendon and fascia lata and

Intra-articular Stabilization   191

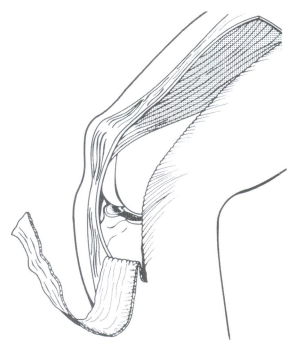

Figure 27.1 Line drawing of the surgical procedure for creation of a fascia lata autograft. The graft has been reflected distally before passing through the stifle joint. The joint capsule is not shown. Reproduced from Shires et al. (1984), with permission from the American Animal Hospital Association.

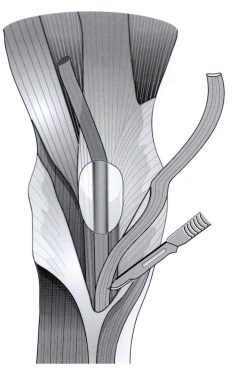

Figure 27.2 The patellar tendon autograft can be collected from the central third of the patellar tendon and patellar bone for subsequent bone-to-bone stabilization using a distal femoral bone tunnel (Dueland 1966). Modifications of the patellar tendon autograft include collection of this graft from the medial third of the patellar tendon, the patellar bone, and a strip of fascia lata for over-the-top stabilization. Reproduced and modified from Arnoczky et al. (1979a), with permission from the American Animal Hospital Association. Copyright © Samantha J. Elmhurst at www.livingart.org.uk.

passed over-the-top rather than through a drill hole in the lateral femoral condyle (Arnoczky et al. 1979a). In 1975, an experimental study was performed using the patellar tendon graft to replace the CrCL in dogs. At 8 weeks after surgery, a vascularized synovial sheath covered the graft, but there was histologic evidence of necrosis and hyalinization of the graft, especially in its central third (Chiroff 1975). The grafts appear to be revascularized through the fat pad and caudal soft tissues and not through the attachment sites or bone tunnel (Arnoczky et al. 1979b, 1982). This addressed the importance of preserving soft tissue structures during surgery. Other studies also demonstrated that the graft became revascularized and grossly resembled normal ligament, but in studies as long as 3 years after surgery, the graft did not reach the structural and mechanical integrity of the native CrCL (McFarland et al. 1986; Ng et al. 1995; Fu et al. 1999; Figure 27.3). In a clinical investigation comparing intra-articular stabilization, extra-articular and tibial osteotomy as treatments for CrCL rupture in the dog, none of the techniques resulted in normal return to function at 6 months after surgery. Furthermore, when the techniques were compared at 2 and 6 months after surgery, the intra-articular technique had inferior results compared with the extra-articular and tibial osteotomy techniques (Conzemius et al. 2005). These results should not be surprising considering the failure of intra-articular grafts to regain structural integrity over time (Figure 27.3). This may be due to a combination of biologic and

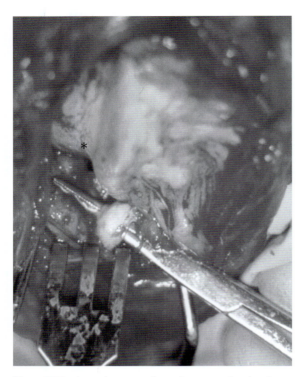

Figure 27.3 Lateral parapatellar arthrotomy of a dog that received an over-the-top fascia lata graft for intra-articular stabilization because of cranial cruciate ligament rupture. Revision surgery was performed because of persistent lameness and joint instability after surgery. During revision surgery, the fascia lata graft (overlying the Kelly forcep) was found to be slack. *Trochlear groove of the distal femur.

mechanical factors that prevent the graft from fully realizing its role as a CrCL substitute. Mechanical failure of the graft may be due to an inability to accurately duplicate the attachment sites and the multiple bundle architecture of the CrCL (Fu et al. 1999). Morbidity of the host graft site has been a problem with both patellar tendon and hamstring grafts in human patients (Fu et al. 1999). A potential solution to the mechanical and morbidity problems might be the use of CrCL allografts.

Allografts

The most commonly described allografts for CrCL replacement are CrCL and Achilles tendon. They can be harvested by sterile technique, but fresh allografts are seldom practical and have been associated with an increased immune-directed inflammatory response. Preservation of the allograft by deep freezing or freeze drying depresses the inflammatory reaction to the graft, but both processes have a negative effect on the mechanical properties of the graft. Alternatively, the allografts can be harvested in a non-sterile environment and secondarily sterilized by either ethylene oxide or gamma irradiation. Ethylene oxide sterilization has a minimal effect on the mechanical properties of the graft, but residues are toxic and potentially carcinogenic. Gamma radiation has adverse effects on the mechanical properties of the graft (Fu et al. 1999). Concerns about the mechanical integrity of the allograft and potential disease transmission from the donor to the recipient have delayed the development of viable allograft replacement of the CrCL.

Prosthetics

Prosthetic ligaments have been described as either primary replacements for CrCL or as augmentation devices for biologic grafts (Knecht 1976; Kdolsky et al. 1997; Mascarenhas & MacDonald 2008). Braided nylon, polytetrafluoroethylene tubes, polytetrafluoroethylene mesh, carbon, and polyethylene terephthalate have all been described and are placed in anatomic positions to replicate the CrCL or less than anatomic positions to augment other grafts (Knecht 1976; Mascarenhas & MacDonald 2008). Although often these synthetic materials have met with acute success, premature wear and deterioration has inevitably led to their failure over time (Mascarenhas & MacDonald 2008). The ideal prosthetic, which has yet to be developed, may be one that acts as a biologic scaffold for ligament differentiation while mechanically protecting the ingrowing tissue until it reaches structural integrity of the CrCL (Murray et al. 2007).

Conclusion

Intra-articular repair of CrCL injuries is the gold standard for treatment in the human patient, but it has not met with enduring success in the canine patient. Premature failure of the grafts, due to mechanical or biologic factors, has relegated this treatment to the back shelf, while other extra-articular treatments have surfaced. Attention to the mechanical nuances of CrCL structure and function may improve the results in canine patients. Additionally, newer biologic scaffolds and disease-modifying therapies may hold promise for intrinsic repair of partially damaged CrCL in dogs.

References

Arnoczky SP. Anatomy of the anterior cruciate ligament. Clin Orthop Relat Res 1983;172:19–25.

Arnoczky, SP, Marshall JL. The cruciate ligaments of the canine stifle: An anatomical and functional analysis. Am J Vet Res 1977;38:1807–1814.

Arnoczky SP, Marshall JL. Pathomechanics of cruciate and meniscal injuries. In: *Pathophysiology of Small Animal Surgery*, Bojrab MJ (ed). Philadelphia: Lea & Febiger, 1981, pp. 590–603.

Arnoczky SP, Tarvin GP, Marshall JL, Saltzman B. The over-the-top procedure: A technique for anterior cruciate ligament substitution in the dog. J Am Anim Hosp Assoc 1979a;15:283–290.

Arnoczky SP, Rubin RM, Marshall JL. Microvasculature of the cruciate ligaments and its response to injury: An experimental study in dogs. J Bone Joint Surg Am 1979b;61:1221–1229.

Arnoczky SP, Tarvin GP, Marshall JL. Anterior cruciate ligament replacement using patellar tendon. J Bone Joint Surg Am 1982;64:217–224.

Bray RC, Rangayyan RN, Frank CB. Normal and healing ligament vascularity: A quantitative histological assessment in the adult rabbit medial collateral ligament. J Anat 1996;188:87–95.

Burnett QM, Fowler PJ. Reconstruction of the anterior cruciate: Historical review. Orthop Clin North Am 1985;16:143–157.

Chiroff RT. Experimental replacement of the anterior cruciate ligament. J Bone Joint Surg Am 1975;57:1124–1127.

Conzemius MG, Evans RB, Besancon MF, et al. Effect of surgical technique on limb function after surgery for rupture of the cranial cruciate ligament in dogs. J Am Vet Med Assoc 2005;226:232–236.

de Rooster H, de Bruin T, van Bree H. Morphologic and functional features of the canine cruciate ligaments. Vet Surg 2006;35:769–780.

Dueland TR. A recent technique for reconstruction of the anterior cruciate ligament. Anim Hosp 1966; 2:1–5.

Fu FH, Bennett CH, Latterman C, Ma CB. Current trends in anterior cruciate ligament reconstruction. Part 1: Biology and biomechanics of reconstruction. Am J Sports Med 1999;27:821–830.

Hulse DA, Michaelson F, Johnson C, et al. A technique for reconstruction of the anterior cruciate ligament in the dog: Preliminary report. Vet Surg 1980;4:135–140.

Kdolsky RK, Gibbons DF, Kwasny O, et al. Braided polypropylene augmentation device in reconstructive surgery of the anterior cruciate ligament: Long-term clinical performance of 594 patients and short-term arthroscopic results, failure analysis by scanning electron microscopy and synovial histomorphology. J Orthop Res 1997;15:1–10.

Knecht CD. Evolution of surgical techniques for cruciate ligament rupture in animals. J Am Anim Hosp Assoc 1976;12:717–726.

Kobayashi S, Hisatoshi B, Uchida K, et al. Microvascular system of anterior cruciate ligament in dogs. J Orthop Res 2006;24:1509–1520.

Lopez MJ, Markel MM, Kalsheur VL, et al. Hamstring graft technique for stabilization of canine cranial cruciate ligament deficient stifles. Vet Surg 2003;32: 390–401.

Mascarenhas R, MacDonald PB. Anterior cruciate ligament reconstruction: A look at prosthetics—past, present and possible future. McGill J Med 2008;11: 29–37.

McFarland EG, Morrey BF, An KN, Wood MB. The relationship of vascularity and water content to tensile strength in a patellar tendon replacement of the anterior cruciate ligament in dogs. Am J Sports Med 1986;14:436–448.

Murray MM, Spindler KP, Devin C, et al. Use of a collagen-platelet rich plasma scaffold to stimulate healing of a central defect in the canine ACL. J Orthop Res 2006;24:820–830.

Murray MM, Spindler KP, Ballard P, et al. Enhanced histologic repair in a central wound in the anterior cruciate ligament with a collagen-platelet-rich plasma scaffold. J Orthop Res 2007;25:1007–1017.

Ng GY, Oakes BW, Deacon OW, et al. Biomechanics of patellar tendon autograft for reconstruction of the anterior cruciate ligament in the goat: Three year study. J Ortho Res 1995;13:602–608.

O'Donoghue DH, Rockwood CA, Frank GR, et al. Repair of the anterior cruciate ligament in dogs. J Bone Joint Surg Am 1966;48:503–519.

Shires PK, Hulse DA, Liu W. The under-and-over fascial replacement technique for anterior cruciate ligament rupture in dogs: A retrospective study. J Am Anim Hosp 1984;20:69–77.

Spindler KP, Murray MM, Devin C, et al. The central ACL defect as a model for failure of intra-articular healing. J Orthop Res 2006;24:401–406.

28 Biomechanics of the Cranial Cruciate Ligament-Deficient Stifle Treated by Tibial Osteotomies

Antonio Pozzi and Stanley E. Kim

Introduction

Normal tibiofemoral motion is constrained by articular surfaces, ligaments, capsule, and menisci. Cranial cruciate ligament (CrCL) deficiency alters these constraints and causes abnormal motion between the articular surfaces (Anderst et al. 2009). The modification in cartilage loading caused by the altered surface interaction initiates progressive osteoarthritis (Tashman et al. 2004; Anderst et al. 2009). Thus, the goal for CrCL reconstruction should be to restore normal stifle mechanics, reestablish biomechanical homeostasis, and cease progression of osteoarthritis.

Much of the current knowledge regarding CrCL repair biomechanics in dogs has been derived from cadaveric studies evaluating normal, CrCL-deficient, and surgically treated stifles under controlled, *ex vivo* conditions, or theoretical analysis. However, cadaveric and theoretical studies cannot replicate functional loading and represent only the "time-zero" condition (immediately after surgical fixation) (Warzee et al. 2001; Shahar & Milgram 2006; Apelt et al. 2007). These investiga-

tions should be interpreted into the clinical setting with much caution.

Most clinical and experimental studies evaluating surgical techniques for CrCL deficiency adopt static stability as a measure of the success of the surgical technique to reestablish normal joint mechanics (Gambardella et al. 1981; Slocum & Slocum 1993; Warzee et al. 2001). For example, a persistent positive cranial drawer test after an extracapsular technique has been traditionally considered a sign of stifle instability and an indication of failure of the procedure. A neutralized cranial tibial thrust following tibial plateau leveling osteotomy (TPLO) has been generally used as an indication for a "stable" stifle after reduction of the tibial plateau slope. However, in both cases, static stability (palpable stability on orthopaedic examination) may not necessarily correlate with dynamic stability (controlled alignment of the stifle during activity *in vivo*).

A key concept is that stifle stability is a dynamic phenomenon, describing the response of the neuromusculoskeletal system to a complex combination of body position, muscle forces, external loads, and sensory inputs. The limited value of palpation tests (cranial drawer and tibial compression tests) for predicting clinical function is likely a reflection of the discrepancy between measures of *joint laxity* versus measures of *dynamic stability*. Laxity tests measure the maximum displacement

---

Advances in the Canine Cranial Cruciate Ligament, Edited by Peter Muir, © 2010 ACVS Foundation, This Work is a co-publication between the American College of Veterinary Surgeons Foundation and Wiley-Blackwell.

of the joint in response to an applied external load, in the absence of muscle forces. Simple laxity elicited by palpation cannot simulate the complexity, directions, and rate of application of muscular forces produced at the stifle during movement. Even the tibial compression test, which attempts to simulate weight-bearing, fails to replicate significant loads transmitted across the stifle such as a quadriceps force. For this reason, it would be more correct to use the term "laxity" when static stability is evaluated, and consider dynamic stability only if stifle kinematics can be evaluated in the whole range-of-motion during different gait patterns *in vivo*.

Biomechanics of tibial osteotomies

In 1983, Slocum described the cranial tibial thrust as a tibiofemoral shear force occurring during weight-bearing (Slocum & Devine 1983). Slocum also presented a theoretical model that proposed that the magnitude of cranial tibial thrust was dependent on the degree of the caudal slope of the tibial plateau (Slocum & Slocum 1993). The compressive forces of weight-bearing, assumed to be parallel to the axis of the tibia, can be resolved into a cranially directed component responsible for cranial tibial translation, and a joint compressive force (Figure 28.1). In the normal stifle, the cranial shear component is opposed by the CrCL and by the muscle forces. In the CrCL-deficient stifle, the uncontrolled cranial shear force results in cranial tibial subluxation.

Based on his model, Slocum proposed that the tibial plateau angle (TPA) was a major factor in stifle biomechanics influencing the magnitude of cranial shear force. In the attempt to dynamically decrease the uncontrolled shear force in the CrCL-deficient stifle, Slocum described in 1984 the cranial tibial closing wedge osteotomy (CTWO) for the treatment of CrCL rupture in dogs (Slocum & Devine 1984). This technique was intended to eliminate cranial tibial thrust during the weight-bearing phase of the stride by reducing the TPA. Its mechanism has been recently investigated in a cadaveric study evaluating the size of the wedge ostectomy necessary to neutralize the tibial thrust (Apelt et al. 2010). An ostectomy with a wedge angle equal to TPA +5° resulted in a stable stifle at

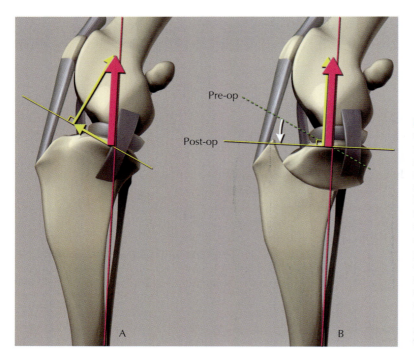

Figure 28.1 Slocum theorized that, during weight-bearing, the joint reaction force (magenta arrow) is approximately parallel the longitudinal axis of the tibia. In the CrCL-deficient stifle (A), the joint reaction force can be resolved into a cranially directed tibiofemoral shear component (parallel to tibial plateau) and a joint compressive force (perpendicular to tibial plateau). By leveling the tibial plateau (B), the joint reaction force is perpendicular to the tibial plateau and thus can only be resolved into a joint compressive force; cranial tibial thrust is eliminated. Reproduced from Kim et al. (2008), with permission from Wiley-Blackwell.

a TPA of approximately 6°. Other factors that influence the postoperative TPA after CTWO include the position of the ostectomy and the cortical alignment after reduction (Bailey et al. 2007). These variables may be responsible for the discrepancies in TPA reported after CTWO (Macias et al. 2002).

A large cranial closing wedge ostectomy can shorten the tibia cranially and alter the femoropatellar joint, lowering the patella relative to the femur leading to hyperextension of the stifle joint (Corr & Brown 2007). Kinematic gait analysis following the CTWO procedure has shown an increase in extension during the swing phase of the stifle and talocrural joints, and an increase in limb extension at paw contact, but no changes in stifle and talocrural joint angles at the stance phase occur (Lee et al. 2007).

The goal of TPLO is to also neutralize cranial tibial thrust and prevent tibial subluxation (Slocum & Slocum 1993). Biomechanical studies have demonstrated that following tibial plateau rotation, the tibiofemoral shear force shifts from cranial to caudal when the limb is loaded (Warzee et al. 2001; Reif et al. 2002). Thus, it has been postulated that joint stability is dependent on the caudal cruciate ligament (CaCL) neutralizing caudal tibial translation following TPLO (Warzee et al. 2001; Reif et al. 2002).

The integrity of the CaCL must be assessed at the time of arthrotomy or arthroscopy before performing TPLO. In the authors' experience, CaCL abnormalities of varying severity can occur concurrently with CrCL rupture (see also Chapter 17). The underlying cause of CaCL degeneration is also unknown, but may be secondary to osteoarthritic change, or due to the same pathologic processes that causes CrCL insufficiency. TPLO increases loads on the CaCL during weight-bearing (Warzee et al. 2001), which may accelerate any preexisting ligamentous degeneration of the CaCL postoperatively. While rare, complete rupture of the CaCL has been documented (Slocum & Slocum 1993), and this complication will result in severe stifle instability. Hence, CaCL abnormalities may preclude the use of TPLO in CrCL-deficient stifles.

Another biomechanical theory argues that the tibia is not axially loaded as proposed by Slocum. Rather, Tepic suggests that the total femorotibial joint forces *in vivo* are directed parallel to the patellar tendon (Tepic et al. 2002). Cranial tibial thrust, according to this model, is then dependent on the angle between the tibial plateau and the patellar tendon (Figure 28.2). This model also predicts that cranial tibial translation should not occur when a CrCL-deficient stifle is flexed beyond 90°. The role of the flexion angle in stifle biomechanics has been investigated in cadaveric studies. As the joint approaches 90° of flexion, the quadriceps mechanism becomes a stabilizer and effectively unloads the CrCL by pulling the tibia caudally (Pozzi et al. 2008; Kim et al. 2010). Likewise, tibial tuberosity advancement aims to impart functional stability by moving the patellar tendon angle to approximately 90° when the stifle is positioned at a standing angle (Montavon et al. 2002). *Ex vivo* studies demonstrated that stifle stability after CrCL transection is attained by tibial tuberosity advancement (TTA) when the patellar tendon angle is 90 ± 9° (Apelt et al. 2007).

The proposed theoretical mechanism of action of the TTA may also explain the mechanism of action for TPLO (Tepic et al. 2002; Drygas et al. 2010). The Tepic model takes into consideration both extensor mechanism anatomy and the geometry of the articulating surfaces of the stifle, and differs from Slocum's theory in that the direction of the joint reaction force is dependent on the inclination of the patellar tendon. By changing the orientation of the tibial plateau relative to the patellar tendon, TPLO may achieve a patellar tendon angle of about 90° in a different way from the TTA (Drygas et al. 2010). The value of using the measurement of patellar tendon angle for TPLO has not yet been clinically evaluated.

Given that craniocaudal stability is directly related to the patellar tendon angle, and therefore the flexion angle of the stifle, it is possible that the degree of cranial tibial subluxation may vary between different activities, or even different breeds. When the stifle is loaded in deep (90° or greater) flexion, cranial tibial subluxation does not occur, as the patellar tendon angle also reaches 90° (Kim et al. 2010). Hence, it could be argued that tibial osteotomies may not benefit dogs with crouched postures, or during activities such as stair-climbing. A recent cadaveric study demonstrated TPLO did not improve joint mechanics when CrCL-deficient stifles were loaded in deep

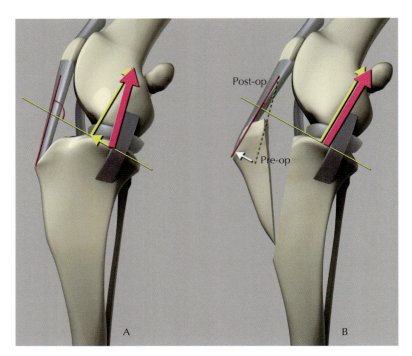

Figure 28.2 An alternate theory, proposed by Tepic, suggests that the joint reaction force (magenta arrow) is approximately parallel to the patella tendon, not the tibial long axis. In the CrCL-deficient stifle (A), the joint reaction force can be resolved into a cranially directed tibiofemoral shear component and a joint compressive force (yellow arrows). By advancing the tibial tuberosity cranially, the patella tendon is perpendicular to the tibial plateau during stance phase of gait (B). The joint reaction force, therefore, becomes perpendicular to the tibial plateau during weight-bearing and thus can only be resolved into a joint compressive force; cranial tibial thrust is eliminated. Reproduced from Kim et al. (2008), with permission from Wiley-Blackwell.

flexion (Kim et al. 2010). Differing stifle joint excursions over a gait cycle may also mean that the amount of tibial plateau rotation (by TPLO) or advancement of the patellar tendon insertion (by TTA) necessary to neutralize subluxation varies between individual dogs. Firm evidence to support specific "tailoring" of postoperative TPAs/patellar tendon angles is lacking; however, it is unlikely that the reported optimal angles (e.g., TPA of 6°) are universal for every dog with CrCL rupture.

Traditional surgical techniques that involve placement of a passive stabilizing structure, such as lateral suture stabilization, hinder full stifle flexion and restrict axial rotational motion of the stifle, as placement of the implant cannot be not perfectly isometric in all three planes. Flexion–extension range-of-motion in stifles treated with TPLO and TTA should not be as diminished as when traditional procedures are used (Chailleux et al. 2007). Full flexion may be slightly decreased after TPLO and CTWO when compared to normal, as they move the distal tibial segment (i.e., the longitudinal axis of the tibia) into slight extension.

The biomechanical models on which TPLO and TTA are based are two-dimensional; hence, tibial osteotomies do not directly attempt to address axial rotational instability caused by CrCL deficiency. Axial rotation of the tibia relative to the femur remains unrestricted, and control of internal–external rotational motion must then rely on muscular forces about the stifle. It is uncertain whether this muscular compensation occurs in dogs, or whether abnormal axial rotation is a clinically significant factor in stifles treated by tibial osteotomies. Persistent axial rotational instability may be one explanation for the progression of osteoarthritis and the subsequent meniscal tears in stifles treated by tibial osteotomies (Lazar et al. 2005; Lafaver et al. 2007). Extracapsular stabilization, on the other hand, creates constant external rotation and abduction of the stifle over a range-of-motion, which may also be detrimental to joint homeostasis (Chailleux et al. 2007).

The primary kinematic abnormality of CrCL deficiency is an increase in cranial tibial translation. Tibial osteotomies have been shown to successfully neutralize cranial tibial thrust and reestablish normal alignment of the stifle in cadaver models. However, it is still unknown if similar results are achieved *in vivo*, during everyday activity. Additional work, particularly *in vivo* investigations, is required to further elucidate the mechanism by which tibial osteotomies improve clinical lameness in dogs.

References

Anderst WJ, Tashman S. The association between velocity of the center of closest proximity on subchondral bones and osteoarthritis progression. J Orthop Res 2009;7:71–77.

Apelt D, Kowaleski MP, Boudrieau RJ. Effect of tibial tuberosity advancement on cranial tibial subluxation in canine cranial cruciate-deficient stifle joints: An in vitro experimental study. Vet Surg 2007;36:170–177.

Apelt D, Pozzi A, Marcellin-Little DJ, Kowaleski MP. Effect of cranial tibial closing wedge angle on tibial subluxation: An ex vivo study. Vet Surg 2010, epub.

Bailey CJ, Smith BA, Black AP. Geometric implications of the tibial wedge osteotomy for the treatment of cranial cruciate ligament disease in dogs. Vet Comp Orthop Traumatol 2007;20:169–174.

Chailleux N, Lussier B, De Guise J, et al. In vitro 3-dimensional kinematic evaluation of 2 corrective operations for cranial cruciate ligament-deficient stifle. Can J Vet Res 2007;71:175–180.

Corr SA, Brown C. A comparison of outcomes following tibial plateau levelling osteotomy and cranial tibial wedge osteotomy procedures. Vet Comp Orthop Traumatol 2007;20:312–319.

Drygas KA, Pozzi A, Goring RL, et al. Effect of tibial plateau leveling osteotomy on patellar tendon angle: A radiographic cadaveric study. Vet Surg 2010, epub.

Gambardella PC, Wallace LJ, Cassidy F. Lateral suture technique for management of anterior cruciate ligament rupture in dogs: A retrospective study. J Am Anim Hosp Assoc 1981;17:33–38.

Kim SE, Pozzi A, Kowaleski MP, Lewis DD. Tibial osteotomies for cranial cruciate ligament insufficiency in dogs. Vet Surg 2008;37:111–125.

Kim SE, Pozzi A, Banks SA, et al. Effect of cranial cruciate ligament deficiency, tibial plateau leveling osteotomy, and tibial tuberosity advancement on contact mechanics and kinematics of the stifle in flexion. Vet Surg 2010;39:363–370.

Lafaver S, Miller NA, Stubbs WP, et al. Tibial tuberosity advancement for stabilization of the canine cranial cruciate ligament-deficient stifle joint: Surgical technique, early results, and complications in 101 dogs. Vet Surg 2007;36:573–586.

Lazar TP, Berry CR, deHaan JJ, et al. Long-term radiographic comparison of tibial plateau leveling osteotomy versus extracapsular stabilization for cranial cruciate ligament rupture in the dog. Vet Surg 2005;34:133–141.

Lee JY, Kim G, Kim JH, et al. Kinematic gait analysis of the hind limb after tibial plateau levelling osteotomy and cranial tibial wedge osteotomy in ten dogs. J Vet Med A Physiol Pathol Clin Med 2007;54:579–584.

Macias C, McKee WM, May C. Caudal proximal tibial deformity and cranial cruciate ligament rupture in small-breed dogs. J Small Anim Pract 2002;43: 433–438.

Montavon PM, Damur DM, Tepic S. Advancement of the tibial tuberosity for the treatment of cranial cruciate deficient canine stifle. *Proceedings of the 1st World Orthopaedic Veterinary Congress.* Munich, Germany, 2002, p. 152.

Pozzi A, Kim SE, Banks SA, et al. Ex-vivo pathomechanics of the Pond-Nuki model. *Proceedings of the Veterinary Orthopedic Society Scientific Meeting.* Big Sky, MT, 2008.

Reif U, Hulse DA, Hauptman JG. Effect of tibial plateau leveling on stability of the canine cranial cruciate-deficient stifle joint: An in vitro study. Vet Surg 2002;31:147–154.

Shahar R, Milgram J. Biomechanics of tibial plateau leveling of the canine cruciate-deficient stifle joint: A theoretical model. Vet Surg 2006;35:144–149.

Slocum B, Devine T. Cranial tibial thrust: A primary force in the canine stifle. J Am Vet Med Assoc 1983;183:456–459.

Slocum B, Devine T. Cranial tibial wedge osteotomy: A technique for eliminating cranial tibial thrust in cranial cruciate ligament repair. J Am Vet Med Assoc 1984;184:564–569.

Slocum B, Slocum TD. Tibial plateau leveling osteotomy for repair of cranial cruciate ligament rupture in the canine. Vet Clin North Am Small Anim Pract 1993;23:777–795.

Tashman S, Anderst W, Kolowich P, et al. Kinematics of the ACL-deficient canine knee during gait: Serial changes over two years. J Orthop Res 2004;22:931–941.

Tepic S, Damur DM, Montavon PM. Biomechanics of the stifle joint. *Proceedings of the 1st World Orthopaedic Veterinary Congress.* Munich, Germany, 2002, pp. 189–190.

Warzee CC, Dejardin LM, Arnoczky SP, et al. Effect of tibial plateau leveling on cranial and caudal tibial thrusts in canine cranial cruciate-deficient stifles: An *in vitro* experimental study. Vet Surg 2001;30: 278–286.

29 Arthroscopic Follow-Up after Surgical Stabilization of the Stifle

Brian S. Beale and Don A. Hulse

Introduction

Cranial cruciate ligament (CrCL) rupture is one of the most common causes of pelvic limb lameness in mature breeds of dogs (Aragon & Budsberg 2005). The majority of veterinary surgeons agree that return to optimal function is best accomplished through surgical treatment. A variety of surgical techniques have been described to stabilize the cruciate-deficient stifle, including extracapsular stabilization, intracapsular CrCL reconstruction, and techniques designed to reduce the force that causes cranial tibial translation (cranial tibial thrust) during the weight-bearing phase of gait (Slocum & Devine-Slocum 1998; Warzee et al. 2001; Reif et al. 2002; Jerram & Walker 2003). Extracapsular stabilization and tibial plateau leveling osteotomy (TPLO) are the most common techniques used by veterinary surgeons to treat CrCL rupture. Although deemed clinically successful in the majority of cases, complications associated with these techniques have been described (Pacchiana et al. 2003; Priddy et al. 2003; Theoret et al. 2003; Stauffer et al. 2006).

Advances in the Canine Cranial Cruciate Ligament, Edited by Peter Muir, © 2010 ACVS Foundation, This Work is a co-publication between the American College of Veterinary Surgeons Foundation and Wiley-Blackwell.

Follow-up arthroscopic evaluation of intra-articular structures of the stifle after surgical stabilization has provided important evidence to assess outcome after surgical stabilization of CrCL tears (Whitney 2003, Rayward et al. 2004; Arthur et al. 2005; Aman & Beale 2009; Hulse et al. 2010).

Surgical recommendations should ideally be made by applying the principles of evidence-based medicine (Aragon & Budsberg 2005). Follow-up arthroscopic evaluation of intra-articular structures is performed as an outcome measurement in experimental studies or in client-owned dogs with clinical signs after a previous surgical procedure. Follow-up arthroscopic evaluation is also occasionally used to assess outcome in patients without clinical signs. Advocates of follow-up arthroscopy in this group of patients cite the low morbidity associated with the technique, frequent discovery of unknown pathology, and the ability to better understand the patient's true outcome after surgery as justification. Follow-up arthroscopy is typically only performed if the patient is having clinical problems or is undergoing general anesthesia for another reason, usually another surgical procedure. A common example would be follow-up arthroscopy performed on a stifle after previous CrCL stabilization at the time of treatment of the contralateral stifle for CrCL rupture. Evidence of changes seen within the joint can influence treatment and activity recommendations for the patient. In addition, simultaneous implant removal can be performed, eliminating the potential necessity for implant removal in the future. Follow-up arthroscopy of the stifle has been used most commonly to assess TPLO patients, but its use has also given valuable information in patients undergoing extracapsular or intracapsular CrCL stabilization and treatment of osteochondritis dessicans (OCD) of the femoral condyle.

Follow-up arthroscopic examination after TPLO

Follow-up arthroscopic examination of the stifle is performed using standard arthroscopic technique (Beale et al. 2003). Typically, the same portals are used as the initial arthroscopy. Exploration of the intra-articular structures is performed, starting in the proximal aspect of the joint, with the stifle held in an extended position. Periarticular osteophytes, cartilage integrity, and synovial membrane character are evaluated. The intercondylar notch region is evaluated with the stifle positioned in flexion. The CrCL and caudal cruciate ligament (CaCL) are assessed for fiber damage, inflammation, remodeling, and vascular proliferation. The menisci are carefully observed and probed for the presence of tears or wear. A Hohmann retractor can be inserted into the joint just lateral to the proximal aspect of the patellar tendon through an accessory instrument portal to separate the joint surfaces and improve the view and access to the menisci. Alternatively, a stifle distractor can be used to improve examination of the menisci. The distractor is secured to the medial femoral condyle and the medial aspect of the proximal tibia using threaded fixator pins. Bucket-handle tears of the medial meniscus are the most common type of meniscal tear seen and are typically treated by partial meniscectomy. Radial tears are also common and are treated by partial meniscectomy at the discretion of the surgeon. Large radial tears are generally treated while small radial tears, and small frays are left untreated. Small frays of the axial border of the lateral meniscus are common in normal dogs without clinical signs. Small frays may increase the susceptibility to larger radial tears in the future in stifles experiencing instability. A medial meniscal release (MR) can also be performed if deemed necessary by the surgeon.

Follow-up arthroscopy was found to be valuable in assessing patients treated with TPLO (Chandler et al. 2002; Arthur et al. 2005; Aman & Beale 2009; Hulse et al. 2010). Hulse et al. (2010) used second-look arthroscopic examination to evaluate dogs with partial and complete CrCL tears after TPLO. Intra-articular structures appeared normal or near normal at long-term follow-up after a TPLO procedure in early partial tears of the CrCL in this study, as well as others (Chandler et al. 2002; Arthur et al. 2005; Hulse et al. 2010). The CrCL did not continue to fail after the plateau was leveled to approximately 6° (Figure 29.1). The lack

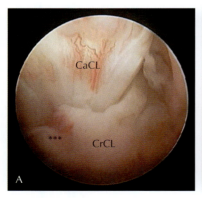 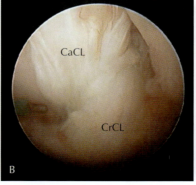 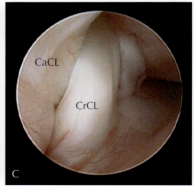

Figure 29.1 (A) The insertion of the craniomedial band is torn (***) in this dog with a partial tear of the cranial cruciate ligament (CrCL). This patient has a normal amount of cranial tibial translation. The caudal cruciate ligament (CaCL) is also visible. (B) The torn fibers of the ligament have been carefully debrided before performing a TPLO. The intact fibers of the CrCL were probed and found to have normal integrity and were left intact. (C) The CrCL appears healthy and functional at follow-up arthroscopic exam of the same patient 2 years later.

of continuing rupture of the CrCL was assumed by the authors to be a result of decreased stress experienced by the CrCL following rotation of the tibial plateau. This would be in accordance with the *in vitro* findings of Warzee et al. (2001) and Reif et al. (2002), and clinical studies of Chandler et al. (2002) and Wolf et al. (2008). When the tibial plateau is rotated to approximately 6° relative to the weight-bearing axis, cranial tibial thrust is transformed to a caudal tibial thrust (Warzee et al. 2001; Reif et al. 2002). Eliminating cranial tibial thrust would likely lower strain within the CrCL, reducing the possibility of further fiber tearing. This supports other clinical work that suggests that TPLO has a protective effect on the CrCL in dogs having an early partial CrCL tear (Chandler et al. 2002; Wolf et al. 2008). As such, the authors do not recommend debridement of intact functional CrCL fibers due to good functional outcome and the potential protective effect on the menisci and cartilage. The articular cartilage of the femur and tibia, the medial and lateral menisci, and synovial joint capsule all appeared normal in all joints in this group of dogs (Figure 29.2). These observations were true at 4 years after surgery, the longest interval from initial surgery to second-look arthroscopy in this group of dogs.

Conversely, the majority of dogs having a partial tear with an incompetent remaining CrCL and cranial drawer or a completely ruptured CrCL ligament had significant intra-articular changes. Of interest were articular cartilage lesions involving the medial or lateral femoral condyle or tibial plateau (Figure 29.3). Lesions included chondromalacia, fibrillation, and erosion (Figure 29.4). The lesions are thought to be secondary to abnormal joint contact mechanics or increased contact with cranial soft tissue after rotation of the tibial plateau to eliminate cranial tibial thrust. Eighty-five percent of the stifles in this group (39 of 46 stifles) had visible cartilage lesions, with the majority (28 of 39 stifles) having Grade 3 or Grade 4 lesions (see Beale et al. 2003 for grading system). Cartilage lesions appeared in the medial femoral condyle (13 joints), lateral femoral condyle (12 joints), and tibial plateau (3 joints) (Figure 29.5). Abaxial nonarticular cartilage abrasion was most common, but

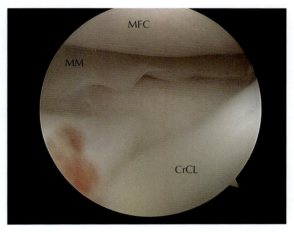

Figure 29.2 The cartilage of the medial femoral condyle (MFC) and tibial plateau and the medial meniscus (MM) appear healthy in dogs with early partial tears of the cranial cruciate ligament (CrCL) at follow-up arthroscopy.

Figure 29.3 (A) The cartilage of the medial femoral condyle (MFC) and tibial plateau (TP) and the medial meniscus (MM) appear normal at the time of TPLO in this patient with an unstable partial CrCL tear. (B) The cartilage of the MFC and TP has fibrillation at the time of follow-up arthroscopy in this patient 12 months later. The MM also has small radial tears.

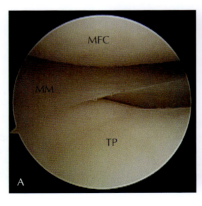 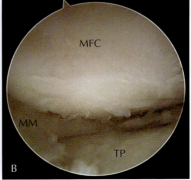

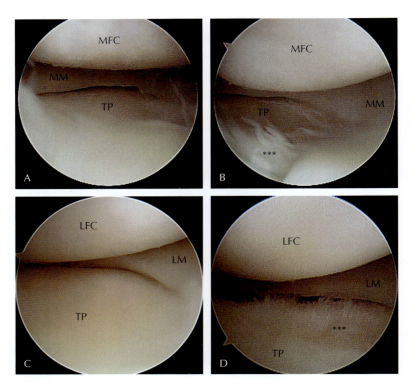

Figure 29.4 (A) The cartilage of the medial femoral condyle (MFC) and tibial plateau (TP) appears healthy in this patient with a complete CrCL tear. Small radial tears of the medial meniscus (MM) are present in this patient treated with a TPLO. (B) The majority of the cartilage of the medial compartment continues to appear healthy in this patient 18 months later. A focal area of fibrillation is seen at the cranial aspect of the TP (***). Small radial tears of the MM have progressed slightly. (C) The cartilage of the lateral femoral condyle (LFC) and tibial plateau (TP) appears healthy in this patient with a complete CrCL tear. (D) The majority of the cartilage of the lateral compartment continues to appear healthy in this patient at follow-up arthroscopy. A focal area of fibrillation is seen at the caudal aspect of the TP (***). LM: lateral mensicus.

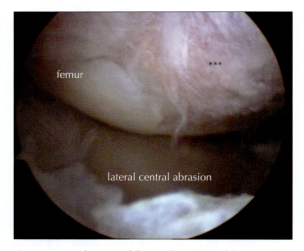

Figure 29.5 Abrasion of the cartilage (***) of the central weight-bearing region of the lateral femoral condyle can be seen in this TPLO patient 28 months after surgery.

axial lesions of the weight-bearing surface were also noted (Figures 29.6 and 29.7). In the majority of dogs, mild fraying of the CaCL was noted; in three dogs there was complete rupture of the CaCL. In one of the three dogs, there was over-rotation of the tibial plateau at revision surgery (initial postoperative slope 6°; postoperative slope after revision 0°); in the other two dogs, the tibial plateau was rotated to 7° in one case, and to 10° in the other case. The history and acute nature of lameness in the latter two dogs was suggestive of a traumatic episode. Eight dogs developed a bucket-handle tear in the caudal horn of the medial meniscus (postliminary meniscal tear). Commonly, the only clinical finding was the onset of decreased limb function. Without specific intra-articular inspection, clinical findings in these cases may be mistakenly diagnosed with overuse injury or progression of osteoarthritis.

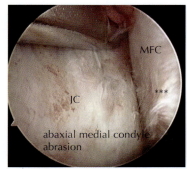 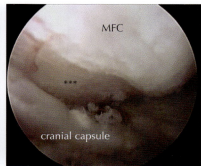

Figures 29.6 (A,B) Abrasion of the cartilage (***) of the abaxial non-weight-bearing region of the medial femoral condyle (MFC) adjacent to the cranial joint capsule (JC) can be seen in these TPLO patients at long-term follow-up arthroscopy. The JC is thickened and has increased stiffness in both patients.

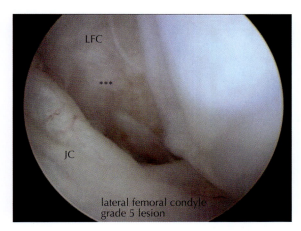

Figure 29.7 Abrasion of the cartilage (***) of the abaxial non-weight-bearing region of the lateral femoral condyle (LFC) adjacent to the cranial joint capsule (JC) can be seen in this TPLO patient at follow-up arthroscopy.

Arthur et al. (2005) evaluated the synovium, CrCL, CaCL, medial meniscus, lateral meniscus, femoral trochlea, femoral condyles, and tibial plateau using follow-up arthroscopy in 40 dogs (45 stifles) previously treated with TPLO. Pathologic changes were identified at the time of initial surgery and followed over time. Radiographic evidence of periarticular osteophytes (PAOs) was unchanged or only minimally increased at the time of follow-up in 36 stifles and markedly increased in 9 stifles. Progression of PAOs was evident arthroscopically in 25% of stifles at follow-up. Cartilage wear was unchanged in 15 stifles and increased in 20 stifles. Small radial tears of the lateral meniscus treated by radiofrequency partial meniscectomy had increased cartilage wear in 67% of treated stifles. Increased cartilage wear was evident in 50% of stifles with similar meniscal tears left untreated. Treatment of small radial tears of the lateral meniscus with radiofrequency partial meniscectomy was associated with a greater frequency of progressive cartilage wear compared with no treatment of the meniscus. Cartilage wear was evident arthroscopically in eight stifles without radiographic evidence of increased osteoarthritis. Synovitis was unchanged in 15, increased in 2, and decreased in 18 stifles. Medial and lateral meniscal tears were present at follow-up in 16 and 8 stifles, with increased cartilage wear in 8 stifles (Figures 29.8 and 29.9). Sites of partial meniscectomies at initial arthroscopy were intact and unchanged in 12 cases, while further meniscal tearing had developed in 6 cases. The CaCL was initially intact in all stifles; however, lesions such as hyperemia and mild fraying were seen at this time in 13 stifles and progressed in 9 cases (Figure 29.10). With the exception of one case of complete rupture, CaCL lesions at follow-up were limited to mild increases in fraying, stretching, and hyperemia (Figures 29.11–29.13). In 10 dogs, gross lesions such as fraying, remodeling, or hyperemia of the CaCL developed subsequent to grossly normal appearance at the time of TPLO.

Important findings in the study included the observation that arthroscopic evaluation of the stifle allowed diagnosis of joint disease not evident radiographically. The CrCL remained intact when early partial tears were treated with TPLO in patients having no palpable instability. Partial tears of the CrCL having instability at the time of

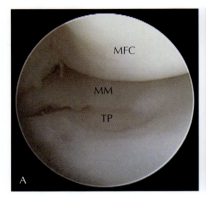
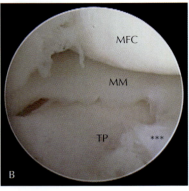

Figure 29.8 (A) The medial femoral condyle (MFC), tibial plateau (TP), and medial meniscus (MM) appear normal at the time of TPLO. (B) The MFC and TP appear normal, but the cranial horn of the medial meniscus has mild radial tears at follow-up arthroscopic examination (***).

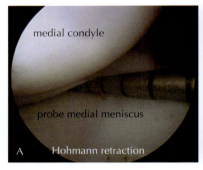
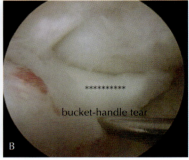

Figure 29.9 (A) The medial meniscus of this patient with a complete CrCL tear has a latent bucket-handle meniscal tear at follow-up arthroscopy. (B) The meniscal tear is not visible until probed (asterisks).

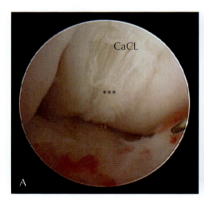
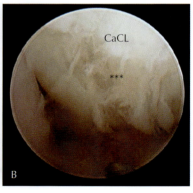

Figure 29.10 (A) The caudal cruciate ligament (CaCL) shows mild wear (***) before TPLO and mild progression of wear at 20 months after surgery (B).

TPLO typically remained intact at follow-up, but the ligament remained stretched (Figure 29.14). Arthroscopic and radiographic evidence of increased PAO formation indicates the potential for progressive osteoarthritis in some cases after TPLO (Figure 29.15). Synovitis was generally decreased at follow-up examination (Figure 29.16).

Cases in which gross changes in the appearance of the CaCL were present lend credence to the potentially detrimental increases in caudal translation after TPLO. Small radial tears of the lateral meniscus may not require treatment, and radio-frequency for partial meniscectomy should be used judiciously.

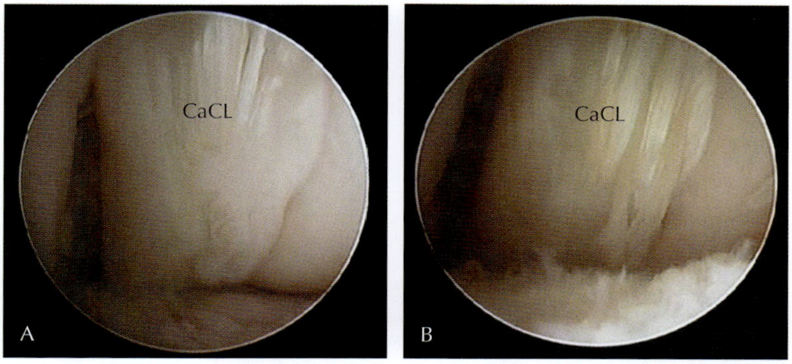

Arthroscopic Follow-Up after Surgical Stabilization of the Stifle   207

Figure 29.11 (A) The caudal cruciate ligament (CaCL) appears normal before TPLO, and normal at 22 months after TPLO (B).

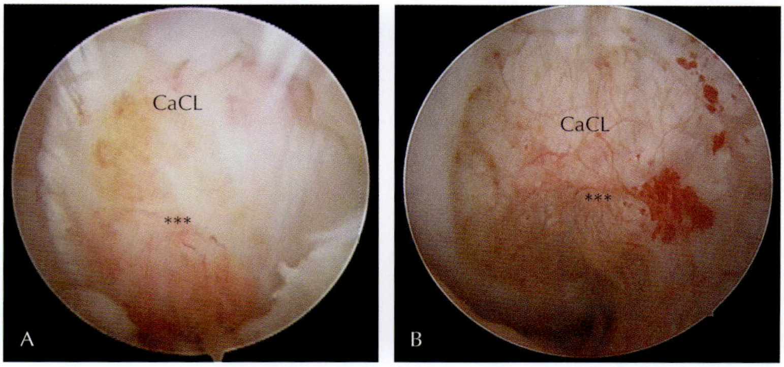

Figure 29.12 (A) The caudal cruciate ligament (CaCL) appears inflamed with loss of detail (***) at the time of TPLO. Normal longitudinal fibers of the CaCL can be seen at the origin of the ligament. (B) The CaCL appears to have progressive inflammation and loss of fiber detail (***) 11 months after surgery. No normal appearing CaCL fibers are visible.

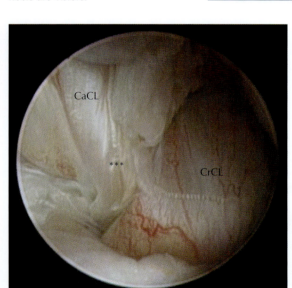

Figure 29.13 The caudal cruciate ligament (CaCL) has substantial tearing (asterisks) in this patient with an incompetent cranial cruciate ligament (CrCL) tear treated with a TPLO. This is an uncommon finding at follow-up arthroscopic examination.

Canine meniscal injuries are often found in conjunction with CrCL rupture or after surgical stabilization of the CrCL-deficient stifle. Meniscal tears may be displaced and easily identified. Others may be latent and require careful palpation with a probe to identify. Meniscal tears that occur subsequent to CrCL repair are termed postlimimary tears. Follow-up arthroscopy has provided valuable information toward the understanding of the impact of progressive cruciate rupture and its treatment on the menisci over time. MR at the time of stabilization of the CrCL-deficient stifle has been recommended to prevent further injury to the caudal pole of the medial meniscus after TPLO surgery (Slocum & Devine-Slocum 1998). Conversely, MR may result in joint instability and impairment of load transmission, which may accelerate the progression of osteoarthritis (Pozzi et al. 2008). Meniscectomy, which has similar mechanical results to MR on the stifle, leads to osteoarthritis in both humans and animals. Kim et al. (2009) suggested that the risk of postlimimary meniscal injury is smaller after TPLO due to the neutralization of cranial tibial thrust; thus, the need for MR is controversial. In addition, Luther et al. (2009) reported that MR alone in CrCL-intact stifles was associated with articular cartilage loss and further meniscal pathology. These studies would tend to suggest that MR is contraindicated at the time of surgical stabilization of a cruciate-deficient stifle. These findings, however, are based on *in vitro* or *ex vivo* work, or in dogs that had intact CrCL. Aman et al. (2009) used follow-up arthroscopy to assess clinical patients with CrCL rupture. Their study compared CrCL-deficient stifles of dogs having undergone TPLO with MR with dogs having undergone TPLO with no MR. Follow-up arthroscopy was used to assess the stifles at long-term follow-up. The findings of Aman et al.'s (2009) study suggested that there may not be a significant difference in progression of osteoarthritis between dogs receiving TPLO with MR and dogs receiving TPLO without MR. They found a risk of postliminary meniscal injury with or without MR, but severe meniscal injury was much more likely without MR. A higher incidence of bucket-handle tears was seen in dogs not receiving a MR. Small radial tears were the predominant type of tear seen if a MR was performed. Meniscal tears were more common in the dogs having a MR at the meniscotibial ligament than in the dogs having a mid-body incision. MR at the meniscotibial ligament or mid-body appeared to remain functional in all dogs having the procedure performed. The meniscotibial ligament did not appear to reattach. The mid-body MR incisions appeared to heal with great variation (Figure 29.17). Some of the mid-body MR incisions healed with a smooth axial border. Others healed with irregular fibrous tissue, and some showed no healing response. The MR appears to remain functional despite variation in healing patterns. Evidence of continued function of the MR includes

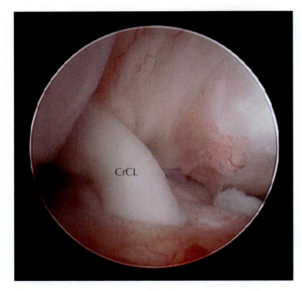

Figure 29.14 Appearance of an incompetent partial cranial cruciate ligament (CrCL) 2 years after TPLO surgery. Instability of the stifle was present due to stretching of the CrCL before TPLO. The ligament continues to have mild laxity, but inflammation has subsided and no further damage to the ligament is seen after TPLO. The TPLO procedure appears to have protected the CrCL from progressive damage.

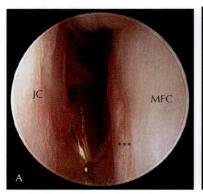
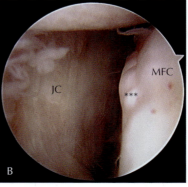

Figure 29.15 (A) Periarticular osteophytes (PAOs) typically remain the same size or become slightly larger over time after TPLO. This patient with a complete CrCL tear had mild PAOs (***) in the medial gutter at the time of TPLO. (B) The PAOs increased little in size over 34 months. JC: joint capsule; MFC: medial femoral condyle.

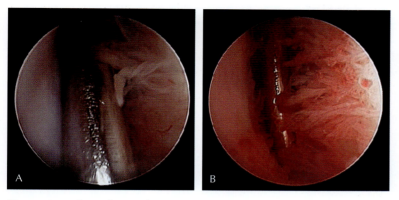

Figure 29.16 Some degree of synovitis was typically seen at follow-up arthroscopy in patients after TPLO. These patients had mild (A) and moderate (B) synovitis, although both patients were subclinical.

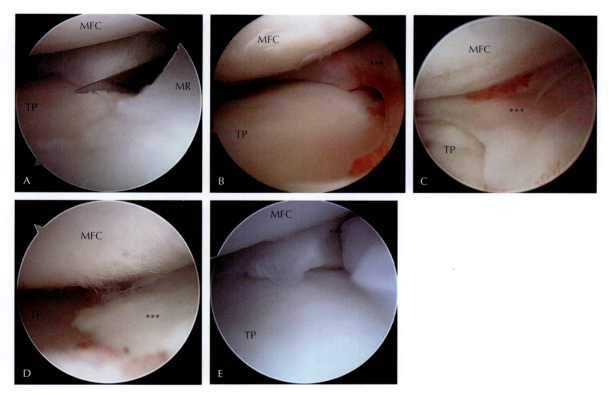

Figure 29.17 (A) A mid-body medial meniscal release (MR) is performed under arthroscopic observation. Follow-up arthroscopic evaluation revealed inconsistent findings at the MR incision site. (B,C) The site of MR healed (***) with a smooth axial border in most patients. (D) The gap at the MR incision was filled with irregular fibrous tissue (***) in some patients. (E) Occasionally, a patient may show no sign of healing at the MR site (***). Interestingly, minimal signs of cartilage wear of the medial femoral condyle (MFC) and tibial plateau (TP) were seen. The MR appears to remain functional, despite variation in healing patterns. Evidence of continued function of the MR includes the caudal position of the medial meniscus (asterisks) and the dramatic reduction in the prevalence of postliminary meniscal tears.

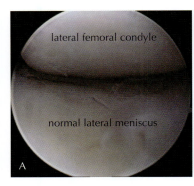 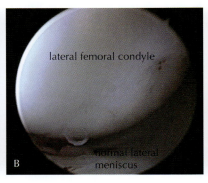 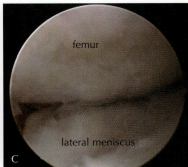

Figure 29.18 The cartilage of the femoral condyle and tibial plateau had an inconsistent appearance at the time of follow-up arthroscopic examination after extracapsular stabilization among patients with cranial cruciate ligament rupture. The cartilage appeared to be normal (A), have mild wear (B), or have moderate wear (C).

the caudal position of the medial meniscus and the dramatic reduction in the prevalence of postliminary meniscal tears. The caudal horn of the medial meniscus appeared to sit in a more caudal position, and the meniscus did not appear to shift forward during a tibial compression test or a cranial drawer test while the meniscus was viewed arthroscopically.

Follow-up arthroscopic examination after extracapsular stabilization

Follow-up arthroscopy has also been used to assess the stifle joint after extracapsular stabilization of the CrCL-deficient stifle. Most of the dogs examined in this group had undergone complete debridement of the CrCL at the time of stabilization. Periarticular osteophytes typically enlarge over time. Mild to moderate synovitis is seen. Cartilage erosion is variable (Figure 29.18). Some dogs show progressive cartilage erosion of the medial and lateral compartment (Figure 29.19). Erosion primarily involves the articular cartilage of the weight-bearing regions of the medial and lateral femoral condyle and tibial plateau. Cartilage damage is often more severe in the lateral compartment. Increased cartilage damage in the lateral compartment may be secondary to increased forces generated by the placement of a lateral extracapsular suture. Cartilage erosion does not appear to commonly involve non-weight-bearing regions, unlike that seen after TPLO. Some dogs show very little evidence of articular cartilage damage. Meniscal tears are also common at the time of follow-up arthroscopic exam in this group of patients (Figure 29.20). Interestingly, many dogs identified as having bucket-handle tears of the medial meniscus were not observed to have significant lameness by the owners. Physical exam, however, tended to show a stiff pelvic limb gait, reluctance to sit square, or a slight click when flexing the stifle. It appears that some dogs are quite effective in minimizing clinical signs of pain associated with a meniscal tear. Medial patellar luxation has also been observed at the time of follow-up arthroscopic exam after extracapsular stabilization for CrCL insufficiency. Arthroscopic evaluation of infected joints secondary to an infected extracapsular suture gives valuable information regarding the intensity of the synovitis and degree of cartilage damage.

Follow-up arthroscopic examination after intracapsular stabilization

Intracapsular repairs are most commonly performed in medium and large breed dogs. Follow-up arthroscopy after intracapsular stabilization has revealed similar findings to extracapsular stabilization. Periarticular osteophytes typically enlarge over time. Mild to moderate synovitis is seen. Cartilage erosion is variable. Some dogs show progressive cartilage erosion of the medial and lateral compartment. Erosion is seen to involve

Figure 29.19 Some patients show severe cartilage damage at follow-up evaluation after extracapsular stabilization. Erosion of the lateral femoral condyle (***) in the region opposite the lateral tibial eminence is seen in this patient (A). This lesion is thought to occur due to excessive shear force. Full thickness erosion (***) of weight-bearing regions of the medial femoral condyle (MFC) are occasionally seen (B).

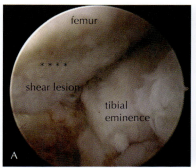 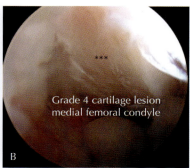

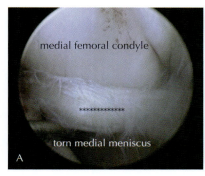 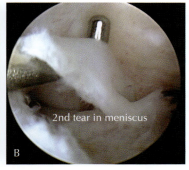

Figure 29.20 Bucket-handle tears of the medial meniscus were commonly seen at follow-up arthroscopic examination of patients treated with extracapsular stabilization of cranial cruciate ligament tears in both dogs with clinical signs and dogs thought to be without clinical signs. (A) Some meniscal tears were displaced and easily identified (asterisks). Other bucket-handle tears were latent and identified only after careful probing. This patient had two bucket-handle tears of the medial meniscus. The first tear was displaced and easily identified. Partial meniscectomy was performed. The second bucket-handle tear was latent and was identified after carefully probing the medial meniscus after removal of the first tear (B).

the articular cartilage of the weight-bearing regions of the medial and lateral femoral condyles and tibial plateau. On the other hand, some dogs show very little change in appearance of the articular cartilage. Intracapsular stabilization techniques may be performed using a prosthetic or a biological ligament replacement. Prosthetic ligament replacements have a high rate of failure. Follow-up arthroscopy has found fibers of the ligament to have significant wear leading to stretching, partial tear or complete tear of the prosthetic ligament. Biological replacement ligaments have also been found to experience fiber tearing at follow-up arthroscopic exam. Fibers of the ligament are often stretched or the ligament may have a partial or complete tear. A minority of patients have a healthy-appearing replacement ligament (Figure 29.21). Meniscal tears are also

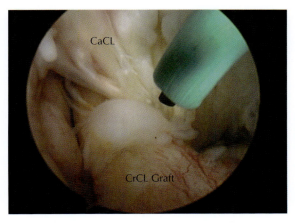

Figure 29.21 The fascial lata graft appears healthy and functional at follow-up arthroscopic examination in this patient treated with intracapsular stabilization after CrCL. CaCL: caudal cruciate ligament.

common at the time of follow-up arthroscopic exam in this group of patients. This group of dogs typically has persistent or intermittent lameness and often will have a meniscal click if a bucket-handle tear of the medial meniscus is present.

Conclusion

Follow-up arthroscopy has provided much needed evidence of outcome after cruciate stabilization surgery. Follow-up arthroscopy was associated with minimal morbidity. Many changes in the intra-articular environment of the stifle have been identified, including meniscal tears, CaCL fiber wear, chronic synovitis, cartilage wear, and osteophyte production. Many of the pathologic changes were evident in dogs that were thought to be without clinical signs. Many of the arthroscopic findings are not easily assessed by imaging techniques. Follow-up arthroscopy is an excellent method of assessing the intra-articular condition of the canine stifle joint months to years after stifle surgery.

References

Aman A, Beale BS. Follow-up arthroscopic evaluation of canine stifles having undergone tibial plateau leveling osteotomy with and without meniscal release. *Proceedings of the 36th Annual Conference of the Veterinary Orthopedic Society*. Steamboat Springs, CO, 2009, p. 21.

Aragon CL, Budsberg SC. Applications of evidence-based medicine: Cranial cruciate ligament injury repair in the dog. Vet Surg 2005;34:93–98.

Arthur EG, Beale BS, Whitney WO. Second-look arthroscopic evaluation of the canine stifle following tibial plateau osteotomy. *Proceedings of the 32nd Annual Conference of the Veterinary Orthopedic Society*. Snowmass CO, 2005, p. 45.

Beale BS, Hulse DA, Schulz KS, Whitney WO. Small Animal Arthroscopy. Philadelphia: WB Saunders, 2003.

Chandler JC, Whitney WO, Beale BS. Management of partial cranial cruciate ligament ruptures with arthroscopic assisted tibial plateau leveling osteotomy. *Proceedings of the 29th Annual Conference Veterinary Orthopedic Society*. The Canyons, UT, 2002, p. 31.

Hulse DA, Beale BS, Kerwin S. Second look arthroscopic findings after tibial plateau leveling osteotomy. Vet Surg 2010;39:350–354.

Jerram RM, Walker AM. Cranial cruciate ligament injury in the dog: Pathophysiology, diagnosis and treatment. N Z Vet J 2003;51:149–158.

Kim S, Pozzi A, Banks SA, et al. Effect of tibial plateau leveling osteotomy on femorotibial contact mechanics and stifle kinematics. Vet Surg 2009;38:23–32.

Luther JK, Cook CR, Cook JL. Meniscal release in cruciate ligament intact stifles causes lameness and medial compartment cartilage pathology in dogs 12 weeks postoperatively. Vet Surg 2009;38:520–529.

Pacchiana PD, Morris E, Gillings SL, et al. Surgical and postoperative complications associated with tibial plateau leveling osteotomy in dogs with cranial cruciate ligament rupture: 397 cases (1998–2001). J Am Vet Med Assoc 2003;222:184–193.

Pozzi A, Litsky AS, Field J, et al. Pressure distributions on the medial tibial plateau after medial meniscal surgery and tibial plateau levelling osteotomy in dogs. Vet Comp Orthop Traumatol 2008;21:8–14.

Priddy NH, Tomlinson JL, Dodam JR, et al. Complications with and owner assessment of the outcome of tibial plateau leveling osteotomy for treatment of cranial cruciate ligament rupture in dogs: 193 cases (1997–2001). J Am Vet Med Assoc 2003;222:1726–1732.

Rayward RM, Thomson DG, Davies JV, et al. Progression of osteoarthritis following TPLO surgery: A prospective radiographic study of 40 dogs. J Small Anim Pract 2004;45:92–97.

Reif U, Hulse DA, Hauptman JG. Effect of leveling on stability of the canine cranial cruciate-deficient stifle joint: An *in-vitro* study. Vet Surg 2002;31:147–154.

Slocum B, Devine-Slocum T. Tibial plateau leveling osteotomy for cranial cruciate ligament rupture. In: *Current Techniques in Small Animal Surgery*, Bojrab MJ (ed.), fourth edition. Philadelphia: Lea & Febiger, 1998, pp. 1209–1215.

Stauffer K, Tuttle T, Elkins D. Complications associated with 696 tibial plateau leveling osteotomies (2001–2003). J Am Anim Hosp Assoc 2006;42:44–50.

Theoret MC, Withney WO, Beale BS. Complications associated with tibial plateau leveling osteotomy. *Proceedings of the 30th Annual Conference Veterinary Orthopaedic Society*. Steamboat Springs, CO, 2003, p. 80.

Warzee CC, Dejardin LM, Arnoczky SP, et al. Effect of tibial plateau leveling on cranial and caudal tibial thrusts in canine cranial cruciate-deficient stifles: An in-vitro experimental study. Vet Surg 2001;30:278–286.

Whitney WO. Arthroscopically assisted surgery of the stifle joint. In: *Small Animal Arthroscopy*, Beale BS, Hulse DA, Schulz KS, Whitney WO (eds). Philadelphia: WB Saunders, 2003, pp. 117–157.

Wolf R, Beale BS, Whitney WO. Effect of debridement of the cranial cruciate ligament in dogs having early partial tears of the cranial cruciate ligament at the time of TPLO. Vet Surg 2008;37:E2.

30 Cranial Cruciate Ligament Debridement

David E. Spreng

Introduction

Before the widespread use of arthroscopy, stifle arthrotomy had long been considered "the standard of care" during treatment of cranial cruciate ligament (CrCL) rupture. Debridement of the torn ends of the ligament was considered necessary to decrease the inflammatory response during the postoperative period. Some publications also advocated that partially ruptured ligaments should be completely removed, again to decrease postoperative inflammation. Meanwhile, new important information published on the function of the CrCL has led to new developments in the approach to ligament debridement.

The CrCL has a primarily mechanical function. It is the main restraint mechanism for cranial tibial translation throughout the whole range-of-motion and is also responsible for limitation of the internal rotation of the tibia (Vasseur 2002). Most surgeons consider ligaments only to be passive stabilizers of the joint. However, there is good evidence that the CrCL also plays an important role in proprioception and neuromuscular function.

Advances in the Canine Cranial Cruciate Ligament,
Edited by Peter Muir, © 2010 ACVS Foundation, This Work is a co-publication between the American College of Veterinary Surgeons Foundation and Wiley-Blackwell.

Mechanoreceptors within the CrCL might be responsible for signaling muscle stiffness of the pelvic limb (Adachi et al. 2002).

Many human patients who have had an injury of the lower extremity describe vague symptoms such as unsteadiness (giving-way) of the joint (Noyes et al. 1989). It seems likely that at least some aspects of these symptoms are related to mechanoreceptors. However, this is difficult to document due to the lack of sufficiently sensitive yet measurable parameters. A tear or removal of the anterior cruciate ligament in humans has been associated with neuromuscular changes such as loss of proprioception, alterations in muscle reflexes initiated by the ligament, alterations in muscle stiffness, quadriceps-force deficits, and changes in gait and electromyographic measurements (DeFranco & Bach 2009). It is not clear whether these changes are caused by the loss of mechanoreceptors in the torn ligament or by altered stimulation of the remaining receptors in other articular tissue such as the joint capsule.

Mechanoreceptors have been identified within the canine CrCL. The receptors are pressure-sensitive corpuscles including Ruffini receptors, Pacini receptors, and free nerve endings, which are responsible for pain perception and autonomic nervous system regulation of blood flow (Cole et al. 1996). Considering the innervation of the entire stifle, the receptors in the CrCL constitute only a small minority. It seems, however, that canine CrCL have more mechanoreceptors than other species. According to Arcand (Arcand et al. 2000), more than 450 receptors could be identified in the canine CrCL compared with very few receptors in humans (<20) (Hogervorst & Brand 1998) and cats (<50) (Madey et al. 1997). The comparison should be interpreted with caution due to different study designs and detection techniques. It is, however, an interesting observation as cats and humans produce less severe osteoarthritis after CrCL rupture compared with dogs. Free nerve endings are mainly nociceptors, which react to inflammation and pain stimuli (Cole et al. 1996). Vasoactive neuropeptides, such as substance P, have been reported in free nerve endings and they are thought to behave as vasoactive substances. Therefore, free nerve endings do not only transfer information but also have effector functions such as vasodilation, vascular permeability, and effects on the immune system (Hogervorst & Brand 1998). Considering this information and the fact that the CrCL helps to maintain joint stability and is beneficial in preventing meniscal tears, it seems that total debridement of the partially ruptured CrCL should be used cautiously.

Since the introduction of arthroscopy, the diagnostics and surgical treatments for CrCL rupture have been performed much earlier during the disease process. Early detection of partially ruptured CrCL has consequently increased. This is documented by the fact that before introduction of arthroscopy in CrCL therapy, an incidence of 8% of partially ruptured CrCL diagnosed during surgery was published in the 1990s (Scavelli et al. 1990) compared with 21% in 2000 (Ralphs & Whitney 2002) and 44% observed during a period in which arthroscopy has become a routine procedure (unpublished data from the author's hospital 2009). With this evolution in mind, it has become very important to assess the different possibilities of CrCL debridement. Intraoperative decisions of how much to debride can be very difficult. Accurate visual grading of the percentage of torn CrCL is difficult because ligament tissue that appears to be intact may mask a substantial injury. Plastic deformation is possible and leads to a lax nonfunctional ligament. Electrothermal shrinkage of collagen fibers of a lax ligament is potentially possible and has been used in the treatment of lax anterior cruciate ligaments in humans (Lamar et al. 2005). After initial promising results, however, a multicenter study showed a high failure rate for thermal shrinkage, with the conclusion that this was not an appropriate treatment (Smith et al. 2008).

Ligament debridement in complete CrCL rupture

It is well known that ruptured cruciate ligaments do not heal spontaneously (Hefti et al. 1991) and mechanoreceptors probably do not regenerate and have a questionable function without physiologic tension (Hogervorst & Brand 1998). Furthermore, some believe that remnants of the ligament might be an inflammatory trigger and increase OA. Experimentally, it has been shown that CrCL remnants disappear 3 months after CrCL transection in rabbits (Hefti et al. 1991). In canine clinical and experimental cases, resorption of the torn ligament is also possible. However, in contrast, also nodular, vascularized swellings (Figure 30.1), or drumstick formations of the free ends of the torn ligament (Figure 30.2) are often present and might disturb normal motion. Therefore, debridement of totally ruptured ligaments is an appropriate and indicated therapy usually performed before meniscal inspection with a motorized shaver during arthroscopy or with a scalpel blade in open arthrotomy.

Ligament debridement in partial CrCL rupture

Partial debridement of the partially ruptured CrCL is indicated (Figure 30.2). Short-term negative consequences of partial debridement compared with total debridement could not be demonstrated (Wolf et al. 2008). Especially with small partial tears, it is indicated to debride visibly torn fibers using a motorized shaver (Figure 30.3). A radiofrequency energy probe can be used if the shaver debridement is not satisfactory. Punctual application using the lowest possible energy is advised to reduce the risk of thermal injury in the remaining tissue (Lu et al. 2007). During debridement of the partially ruptured CrCL, it is impor-

Cranial Cruciate Ligament Debridement

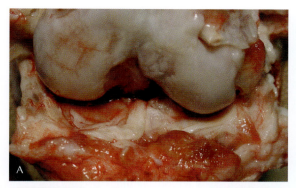

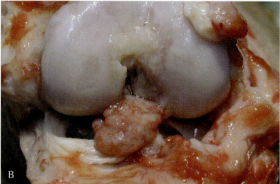

Figure 30.1 Macroscopic view of two canine stifle joints after experimental CrCL transection 12 months earlier. Note the marked cartilage degeneration, meniscal damage, and CrCL resorption (A) versus CrCL vascularized proliferation (B).

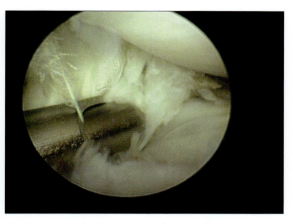

Figure 30.3 Arthroscopic view of a partially ruptured cranial cruciate ligament during debridement of torn fibers with a motorized shaver using a 2.0-mm full radius resector blade. The blade is positioned with the back of the shaver lying against the intact ligament part to protect viable fibers.

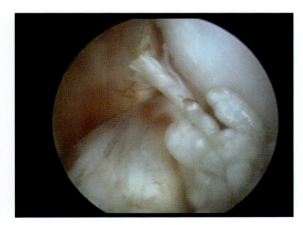

Figure 30.2 Arthroscopic view of a chronic partially ruptured cranial cruciate ligament with visible torn fibers. Note the formation of a "drumstick" proliferation of the ruptured fibers.

tant to save the fat pad as much as possible as it is one of the major origins of vascular supply of the CrCL (Kobayashi et al. 2006).

Dogs with partial CrCL rupture have a lower incidence of meniscal injury compared with dogs with complete rupture (Ralphs & Whitney 2002). One of the reasons could be that the remaining ligament inhibits tibial translation to a certain degree which decreases the risk of meniscal injury. Clinical observations have shown that surgical interventions that dynamically stabilize the stifle joint have an influence on the remnants of the ligament. Dogs with palpably stable stifle joints that have an arthroscopically diagnosed partial CrCL rupture seem to benefit from debridement of visible torn fibers followed by a dynamic stabilization procedure such as tibial plateau leveling osteotomy (TPLO). Subsequent meniscal injuries seem to be uncommon in this patient group, supporting the theory that CrCL remnants maintain better stability of the joint. Second-look arthroscopies have shown an improved appearance of the intact part of the CrCL, probably because the TPLO procedure reduces strain on the CrCL.

References

Adachi N, Ochi M, Uchio Y, et al. Mechanoreceptors in the anterior cruciate ligament contribute to the joint position sense. Acta Orthop Scand 2002;73:330–334.

Arcand MA, Rhalmi S, Rivard CH. Quantification of mechanoreceptors in the canine anterior cruciate ligament. Int Orthop 2000;24:272–275.

Cole KJ, Daley BJ, Brand RA. The sensitivity of joint afferents to knee translation. Sportverletz Sportschaden 1996;10:27–31.

DeFranco MJ, Bach BR, Jr. A comprehensive review of partial anterior cruciate ligament tears. J Bone Joint Surg Am 2009;91:198–208.

Hefti FL, Kress A, Fasel J, et al. Healing of the transected anterior cruciate ligament in the rabbit. J Bone Joint Surg Am 1991;73:373–383.

Hogervorst T, Brand RA. Mechanoreceptors in joint function. J Bone Joint Surg Am 1998;80:1365–1378.

Kobayashi S, Baba H, Uchida K, et al. Microvascular system of anterior cruciate ligament in dogs. J Orthop Res 2006;24:1509–1520.

Lamar DS, Bartolozzi AR, Freedman KB, et al. Thermal modification of partial tears of the anterior cruciate ligament. Arthroscopy 2005;21:809–814.

Lu Y, Meyer ML, Bogdanske JJ, et al. The effects of radiofrequency energy probe speed and application force on chondrocyte viability. Vet Comp Orthop Traumatol 2007;20:34–37.

Madey SM, Cole KJ, Brand RA. Sensory innervation of the cat knee articular capsule and cruciate ligament visualised using anterogradely transported wheat germ agglutinin-horseradish peroxidase. J Anat 1997;190:289–297.

Noyes FR, Mooar LA, Moorman CT, 3rd, et al. Partial tears of the anterior cruciate ligament. Progression to complete ligament deficiency. J Bone Joint Surg Br 1989;71:825–833.

Ralphs SC, Whitney WO. Arthroscopic evaluation of menisci in dogs with cranial cruciate ligament injuries: 100 cases (1999–2000). J Am Vet Med Assoc 2002;221:1601–1604.

Scavelli TD, Schrader SC, Matthiesen DT, et al. Partial rupture of the cranial cruciate ligament of the stifle in dogs: 25 cases (1982–1988). J Am Vet Med Assoc 1990;196:1135–1138.

Smith DB, Carter TR, Johnson DH. High failure rate for electrothermal shrinkage of the lax anterior cruciate ligament: A multicenter follow-up past 2 years. Arthroscopy 2008;24:637–641.

Vasseur PB. Stifle joint. In: *Textbook of Small Animal Surgery*, Slatter D (ed.), third edition. Philadelphia: WB Saunders, 2002, pp. 2090–2132.

Wolf R, Beale B, Whitney W. Effect of debridement of the cranial cruciate ligament in dogs having early partial tears of the cranial cruciate ligament at the time of TPLO. Vet Surg 2008;37:E2.

31 Surgical Treatment of Concurrent Meniscal Injury

James L. Cook and Antonio Pozzi

Introduction

Meniscal pathology in conjunction with cranial cruciate ligament (CrCL) rupture is recognized in 20%–77% of cases (Flo 1993; Williams et al. 1994; Ralphs & Whitney 2002; Mahn et al. 2005; Luther et al. 2007). When CrCL rupture is present in dogs, the medial meniscus, specifically the caudal aspect, is most predisposed to clinically significant injury. The types of injuries commonly seen in dogs include longitudinal, bucket-handle, radial, horizontal, caudal peripheral and complex tears (Figure 31.1). It is imperative that meniscal problems are diagnosed and treated at the time of index surgery in order to ensure optimal relief of pain, debridement of abnormal tissue causing inflammation and degradation, patient recovery, and functional outcomes while minimizing morbidity and the potential need for additional surgeries.

Preoperative diagnosis of meniscal pathology including complete physical examination, joint palpation, and imaging should be comprehensively pursued. These diagnostic approaches are

Advances in the Canine Cranial Cruciate Ligament, Edited by Peter Muir, © 2010 ACVS Foundation, This Work is a co-publication between the American College of Veterinary Surgeons Foundation and Wiley-Blackwell.

addressed in Chapters 15, 19, 20, and 21. Arthroscopy with probing is reported to be the "gold standard" for definitive diagnosis of meniscal pathology because it allows for complete examination with magnification, manipulation of the tissue, and is minimally invasive with low morbidity (Mahn et al. 2005; Pozzi et al. 2008a). Arthrotomy via medial, lateral, or caudomedial approaches with probing is recommended if arthroscopy of the stifle is not possible. Various instruments are available to aid in exposure and access for meniscal assessment and treatment for both arthroscopic and open approaches to stifle surgery. The instruments include probes, Hohmann retractors, micropicks, self-retaining retractors, and distraction devices. The authors highly recommend use of one or more of these instruments for evaluation of the stifle joint. In addition, assessment of the menisci with the joint in flexion and extension, with varus and valgus stress of the joint, and with internal and external rotation of the stifle can improve diagnostic accuracy. Accurate and comprehensive assessment of the menisci is the critical first step in appropriate surgical treatment of meniscal pathology in dogs.

Once meniscal pathology is identified and characterized, three major treatment options can be considered: repair, resection, or release (radial transection). While repair of longitudinal, bucket-

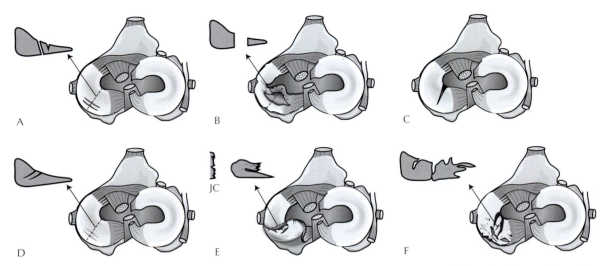

Figure 31.1 Illustrations of longitudinal (A), bucket-handle (B), radial (C), horizontal (D), caudal peripheral (E), and complex (F) tears. JC: joint capsule. Copyright © Samantha J. Elmhurst at www.livingart.org.uk.

handle, and horizontal tears is technically feasible by open or arthroscopic placement of sutures and may be indicated in selected cases (Cook & Fox 2007; Luther et al. 2007; Thieman et al. 2009), the majority of meniscal pathology in dogs is currently treated via resection or release. The lack of success for meniscal repair in most cases in dogs is based on both biologic and biomechanical factors. The primary biologic factors involved are:

1. The majority of tears occur in the axial (inner) 75% of the meniscus, which has no or poor inherent blood supply and low cell density.
2. The majority of dogs with CrCL rupture and meniscal pathology have active osteoarthritis with associated inflammation and degradation processes at work.
3. Meniscal tears in dogs are typically chronic with associated microstructural changes present in the tissue.

The biomechanical issues center on the surgeon's inability to restore normal joint kinematics to the CrCL-deficient stifle. Combined, these detriments to successful healing and restoration of function to damaged menisci suggest that careful decision making regarding meniscal repair in dogs is needed, even when it is technically feasible to accomplish.

Resection of pathologic meniscal tissue is the most commonly recommended and performed treatment for meniscal injuries in dogs at this time. Partial meniscectomy, segmental meniscectomy (or caudal hemimeniscectomy), and total meniscectomy are the three types of resection procedures typically used for dogs (Table 31.1). These can be accomplished arthroscopically or after arthrotomy. Scalpel blades (#11, #15, or Beaver blades), meniscal knives, and arthroscopic basket forceps, scissors, and shavers can be used to perform the resections.

Partial meniscectomy is indicated for longitudinal, bucket-handle, radial, horizontal, and complex tears for which an intact "rim" (peripheral circumferential collagen fiber integrity) can be preserved after resection. Segmental meniscectomy is indicated for all types of tears in the caudal aspect of the meniscus when an intact "rim" cannot be preserved in conjunction with complete resection of pathologic tissue. Total meniscectomy is indicated for tears extending beyond the caudal aspect of the meniscus and for which an intact "rim" cannot be maintained.

There are several key factors to consider for optimizing meniscal resection procedures. First, exposure and access must be achieved such that adjacent structures (articular cartilage, ligaments, etc.) are not damaged during resection. Instru-

Table 31.1 Meniscal resection procedures used in dogs

Procedure	Illustration	Indication
Partial meniscectomy		All meniscal tears that allow for a peripheral rim to be preserved
Segmental meniscectomy (caudal hemimeniscectomy)		Caudal meniscal tears where a functional rim cannot be preserved
Total meniscectomy		All meniscal tears involving more than caudal aspect and rim that cannot be preserved

Note: Images have been reproduced from Johnson et al. (2004), with permission from the American Veterinary Medical Association.

mentation specifically designed for meniscal surgery is recommended for minimizing iatrogenic damage to the articular cartilage during assessment and treatment. Then, two important goals must be balanced in performing the resection:

1. Remove all grossly damaged, displaced, and pathologic meniscal tissue.
2. Preserve as much functional meniscal tissue as possible.

Damaged, displaced, unstable, and pathologic meniscal tissue can cause mechanical dysfunction in the joint, direct articular cartilage damage, inflammation and degradation, with resultant pain, lameness, and progression of osteoarthritis. However, loss or removal of meniscal tissue, especially the peripheral "rim," severely diminishes load bearing, shock absorption, congruency, stability, lubrication, tissue nutrition, and chondro-

protection functions of the meniscus for the joint (see Chapter 4). Clearly, the two goals for treatment of meniscal injuries can be at odds to one another and so careful evaluation and decision making with judicious resection are critical to striking the optimal balance for the patient. The evaluation is based on preoperative imaging in conjunction with careful inspection of the entirety of the meniscus, probing and palpation of meniscal tissue and its attachments, and assessment of the articular cartilage of the femoral condyle and tibial plateau. Healthy, functional meniscal tissue should appear smooth, white, and glistening and not be readily displaced, folded, separated, or penetrated with a blunt meniscal probe. Abnormal meniscal tissue is typically soft, fibrillated, discolored, and abnormal in location, architecture, and/or integrity, and is often associated with local articular cartilage damage. Taken together, these variables help distinguish pathologic from functional meniscal tissue and guide the surgeon in

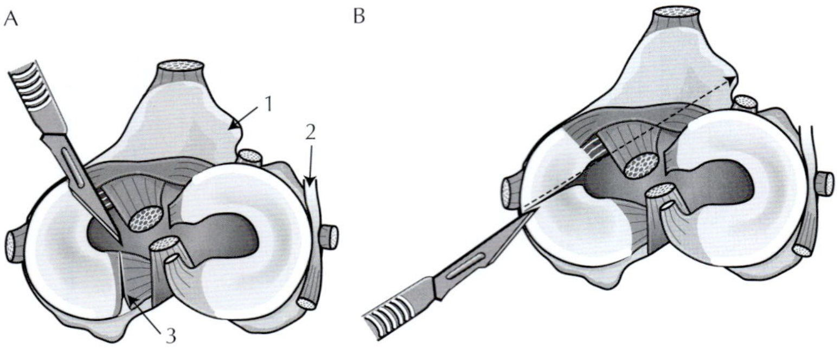

Surgical Treatment

Figure 31.2 Illustrations of caudal (A) and central radial (B) transections of the medial meniscus for meniscal release in dogs. 1: Gerdy's tubercle; 2: popliteal tendon; 3: caudal meniscotibial ligament of the medial meniscus. The radial incision for the central release is made just behind the medial collateral ligament, with the blade aligned with Gerdy's tubercle. Copyright © Samantha J. Elmhurst at www.livingart.org.uk.

determining what to resect and what to preserve.

Meniscal release, or radial transection, is the other procedure commonly performed in dogs for treatment or attempted prevention of meniscal injuries in dogs. This procedure was initially developed and advocated in conjunction with tibial plateau leveling osteotomy (TPLO) based on the high incidence of subsequent medial meniscal injuries diagnosed after initial clinical introduction of TPLO in dogs (Slocum & Slocum 1998). The rationale provided for meniscal release was that because of the inability of TPLO to sufficiently protect the medial meniscus from injury postoperatively, the meniscus should be "released," allowing it to displace, or subluxate, and avoid the damage and clinical problems that were reported to occur after TPLO. In this way, the need for additional surgeries after TPLO could be minimized. It is important to note that it has been suggested that many meniscal injuries diagnosed after the initial surgery for CrCL rupture may instead be tears that were present, but undetected, at the index surgery (Metelman et al. 1995; Thieman et al. 2006). This further highlights the importance of careful observation, inspection, and probing of the menisci during the first surgical procedure.

The radial transection for medial meniscal release can be performed at the caudal meniscal horn–caudal meniscotibial ligament junction (caudal release) or at the mid-body of the meniscus (central release) via arthroscopy or arthrotomy using scalpel blades (#11, #15, or Beaver blades) or meniscal knives (Figure 31.2). While meniscal releases can be associated with significantly lower

risk for clinically apparent subsequent meniscal tears (Thieman et al. 2006), radial transection of the meniscus, regardless of location, completely disrupts the circumferential collagen fiber integrity ("rim") and destroys critical meniscal functions (Pozzi et al. 2006, 2008b; Luther et al. 2009). Released menisci will not functionally heal and will remain biomechanically deficient. Meniscal release alone (in CrCL-intact stifles) in dogs results in articular cartilage loss, further meniscal pathology, osteoarthritis, and lameness within 12 weeks (Luther et al. 2009). In clinical patients with CrCL rupture, however, statistically or clinically significant differences in outcome between groups receiving or not receiving meniscal release have not been noted based on subjective assessments (Thieman et al. 2006). As such, the authors suggest that meniscal release can be justified when the meniscus cannot be fully assessed for pathology and cannot be sufficiently resected safely, or the subsequent meniscal tear rate is unacceptably high to the surgeon and/or clientele. The options, decision-making process, and ramifications associated with meniscal release should be discussed with the client during the preoperative consult and consent to treatment (Table 31.2).

Meniscal injuries concurrent with CrCL rupture in dogs are extremely common. As a good rule of thumb, if you are not recognizing meniscal pathology in at least 50% of your patients with CrCL rupture, it is very likely that you are missing tears. Preoperative assessment by palpation and imaging combined with careful and meticulous intraoperative assessment with probing and palpation of meniscal tissue are the keys to comprehensive diagnosis of meniscal pathology. Once accurate

Table 31.2 Current best evidence for and against use of meniscal release in dogs

Evidence for meniscal release	Evidence against meniscal release
Significantly reduces the rate of subsequent meniscal tears (Thieman et al. 2006)	Does not eliminate subsequent tears (Thieman et al. 2006)
No clinically significant differences in subjective outcome(Thieman et al. 2006)	Eliminates biomechanical functions of meniscus equivalent to total meniscectomy (Pozzi et al. 2006, 2008)
	Released menisci will not functionally heal (Luther et al. 2009)
	Release alone associated with full-thickness cartilage loss, radiographic osteoarthritis, and lameness (Luther et al. 2009)

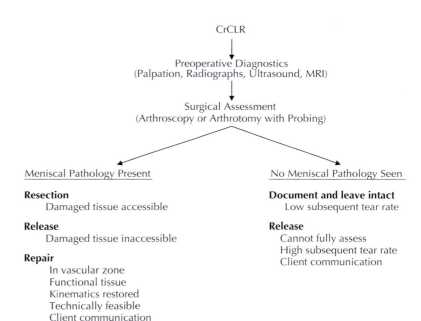

Figure 31.3 Algorithm for decision making regarding surgical treatment of meniscal injuries in dogs. CrCLR: cranial cruciate ligament rupture.

and complete assessment has been performed, a treatment algorithm for meniscal injury concurrent with CrCL rupture can be applied based on the location and severity of the pathology, technical aspects of the various procedures, and subsequent tear rates for the surgeries performed in the individual practice setting (Figure 31.3). Informing the client of the risks and benefits associated with the various options and involving them in the decision-making process is not only appropriate, but imperative, for optimal delivery of care in a patient- and client-based approach to small animal orthopaedic surgery.

References

Cook JL, Fox DB. A novel bioabsorbable conduit augments healing of avascular meniscal tears in a dog model. Am J Sports Med 2007;35:1877–1887.

Flo GL. Meniscal injuries. Vet Clin North Am 1993;23:831–843.

Johnson KA, Francis DJ, Manley PA, et al. Comparison of the effects of caudal pole hemi-meniscectomy and complete medial meniscectomy in the canine stifle joint. Am J Vet Res 2004;65:1053–1060.

Luther JK, Cook CR, Constantinescu IA, et al. Clinical and anatomical correlations of the canine meniscus. J Exp Med Surg Res 2007;14:5–14.

Luther JK, Cook CR, Cook JL. Meniscal release in cruciate ligament intact stifles causes lameness and medial compartment cartilage pathology in dogs 12 weeks postoperatively. Vet Surg 2009;38:520–529.

Mahn MM, Cook JL, Cook CR, Balke MT. Arthroscopic verification of ultrasonographic diagnosis of meniscal pathology in dogs. Vet Surg 2005;34:318–323.

Metelman LA, Schwarz PD, Salman M, et al. An evaluation of three different cranial cruciate ligament surgical stabilization procedures as they relate to postoperative meniscal injuries. Vet Comp Orthop Traumatol 1995;8:118–123.

Pozzi A, Kowaleski MP, Apelt D, et al. Effect of medial meniscal release on tibial translation after tibial plateau leveling osteotomy. Vet Surg 2006;35:486–494.

Pozzi A, Hildreth BE, 3rd, Rajala-Schultz PJ. Comparison of arthroscopy and arthrotomy for diagnosis of medial meniscal pathology: An *ex vivo study*. Vet Surg 2008a;37:749–755.

Pozzi A, Litsky AS, Field J, et al. Pressure distributions on the medial tibial plateau after medial meniscal surgery and tibial plateau levelling osteotomy in dogs. Vet Comp Orthop Traumatol. 2008b;21:8–14.

Ralphs SC, Whitney WO. Arthroscopic evaluation of menisci in dogs with cranial cruciate ligament injuries: 100 cases (1999–2000). J Am Vet Med Assoc 2002;221:1601–1604.

Slocum B, Slocum TD. Meniscal release. In *Current Techniques in Small Animal Surgery*, Bojrab M (ed.), fourth edition. Baltimore: Williams & Wilkins. 1998, pp. 1197–1199.

Thieman KM, Tomlinson JL, Fox DB, et al. Effect of meniscal release on rate of subsequent meniscal tears and owner-assessed outcome in dogs with cruciate disease treated with tibial plateau leveling osteotomy. Vet Surg 2006;35:705–710.

Thieman KM, Pozzi A, Ling H, Lewis DD. The contact mechanics of meniscal repairs and partial meniscectomy as treatment for simulated bucket handle tears in the stifle of dogs. *Proceedings of the Veterinary Orthopedic Society Annual Conference*. Steamboat Springs, CO, 2009, p. 18.

Williams J, Tomlinson J, Constantinescu GM. Diagnosing and treating meniscal injuries in the dog. Vet Med 1994;89:42–47.

32 Meniscal Release

Antonio Pozzi and James L. Cook

Introduction

Meniscal pathology is commonly reported in conjunction with cranial cruciate ligament (CrCL) rupture (Flo 1993; Williams et al. 1994; Ralphs & Whitney 2002; Luther et al. 2007) or at some point after surgical treatment of the CrCL-deficient stifle joint (Metelman et al. 1995; Thieman et al. 2006; Lafaver et al. 2007; Case et al. 2008). Chronic stifle instability from CrCL rupture causes supraphysiologic loading of the menisci, particularly shear and compression of the caudal pole of the medial meniscus, resulting in meniscal tears. When surgical treatments do not fully restore stifle kinematics, as is the case for the majority of surgical procedures, the menisci are still at risk after treatment. Meniscal pathology noted at the time of initial surgery is termed concurrent or coincident, and when diagnosed after surgery it is said to be subsequent, latent, or postliminary. Concurrent meniscal pathology is recognized in 20%–77% of cases (Flo 1993; Williams et al. 1994; Ralphs & Whitney. 2002; Mahn et al. 2005; Luther et al. 2007), while subsequent meniscal injury is recognized in 3%–

Advances in the Canine Cranial Cruciate Ligament,
Edited by Peter Muir, © 2010 ACVS Foundation, This Work is a co-publication between the American College of Veterinary Surgeons Foundation and Wiley-Blackwell.

100% of cases (Metelman et al. 1995; Slocum & Slocum 1998; Thieman et al. 2006; Lafaver et al. 2007; Case et al. 2008). It has been suggested that some cases diagnosed as subsequent meniscal tears may in fact have been concurrent tears that were misdiagnosed (latent tears). The rest of subsequent tears that occur after CrCL surgery are called postliminary tears. Because subsequent tears are often associated with pain and lameness and may necessitate a second surgery, veterinary surgeons have aimed for improved diagnostic approaches to meniscal disease in dogs (see Chapters 19, 20, 21, and 22) and strategies for prevention of subsequent meniscal pathology in a comprehensive approach to CrCL rupture.

One strategy designed to prevent subsequent meniscal injuries is release of the medial meniscus by radial transection. Medial meniscal release is theorized to free the caudal pole from exposure to the abnormal loads delivered during weight-bearing in the CrCL-deficient canine stifle joint (Slocum & Slocum 1998; Kennedy et al. 2005; Pozzi et al. 2006). The clinical goal of meniscal release is to eliminate impingement of the meniscus between femoral and tibial condyles, described as the "wedging phenomenon" (see Chapter 4) and in doing so decrease the likelihood of subsequent meniscal pathology. The theoretical mechanism and clinical goal seem to be realized in most cases. However, the biomechanical and biological consequences are significant, and the procedure is not always effective in accomplishing its objective. Therefore, the pros and cons of meniscal release should be carefully weighed in determining indications and communicating options and prognoses to clients.

Effect of meniscal release on joint biomechanics and biology

Medial meniscal release involves a complete radial transection of the tissue. Several studies have investigated the effects of release on meniscal function to determine if this procedure has detrimental effects on the joint (Pozzi et al. 2006, 2008a, 2010; Luther et al. 2009). The complex material properties and functional anatomy of the meniscus allow it to absorb energy by undergoing constrained elongation, as a load is applied through the stifle (see Chapter 4). As the joint compresses, the wedge-shaped meniscus will normally slightly extrude peripherally as its circumferentially oriented collagen fibers elongate. Extrusion and elongation are limited by the large tensile hoop stress developed within the strong circumferential collagen fiber bundles of the menisci and their cranial and caudal attachments to tibial bone. This hoop stress is critical to normal meniscal functions and joint health. Meniscal release eliminates the ability of the meniscus to develop necessary hoop tension. Similar to a hammock that has lost its anchor points, a released meniscus "collapses"; that is, it undergoes unconstrained extrusion under weight-bearing because of the lack of continuous circumferential fibers with cranial and caudal attachments (see also Chapter 4, Figure 4.4). The radial transection renders the meniscus functionally equivalent to a hemi- or a complete meniscectomy in humans (Pozzi et al. 2008a). Cadaveric studies have shown that radial transections at various locations redistribute and concentrate weight-bearing load to a small area in the caudal aspect of the femorotibial articulation (Figure 32.1; Pozzi et al. 2008a, 2010). As expected, complete radial transection causes a 50% decrease in contact area, a caudal shift in contact pressure, and a 40% increase in the magnitude of articular surface stress in the medial compartment of CrCL-deficient stifles treated with a tibial plateau leveling osteotomy (TPLO;

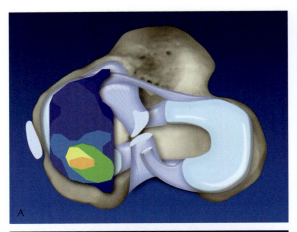

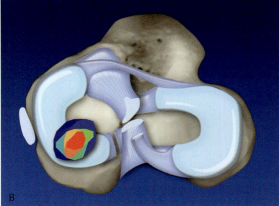

Figure 32.1 Illustration of contact pressures obtained from the Tekscan software (South Boston, MA) in the tibial plateau leveling osteotomy-treated cranial cruciate ligament-deficient stifle with an intact meniscus (A) and after transection of the caudal meniscotibial ligament (B). The caudal meniscal release resulted in reduced area and increased pressure; the load across the medial compartment shifted completely to the caudal half of the compartment. The caudal meniscotibial ligament release and the mid-body release are equivalent because they eliminate the hoop tension and the ability of the meniscus to control the radially directed force developing from axial compression. Reproduced from Pozzi et al. (2010), with permission from Wiley-Blackwell.

Pozzi et al. 2008a, 2010). The contribution of the meniscus to joint stability is also crucial (Pozzi et al. 2006). By effectively deepening the tibial contact surface, the meniscus improves joint congruity and acts as a secondary stabilizer. This role of the intact meniscus is especially important after surgical treatment of the CrCL-deficient stifle since no current modality affords restoration of normal stifle kinematics. Functional menisci may contribute to improved stifle kinematics and contact mechanics after surgery, while meniscal release effectively eliminates the stabilizing properties of the tissue. Loss of these critical functions after meniscal release has severe ramifications for health and function of the stifle joint. Since meniscal release is functionally equivalent to meniscectomy, severe cartilage degeneration can be expected (Fairbank 1948), and an *in vivo* experimental study in dogs showed that meniscal release in CrCL-intact stifles resulted in severe articular cartilage pathology as early as 12 weeks after surgery (Luther et al. 2009; Figures 32.2 and 32.3). In addition, meniscal release alone was associated with lameness, radiographic changes consistent with osteoarthritis, and further meniscal damage in these dogs (Luther et al. 2009). The effect of meniscal release in a CrCL-deficient stifle may be less evident, considering the abnormal joint biomechanics caused by CrCL insufficiency. However, it could be argued that for this reason the meniscus should be preserved at any cost, despite the risk of reoperation because of a subsequent meniscal tear.

Surgical technique

Two types of meniscal release are routinely performed. The abaxial or mid-body or central meniscal release is performed by radial transection of the meniscus immediately caudal to the medial collateral ligament. The axial or meniscotibial ligament or caudal meniscal release is characterized by a radial transection at the junction of the meniscotibial ligament and the caudal pole of the medial meniscus (Kennedy et al. 2005; see Chapter 31). Meniscal release can be performed through an open approach or arthroscopically (Slocum & Slocum 1998; Luther et al. 2009). Regardless of approach, the basic principles of meniscal surgery should be followed:

1. Optimize exposure and joint distraction before performing the release.
2. Use atraumatic surgical technique.

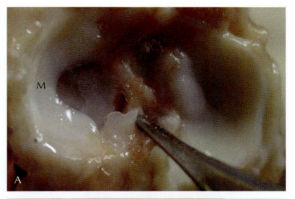
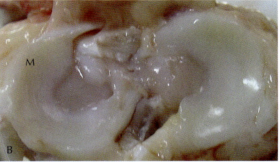

Figure 32.2 Photograph of right tibial plateau of disarticulated right stifle 12 weeks after experimental caudal meniscotibial release (MR) in a stifle with an intact cranial cruciate ligament (A) and sham surgery (B). The metallic probe indicates the junction of the caudal horn and the caudal meniscal ligament of the medial meniscus, where MR was performed. Healing of the caudal horn MR site was minimal and limited to the abaxial region. Notice the gross articular fibrillation on the medial aspect of the tibial plateau. M: medial meniscus. Reproduced from Luther et al. (2009), with permission from Wiley-Blackwell.

Exposure and assessment of the meniscus is a crucial step in performing any meniscal treatment, including meniscal release. For arthrotomy and arthroscopy, the combination of joint distraction, femorotibial subluxation, and varus and valgus stress applied to the stifle allows examination of the entire meniscus in most cases (Pozzi et al. 2008b). Tibial subluxation can be achieved by placing the tip of a Hohmann retractor in the medial aspect of the popliteal notch, caudal to the meniscotibial ligament, and by levering the tibia against the femur. Some surgeons prefer a self-retaining joint distractor placed across the joint to

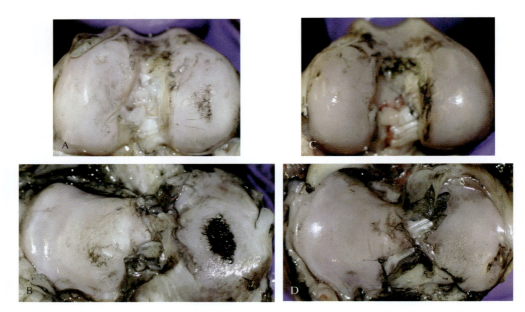

Figure 32.3 Representative gross appearances of India ink-stained articular cartilage surfaces in meniscal release (MR) (A,B) and sham-operated stifle joints (C,D). The photographs were taken immediately after tracings of the articular surfaces and lesions were made. Percent area of cartilage damage was significantly greater in MR than in sham stifles, as indicated here by the darkly stained regions on the medial femoral condyle and tibial plateau. Reproduced from Luther et al. (2009), with permission from Wiley-Blackwell.

achieve more distraction than subluxation. Exposure of the meniscus is more challenging in the stable stifle with a partial CCL rupture. In these cases, debridement of the entire CrCL or exposure of the caudal pole of the meniscus through a caudomedial approach should be considered (Pozzi et al. 2008b). After exposure, every region of the meniscus is accurately probed to evaluate its firmness and smoothness, and for the presence of tears (Pozzi et al. 2008b). Latent tears may occur due to misdiagnosis at the time of the initial joint evaluation (Thieman et al. 2006; Case et al. 2008). Therefore, complete and careful inspection for all types of pathology potentially present is mandatory for comprehensive management of CrCL rupture in dogs. A meticulous surgical technique with an optimal view of the meniscus (arthroscopy, headlamp, appropriate surgical lights) is also necessary to avoid iatrogenic damage to the cartilage, the medial collateral ligament, and the caudal cruciate ligament (Austin et al. 2007).

The mid-body release can be performed using an inside-to-outside or an outside-to-inside technique. For the inside-to-outside technique, a needle is inserted into the joint from outside at the level of the caudal edge of the medial collateral ligament. The needle guides the blade inserted from inside the joint through the entire meniscus. In the outside-to-inside technique, the #11 blade is inserted just caudal to the medial collateral ligament in a direction toward Gerdy's tubercle. Aiming at Gerdy's tubercle should allow the surgeon to transect the meniscus at a 30° craniomedial angle, which is necessary to accomplish a complete release (Slocum & Slocum 1998). To confirm that a complete release has been performed, a probe is used to evaluate the extent of radial transection.

Meniscotibial release is used more commonly in conjunction with craniomedial arthrotomy or arthroscopy. The meniscotibial ligament can be transected with a #11, #15, or Beaver scalpel blade, meniscal knives, or arthroscopic basket forceps or scissors. Radiofrequency probes and electrosurgical devices have also been used but are not recommended by the authors due to the potential for thermal damage to adjacent tissues. The meniscal probe can be used while releasing the meniscus to

Meniscal Release 227

hooked after transection. Another technique entails using a pull-meniscal knife. This instrument allows "hooking" and transecting the whole ligament (Figure 32.4B) and facilitates performing a complete release, potentially decreasing the risk of iatrogenic damage to the joint.

Clinical decision making

Optimal treatment of meniscal injury should alleviate pain while preserving meniscal function. If this principle is applied to clinical decision making regarding an intact meniscus, meniscal release should not be performed because of its impact on meniscal function and consequently joint function (Pozzi et al. 2006, 2008a, 2010; Thieman et al. 2006; Luther et al. 2009). This conservative approach is further supported by the evidence that dogs without meniscal injury and without release have a better short- and long-term outcome (Innes et al. 2000; Luther et al. 2009).

Thorough evaluation of the meniscus should be performed, especially if the meniscus is not released. Latent tears represent a failure of diagnosis at surgery and may result in persistent lameness and require additional surgical treatment. To decrease the risk of latent tears, arthroscopy and meniscal probing are recommended for their high sensitivity and specificity (Mahn et al. 2005; Pozzi et al. 2008b). By improving the diagnosis of tears at the initial joint exploratory surgery, it may be possible to decrease the incidence of late injuries to a point that a release procedure may not be necessary.

Subsequent meniscal tears cause discomfort to the patient and may require costly reoperation. Meniscal release decreases the rate of these tears, thus eliminating the need for revision surgeries in some dogs (Thieman et al. 2006). For this reason, meniscal release could be considered in cases of where there is a high rate of subsequent meniscal injury and when a revision surgery is not acceptable for the owner. However, in these cases, consideration should be given to hemimeniscectomy in place of meniscal release because meniscal tears may still occur despite a meniscal release. The decision of releasing an intact meniscus is complex and should be made after considering several factors including diagnostic approach, type of

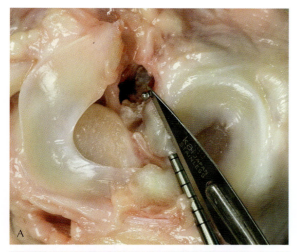
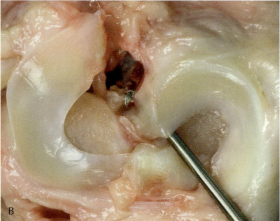

Figure 32.4 (A) Photograph of right tibial plateau illustrating the caudal meniscotibial release using a meniscal probe as a guide for the blade. The meniscal release is completed as the tip of the probe is freed by the meniscal ligament. (B) Photograph of right tibial plateau illustrating the caudal meniscotibial release using a pull-meniscal knife. After hooking the ligament with the knife, traction is applied until the ligament is transected. Care should be taken to avoid hooking the caudal cruciate ligament. The meniscal–tibial ligament should be probed to confirm that the meniscal release is complete. Both techniques can be performed via arthrotomy or arthroscopy.

assure that the whole ligament is transected. The tip of the probe is hooked onto the ligament and the probe is used as a guide for the blade (Figure 32.4A). An incomplete release is recognized using this technique if the tip of the probe remains

CrCL stabilization technique, and client communication (see also Chapter 31, Table 31.1, and Figure 31.3).

References

Austin B, Montgomery RD, Wright J, et al. Evaluation of three approaches to meniscal release. Vet Comp Orthop Traumatol 2007;20(2):92–97.

Case JB, Hulse D, Kerwin SC, et al. Meniscal injury following initial cranial cruciate ligament stabilization surgery in 26 dogs (29 stifles). Vet Comp Orthop Traumatol 2008;21:365–367.

Fairbank TJ. Knee joint changes after meniscectomy. J Bone Joint Surg Br 1948;30:664–670.

Flo GL. Meniscal injuries. Vet Clin North Am 1993;23:831–843.

Innes JF, Bacon D, Lynch C, et al. Long-term outcome of surgery for dogs with cranial cruciate ligament deficiency. Vet Rec 2000;147:325–328.

Kennedy SC, Dunning D, Bischoff MG, et al. The effect of axial and abaxial release on meniscal displacement in the dog. Vet Comp Orthop Traumatol 2005;18:227–234.

Lafaver S, Miller NA, Stubbs WP, et al: Tibial tuberosity advancement for stabilization of the canine cranial cruciate ligament-deficient stifle joint: Surgical technique, early results, and complications in 101 dogs. Vet Surg 2007;36:573–586.

Luther JK, Cook CR, Constantinescu IA, et al. Clinical and anatomical correlations of the canine meniscus. J Exp Med Surg Res 2007;14:5–14.

Luther JK, Cook CR, Cook JL. Meniscal release in cruciate ligament intact stifles causes lameness and medial compartment cartilage pathology in dogs. Vet Surg 2009;38:520–529.

Mahn MM, Cook JL, Cook CR, et al. Arthroscopic verification of ultrasonographic diagnosis of meniscal pathology in dogs. Vet Surg 2005;34:318–323.

Metelman LA, Schwarz PD, Salman M, et al. An evaluation of three different cranial cruciate ligament surgical stabilization procedures as they relate to postoperative meniscal injuries. Vet Comp Orthop Traumatol 1995;8:118–123.

Pozzi A, Kowaleski MP, Apelt D, et al. Effect of medial meniscal release on tibial translation after tibial plateau leveling osteotomy. Vet Surg 2006;35:486–494.

Pozzi A, Litsky AS, Field J, et al. Pressure distributions on the medial tibial plateau after medial meniscal surgery and tibial plateau levelling osteotomy in dogs. Vet Comp Orthop Traumatol 2008a;21:8–14.

Pozzi A, Hildreth BE, Rajala-Schultz PJ. Comparison of arthroscopy and arthrotomy for the diagnosis of medial meniscal pathology: an ex-vivo study. Vet Surg 2008b;37:23–32.

Pozzi A, Kim SE, Lewis DD. Effect of transection of the caudal menisco-tibial ligament on medial femorotibial contact mechanics. Vet Surg 2010, epub.

Ralphs SC, Whitney WO. Arthroscopic evaluation of menisci in dogs with cranial cruciate ligament injuries: 100 cases (1999–2000). J Am Vet Med Assoc 2002;221:1601–1604.

Slocum B, Slocum TD. Meniscal Release, In: *Current Techniques in Small Animal Surgery* Bojrab M (ed.), fourth edition. Baltimore: Williams & Wilkins, 1998, pp. 1197–1199.

Thieman KM, Tomlinson JL, Fox DB, et al. Effect of meniscal release on rate of subsequent meniscal tears and owner-assessed outcome in dogs with cruciate disease treated with tibial plateau leveling osteotomy. Vet Surg 2006;35:705–710.

Williams J, Tomlinson J, Constantinescu, GM. Diagnosing and treating meniscal injuries in the dog. Vet Med 1994;89:42–47.

33 Progression of Arthritis after Stifle Stabilization

John F. Innes

Introduction

Cranial cruciate ligament (CrCL) rupture and osteoarthritis (OA) of the stifle joint are closely linked disease processes. In fact, transection of the CrCL has been one of the most widely studied models of OA since the early 1970s (Pond & Nuki 1973; Gilbertson 1975; McDevitt et al. 1977). Thus, while it is clear that loss of integrity of the CrCL will inevitably initiate the process of OA, what is of great interest to clinicians is the rate at which this will progress and whether there are treatments that will modify that disease progression.

The natural history of the cruciate-deficient canine stifle joint

Information from canine models of OA

Following transection of the CrCL, there are changes in all tissues of the synovial joint. The articular cartilage undergoes a quite dramatic anabolic response with increased cellular activity and

Advances in the Canine Cranial Cruciate Ligament,
Edited by Peter Muir, © 2010 ACVS Foundation, This Work is a co-publication between the American College of Veterinary Surgeons Foundation and Wiley-Blackwell.

mitosis resulting in increased matrix synthesis and an overall increase in tissue mass (Adams & Brandt 1991). However, this anabolic activity is countered by increased catabolic activity with degradation of the collagen network (Fernandes et al. 1998) and increased activity of enzymes degrading the major proteoglycan, aggrecan (Innes et al. 2005). The result of this proteolytic activity is depletion of the cartilage of aggrecan (Figure 33.1), initially in the superficial zone, and disruption of the collagen network. Thus, the compressive stiffness (Figure 33.2) and the tensile strength of the tissue are both reduced. Continued enzymatic activity over many months leads to loss of tissue, such that there may be full-thickness cartilage lesions within 3–5 years (Brandt et al. 1991).

Information from clinical imaging studies

The time frame of experimentally induced canine stifle OA is relatively long, but one study of a clinical cohort suggests that the progression to end-stage OA in the cruciate-deficient stifle joint is associated with clinical deterioration in dogs as assessed at 50 months after surgical stabilization (Innes et al. 2000). There are only a small number of radiographic studies of clinical canine cohorts that address the progression of OA after surgical intervention for CrCL rupture. Radiographic

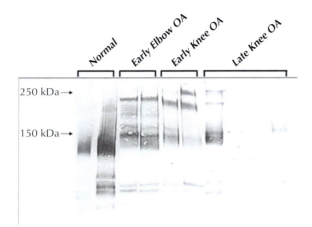

Figure 33.1 Proteoglycan is depleted from canine articular cartilage in osteoarthritis (OA) of the stifle joint through the action of aggrecanase enzymes. In early stifle OA, aggrecanase activity causes release of large aggrecan fragments (approximately 250 kDa), which are not seen in healthy joints. In late-stage stifle OA, there are very few aggrecanase-generated proteoglycan fragments because the tissue has been depleted of aggrecan. Reproduced from Innes et al. (2005), with permission from the American Veterinary Medical Association.

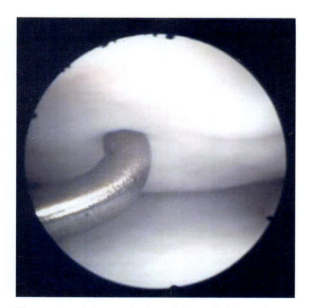

Figure 33.2 Arthroscopic view of the medial femoral condyle in a stifle joint with cranial cruciate ligament rupture. Note the probe sinks easily in to the articular cartilage, indicating loss of compressive stiffness through aggrecan depletion and loss of tensile strength through disruption of the collagen network.

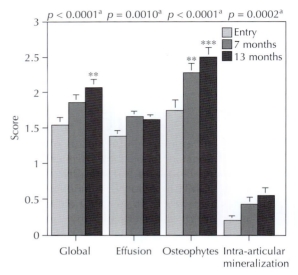

Figure 33.3 Longitudinal changes in mean radiographic scores for 45 stifle joints treated with intracapsular over-the-top fascial graft. Progression in osteophytosis appears most rapid between study entry and 7 months sampling point. [a]Friedman's repeated measures test; Dunnett's post-hoc multiple comparisons test: **, $p < 0.01$; ***, $p < 0.001$. Reproduced from Innes et al. (2004), with permission from Wiley-Blackwell.

assessment of OA is not an ideal method of disease assessment because radiographs only provide information on bony changes such as osteophytosis and sclerosis, and a very limited degree of information regarding soft tissues. Critically, radiographs cannot provide information on femorotibial joint cartilage status. However, all such studies indicate that osteophytosis often continues to progress in the cruciate-deficient stifle joint (Elkins et al. 1991; Vasseur & Berry 1992; Innes et al. 2004; Rayward et al. 2004). One prospective study with three sampling points indicated that osteophyte growth may be more active in the first 7 months after surgery, compared with the period between 7 and 13 months (Innes et al. 2004; Figures 33.3 and 33.4). Interestingly, within this cohort, 45% of dogs were judged not to have progressed on a 4-point global disease severity score. In a similar, but shorter study, 40 dogs that had received tibial plateau leveling osteotomy

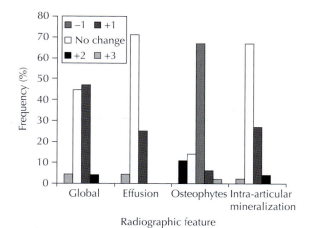

Figure 33.4 Distribution of change over 13 months in the same 45 stifle joints as in Figure 33.3. Reproduced from Innes et al. (2004), with permission from Wiley-Blackwell.

(TPLO) were assessed at entry and 6 months; 57% were judged not to have progressed on a 5-point global scoring system (Rayward et al. 2004). Given the shorter nature of this second study, it is likely that radiographic progression of OA is similar for TPLO when compared with the over-the-top technique, but direct comparison studies are required to investigate this.

One study has evaluated changes in the femoropatellar joint space (FPJS; Innes et al. 2002). The concept behind this study was that, with the stifle joint in flexion and hence the FPJS loaded, one can infer cartilage thickness from measuring the interbone distance at the narrowest point of the FPJS. In a cohort of 53 dogs, the FPJS in the index joint was significantly greater than that in the contralateral stifle joint. The FPJS had a strong independent correlation with bodyweight (bigger dogs have bigger joint spaces) and stifle joint flexion angle (greater flexion decreases the joint space). There is also evidence of a weaker, negative, independent effect of age. This latter finding is interesting in that it suggests that older dogs have less cartilage, or have a less anabolic response in the cartilage, compared with younger dogs. In the temporal analysis of FPJS over a 13-month period, the FPJS width increased significantly in the first 7 months of this prospective study. The results indicate a moderate to strong positive relationship between bodyweight at baseline and change in FPJS from entry to 7 months (i.e., a greater bodyweight tends toward a greater increase in FPJS). To a lesser extent, bodyweight also related positively to FPJS change from 7 to 13 months. Overall, this study concurs with studies in experimentally induced stifle OA, that the articular cartilage undergoes a hypertrophic response in the first months after loss of CrCL function. None of the published imaging studies to date suggest that any of the current surgical treatments are disease-modifying in terms of OA (Sanderson et al. 2009).

Information from biomarker studies

Biochemical markers of joint tissue metabolism are another method with which to probe disease mechanisms in OA. Such biomarkers typically detect macromolecules (or fragments thereof) released from synovial joint tissues, particularly articular cartilage, and they may be measured in synovial fluid, serum, or urine. Clearly, in a local disease such as OA, measurement in synovial fluid is preferred.

The concentrations of markers may increase or decrease following initiation of stifle OA (Thonar et al. 1991; Innes et al. 1998, 1999), and this may reflect increased degradation of certain molecules, increased synthesis of molecules, which are then released in greater quantity, or a change in molecular structure, such as sulfation of aggrecan. All of these factors can influence the amount of a biomarker detected. Probably the more useful markers are those that reflect degradation of key molecules such as type II collagen (Lopez et al. 2006), aggrecan, and cartilage oligomeric matrix protein (COMP) (Carlson et al. 2002; Qi & Changlin 2007). However, studies of such markers in dogs are limited to date and some of the results are conflicting (Hayashi et al. 2009). However, there is evidence that concentrations of certain markers may change after intra-articular CrCL replacement (Innes et al. 1999), but TPLO was found not to alter concentrations of the 5D4 epitope of keratan sulfate, nor COMP (Girling et al. 2006). Further study of biomarkers will hopefully be useful in providing a surrogate method to assess articular cartilage status.

Summary

The continued progression of OA after surgical treatment of the cruciate-deficient stifle joint remains one of the major challenges facing clinicians and scientists. To date, no surgical technique or medical treatment has been demonstrated to halt or slow this progression in the clinical setting.

References

Adams ME, Brandt KD. Hypertrophic repair of canine articular cartilage in osteoarthritis after anterior cruciate ligament transection. J Rheumatol 1991;18:428–435.

Brandt KD, Myers SL, Burr D, et al. Osteoarthritic changes in canine articular cartilage, subchondral bone, and synovium fifty-four months after transection of the anterior cruciate ligament. Arthritis Rheum 1991;34:1560–1570.

Carlson CS, Guilak F, Vail TP, et al. Synovial fluid biomarker levels predict articular cartilage damage following complete medial meniscectomy in the canine knee. J Orthop Res 2002;20:92–100.

Elkins AD, Pechman R, Karrey MT, et al. A retrospective study evaluating the degree of degenerative joint diseases in the stifle joint of dogs following surgical repair of anterior cruciate ligament rupture. J Am Anim Hosp Assoc 1991;27:533–540.

Fernandes JC, Martel-Pelletier JM, Lascau-Coman VL, et al. Collagenase-1 and collagenase-3 synthesis in normal and early experimental osteoarthritic canine cartilage: An immunohistochemical study. J Rheumatol 1998;25:1585–1594.

Gilbertson E. Development of periarticular osteophytes in experimentally induced osteoarthritis in the dog. A study using microradiographic, microangiographic and fluorescent bone-labelling techniques. Ann Rheum Dis 1975;34:12–25.

Girling SL, Bell SC, Whitelock RG, et al. Use of biochemical markers of osteoarthritis to investigate the potential disease-modifying effect of tibial plateau levelling osteotomy. J Small Anim Pract 2006;47:708–714.

Hayashi K, Kim SY, Landsdowne JL, et al. Evaluation of a collagenase generated osteoarthritis biomarker in naturally occurring canine cruciate disease. Vet Surg 2009;38:117–121.

Innes JF, Sharif M, Barr ARS. Relations between biochemical markers of osteoarthritis and other disease parameters in a population of dogs with naturally acquired osteoarthritis of the genual joint. Am J Vet Res 1998;59:1530–1536.

Innes JF, Sharif M, Barr ARS. Changes in concentrations of biochemical markers of osteoarthritis following surgical repair of ruptured cranial cruciate ligaments in dogs. Am J Vet Res 1999;60:1164–1168.

Innes JF, Bacon D, Lynch C, et al. Long-term outcome of surgery for dogs with cranial cruciate ligament deficiency. Vet Rec 2000;147:325–328.

Innes JF, Shepstone L, Holder J, et al. Changes in the canine femoropatellar joint space in the postsurgical, cruciate-deficient stifle joint. Vet Radiol Ultrasound 2002;43:241–248.

Innes JF, Costello M, Barr FJ, et al. Radiographic progression of osteoarthritis of the canine stifle joint: A prospective study. Vet Radiol Ultrasound 2004;45:143–148.

Innes JF, Little CB, Hughes E, et al. Products resulting from cleavage of the interglobular domain of aggrecan in samples of synovial fluid collected from dogs with early- and late-stage osteoarthritis. Am J Vet Res 2005;66:1679–1685.

Lopez MJ, Robinson SO, Quinn MM, et al. In vivo evaluation of intra-articular protection in a novel model of canine cranial cruciate ligament mid-substance elongation injury. Vet Surg 2006;35:711–720.

McDevitt C, Gilbertson E, Muir H. An experimental model of osteoarthritis; early morphological and biochemical changes. J Bone Joint Surg Br 1977;59:24–35.

Pond M, Nuki G. Experimentally induced osteoarthritis in the dog. Ann Rheum Dis 1973;32:387–388.

Qi C, Changlin H. Levels of biomarkers correlate with magnetic resonance imaging progression of knee cartilage degeneration: a study on canine. Knee Surg Sports Traumatol Arthrosc 2007;15:869–878.

Rayward RM, Thomson DG, Davies JV, et al. Progression of osteoarthritis following TPLO surgery: A prospective radiographic study of 40 dogs. J Small Anim Pract 2004;45:92–97.

Sanderson RO, Beata C, Flipo RM, et al. Systematic review of the management of canine osteoarthritis. Vet Rec 2009;164:418–424.

Thonar EJ, Manicourt DM, Williams J, et al. Circulating keratan sulfate: A marker of cartilage proteoglycan catabolism in osteoarthritis. J Rheumatol 1991;27:S24–26.

Vasseur PB, Berry CR. Progression of stifle osteoarthrosis following reconstruction of the cranial cruciate ligament in 21 dogs. J Am Anim Hosp Assoc 1992;28:129–136.

34 Residual Lameness after Stifle Stabilization Surgery

Michael G. Conzemius and Richard B. Evans

Introduction

When deciding what, or even if, surgery should be performed for rupture of the cranial cruciate ligament (CrCL), one needs to understand the probability of success and failure for each treatment option. In addition, it is important to be able to comprehend the outcome measures that are reported in a manuscript and how the data and conclusions might apply to an owner's pet. Several outcome measures can be considered, including gathering information from the pet owner such as using a quality of life owner questionnaire or having them monitor the frequency their pet needs to take anti-inflammatory diets or medications for its best performance. Documenting findings from the veterinarian and objectively measuring the quality and quantity of limb function in the operated leg should also be performed. The purpose of this chapter is to briefly describe various methods of measuring limb function and to review limb function after stifle stabilization surgery.

Advances in the Canine Cranial Cruciate Ligament,
Edited by Peter Muir, © 2010 ACVS Foundation, This Work is a co-publication between the American College of Veterinary Surgeons Foundation and Wiley-Blackwell.

Owner questionnaire

Since the owner spends the most time with the pet and generally pays the bills for surgical repair, it makes perfect sense to establish the owner's perspective on outcome. The opinion of the owner is likely used during everyday practice and has been included in many study designs to determine outcome after surgical treatment of dogs with CrCL rupture (Hoffmann et al. 2006; Corr & Brown 2007; Stein & Schmoekel 2008). In those manuscripts, owners reported that their pets had a "good or excellent" outcome 88.5%–93% of the time. These findings, however, must be interpreted with caution in most studies because the use of questionnaires had not been validated. In addition, comparisons between studies must be avoided because the questions between studies are different, the postoperative follow-up is different, and even the methods of questionnaire delivery (mail, phone, or personnel interview) are different. Publication of the Canine Brief Pain Inventory (CBPI) for dogs with osteoarthritis (OA) provides reasonable evidence that owner questionnaires can be effectively used in clinical research (Brown et al. 2008). In this study, a series of questions were provided to owners of dogs with OA. The dogs were treated with either a nonsteroidal anti-inflammatory drug (NSAID) or a placebo, and owners were blinded to the treatment. Owners completed the questionnaire before and after treatment. Owners of dogs treated with the NSAID reported that their pets, on average, improved, while owners of dogs treated with the placebo reported that their pets, on average, did not improve. The CBPI validation study was based on dogs with chronic OA in one or many joints, so some uncertainty exists with how it can be translated to a pet's recovery from surgical treatment of CrCL rupture. In addition, it is important to remember that owners have innate biases because they are also the client (i.e , paid the bill); they participated in the decision to have surgery performed; they may have chosen what surgery to have; and they have variable experience with dogs. Given this, study design is of paramount importance when using owner questionnaires with particular consideration to patient dropouts, randomization, study power, and effect size.

Additional information that can be gathered from the owner that is commonly overlooked is changes in the pattern of medication use. For example, it would be useful information if in a study comparing two different surgical stabilization techniques for CrCL rupture it were reported that the dogs in one group used nonsteroidal anti-inflammatory medications more often than did dogs in the other group. Although there are obvious reliability issues whenever the owners are involved, investigators can use prescription boxes and mandatory calendars to limit data entry errors. These types of questions are clinically relevant and provide objective data to help detect differences between groups.

One important fact regarding owner questionnaires is that they may not necessarily address limb function, but the owner's perception of the dog's quality of life. If we are specifically interested in quality and quantity of limb function, more objective and sensitive outcome measures exist. Perhaps this is a reasonable explanation why we would suggest that the ideal study include both objective measures of limb function and owner questionnaire.

Veterinary exam

After surgery, a clinician may assign a subjective score to limb function based on his or her assessment of the dog's gait, stance, and posture while sitting. While each clinician differs to some degree, observations when the patient is walking and/or trotting may include a dip in the patient's hip or head, degree of limb carriage, and stride length. During physical exam, the clinician may note the joint's range of motion, the amount of muscle mass, and even whether the leg is positioned "normally" when sitting. All of these can contribute to a determination of the patient's quality of limb function. Findings are generally recorded via a numeric rating score (NRS), where numbers are assigned to each finding, or a visual analog scale (VAS), where limb function is assigned by marking a line with one end representing clinically normal (sound) and the other end representing could not be more lame (i.e., non-weight-bearing) (Waxman et al. 2008). The NRS is limited because there are a restricted number of categories (4 or 5) within a classification, and dogs within a NRS category can have appreciable differences in their lameness severity (Waxman et al. 2008). A VAS does not have this limitation because it provides a continuous scale, which may be easier to handle statistically. Regardless, both provide only the opinion of the observer. Several manuscripts have tried to offset these limitations by including multiple, trained observers. Unfortunately, a recent publication that tried to validate clinician observation of gait reported that neither trained nor untrained observers could reliably identify lameness; that there were large disagreements between individuals; and that untrained observers (first-semester veterinary students) had the same visual acuity for dog lameness as boarded surgeons (Waxman et al. 2008). The only saving grace was a finding that trained clinicians provided repeatable data; that is, they consistently made the same mistake. This would allow a clinician to compare groups over time, but not necessarily comment on outcome of an individual dog.

Pedometers and accelerometers

The greatest limitation to data that are collected at a veterinary hospital is that they measure a moment in time, not the day-to-day level of activity of the dog at home. A pedometer or an accelerometer can be used to measure patient activity level at home over an extended period. In one study, pedometers were successfully used to measure physical activity in dogs over a 14-day period (Chan et al. 2005). Pedometer accuracy varied depending on the patient's size (overestimated walking in large dogs and underestimated walking in small dogs) but correlated well with overall reports of the dog's activity level at home and the dog's condition body score. Accelerometers are a little more sophisticated in that some can measure changes in acceleration in the x-, y-, and z-axes. Thus, body movement in any direction is measured. In one study that determined variability in accelerometer data in companion dogs, it was reported that large day-to-day and even week-to-week variations occurred in dogs, but within dogs, a full 7-day comparison of total activity counts from 1 week to the next provided the least variable estimate of the dogs' activity (Dow et al. 2009). The authors of the study just mentioned also reported that accelerometers may be most useful for documenting changes in the dog's activity over time.

Given the limitations that both pedometers and accelerometers have in their estimates of a patient's activity level, these methods are probably suited for use in studies that seek to compare large groups of dogs that have similar body sizes and shapes. To the authors' knowledge, these methods have not been applied to dogs after CrCL surgery, and their use would be beneficial for outcome comparisons.

Computational gait analysis

Force platform gait analysis provides an objective, sensitive method to measure gait. More specifically, ground reaction forces (GRF) are measured and the clinician can use this tool to check a dog's limb function during a single exam (perhaps to document which leg the dog is using the least) or for change over time. Force platform gait analysis has been used extensively to compare forces before and after surgery for stabilization of the CrCL-deficient stifle in clinical patients (Budsberg et al. 1988; Dupuis et al. 1994; Jevens et al. 1996; Conzemius et al. 2005) and is recognized by many as the gold standard outcome measure for orthopaedic conditions such as CrCL rupture. While documen-

tation of GRFs is a powerful tool in veterinary orthopaedics, it must be performed and interpreted correctly. Careful attention to patient velocity, acceleration, and statistical evaluation of the data is necessary (Evans et al. 2003, 2005). In addition, many investigators have limited the usefulness of the data by only evaluating group means. While this is important information for group comparisons (it has been demonstrated by measuring GRFs that lateral retinacular stabilization and TPLO provide similar outcomes, but over-the-top stabilization outcomes are inferior), it can be lost in translation to an owner that is concerned about his or her individual dog (Conzemius et al. 2005). In one study, GRFs were evaluated to determine the probability that a single patient would return to normal function (Conzemius et al. 2005). When an 80% probability cutoff was used, it was quite uncommon (15%–40% chance) for a dog to return to normal function regardless of which surgical procedure was performed. In addition, the investigators suggested that a dog had a clinically significant improvement if its GRFs were more normal than abnormal. Normal was defined by the GRFs of normal dogs and abnormal by the preoperative GRFs of the patient (Conzemius et al. 2005). While one would assume that the majority of dogs are more normal than abnormal 6 months after surgery, the opposite was found (Figure 34.1 and 34.2). Presenting data in this manner provides information that is clinically relevant to the individual patient and reveals, that as surgeons, we still have quite of bit of room for improvement.

Pressure platform gait analysis can also be used and has specific advantages and disadvantages that are relevant for clinical research. First, it is important to note that the vertical forces measured by Tekscan's Industrial Sensing pressure measurement system (Tekscan, South Boston, MA) has been compared with traditional force platform gait analysis and the data are comparable (Besancon et al. 2003). However, the data are not interchangeable because pressure mats consistently underestimate vertical forces; thus, studies should choose one method or the other. This system has been used successfully to evaluate limb function in dogs after surgery to stabilize the cruciate-deficient stifle (Horstman et al. 2004). Three key advantages of the pressure platform mats include

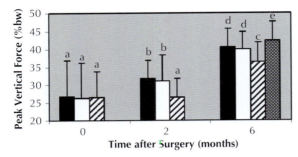

Figure 34.1 Bar graph showing mean peak vertical force (PVF) ± SD of clinically normal dogs (▨ [6 months only]) and dogs with rupture of the cranial cruciate ligament treated with tibial plateau leveling osteotomy (■), lateral suture stabilization (□), or intracapsular stabilization (▨) before surgery and at 2 and 6 months after surgery. Different letter assignments signify statistical difference among groups across all three time points ($p < 0.05$). BW: body weight. Reproduced from Conzemius et al. (2005), with permission from the American Veterinary Medical Association.

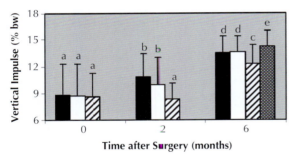

Figure 34.2 Bar graph showing mean vertical impulse (VI) ± SD of clinically normal dogs (▨ [6 months only]) and dogs with rupture of the cranial cruciate ligament treated with tibial plateau leveling osteotomy (■), lateral suture stabilization (□), or intracapsular stabilization (▨) before surgery and at 2 and 6 months after surgery. Different letter assignments signify statistical difference among groups across all three time points ($p < 0.05$). BW: body weight. Reproduced from Conzemius et al. (2005), with permission from the American Veterinary Medical Association.

the fact that they are portable, can measure dogs of very small and large sizes, and, if one uses a pressure platform walkway, they can measure consecutive foot strikes, which dramatically decreases trial variance and the time necessary to collect data. The greatest limitation is that they only measure vertical forces.

Finally, two- or three-dimensional kinematics has been used to evaluate a dog's gait after surgery for a CrCL injury (DeCamp et al. 1996; Marsolais et al. 2003) and represents an excellent noninvasive method to measure joint angles and angular limb velocities. Unfortunately, the power of this methodology is rarely captured in a clinical environment because of the cost of the equipment and the time and expertise necessary to perform it correctly.

Additional consideration regarding residual lameness

Three additional potential contributors to residual lameness in a dog after surgery to stabilize the cruciate-deficient stifle are development of complications, progression of OA, and instability. While many complications are avoidable, their exclusion is impossible. Complication rates have been reported in many studies, and their relative frequency between various stabilization techniques has been estimated by some authors. At this point, however, the definition of a complication (e.g., acute vs. chronic, mild vs. severe) varies enough between authors that comparing surgical techniques is fruitless. Certainly, one can surmise that surgical techniques (arthroscopy vs. arthrotomy, lateral suture vs. tibial plateau leveling osteotomy [TPLO]) that are less invasive would have fewer complications, but until these outcomes are uniformly measured, it remains only a hypothesis. One important concept to accept is that complications (even small complications) are more than just an inconvenience; they affect long-term outcome. Voss et al. used force platform gait analysis to determine outcome in dogs after tibial tuberosity advancement and reported that, while most dogs returned to a function that was 90% of the normal dogs they studied, 25% of the cases had a complication and these dogs had GRFs that were significantly lower than when no complication occurred (Voss et al. 2008).

OA and its progression is inevitable in most cases regardless of the surgical technique used. While the severity of stifle OA is not correlated with the severity of lameness (Gordon et al. 2003), certainly dogs with OA have a greater probability of lameness than their counterparts. Much of this assertion could be related to the limitations of plain radiographs. MRI, using delayed gadolinium-enhanced magnetic resonance imaging of cartilage (dGEMRIC) or T2 mapping, can generate objective information regarding the health of the cartilage and has been shown to be related to OA progression and patient prognosis (Cunningham et al. 2006; Welsch et al. 2009). One aspect of stifle surgery that some surgeons consider routine is release of the medial meniscus. This is done, we assume, so the medial meniscus does not tear after surgery. One fact that surgeons should consider is that release of the medial meniscal rapidly (within 12 weeks) causes OA and lameness even in a stable stifle (Luther et al. 2009). In addition, we should accept that medial meniscal tears occur more commonly in an unstable stifle than in a stable stifle; thus, if the stabilization procedure performed requires a release of the medial meniscus, then an important question is how effective the procedure is at stabilizing the cruciate-deficient stifle joint. Empirically, meniscal pathology and OA are the greatest limitations to outcome after surgery for CrCL rupture. This suggestion is supported by a small study that evaluated dogs with chronic lameness (>3 months) from surgical treatment for CrCL rupture, minimal instability, and a medial meniscal tear (Conzemius 2007). In that study, outcome was measured objectively using GRFs in dogs that had either arthroscopic debridement of the CrCL and medial meniscus or arthroscopic debridement and TPLO stabilization; no differences were found between groups. (Figure 34.3).

For decades veterinary surgeons have debated which surgical procedure provides the best outcome. One component of this debate is establishing that the procedure in question adequately stabilizes the stifle. This is based on the assumption that the degree of instability is related to the degree of lameness. We use the word assumption because the evidence provided to date does not state that instability is good, but does suggest that it may not be all that bad. In one follow-up study after stifle stabilization surgery for CrCL rupture (Hill et al. 1999), dogs were divided into groups, based on owner interview at more than 1 year after surgery, as having either a satisfactory or

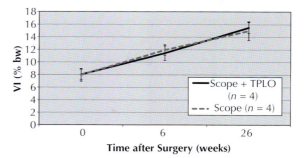

Figure 34.3 Graph showing vertical impulse of dogs before arthroscopic surgery and at 2 and 6 months after surgery. In a group of dogs with cranial cruciate ligament rupture and a medial meniscal tear, dogs treated with only arthroscopic debridement of the ruptured cranial cruciate ligament and medial meniscus were compared with dogs that received arthroscopic debridement together with tibial plateau leveling osteotomy (TPLO). No differences were found between groups.

unsatisfactory outcome. Surprisingly, dogs in the satisfactory outcome group had almost twice the degree of instability and less than half the stifle pain of dogs in the unsatisfactory outcome group on physical exam.

Conclusion

Over the years, our ability to develop sound outcome measures to determine if lameness still persists has improved. While it appears that surgical management can improve lameness in most dogs with CrCL rupture, the unfortunate fact is that we have yet to develop a surgical procedure (whether it includes stabilization or not) that eliminates lameness.

References

Besancon MF, Conzemius MG, Derrick TR, Ritter MJ. Comparison of vertical forces in normal dogs between the AMTI Model OR6-5 force platform and the Tekscan (industrial sensing pressure measurement system) pressure walkway. Vet Comp Orthop Traumatol 2003;16:153–157.

Brown DC, Boston RC, Coyne JC, Farrar JT. Ability of the Canine Brief Pain Inventory to detect response to treatment in dogs with osteoarthritis. J Am Vet Med Assoc 2008;233:1278–1283.

Budsberg SC, Verstraete MC, Soutas-Little RW, et al. Force plate analyses before and after stabilization of canine stifles for cruciate injury. Am J Vet Res 1988;49:1522–1524.

Chan CB, Spierenburg M, Ihle SL, Tudor-Locke C. Use of pedometers to measure physical activity in dogs. J Am Vet Med Assoc 2005;226:2010–2015.

Conzemius MG. Stabilization of the cranial cruciate ligament deficient knee: Do we need it?. *Proceedings of the American College of Veterinary Surgeons Annual Symposium*. Chicago, 2007, p. 332.

Conzemius MG, Evans RJ, Besancon MF, et al. Effect of surgical technique on limb function after surgery for rupture of the cranial cruciate ligament in dogs. J Am Vet Med Assoc 2005;226:232–239.

Corr SA, Brown C. A comparison of outcomes following tibial plateau leveling osteotomy and cranial tibial wedge osteotomy procedures. Vet Comp Orthop Traumatol 2007;20:312–319.

Cunningham T, Jessel R, Zurakowski D, et al. Delayed gadolinium-enhanced magnetic resonance imaging of cartilage to predict early failure of Bernese periacetabular osteotomy for hip dysplasia. J Bone Joint Surg Am 2006;88:1540–1548.

DeCamp CE, Riggs CM, Olivier NB, et al. Kinematic evaluation of gait in dogs with cranial cruciate ligament rupture. Am J Vet Res 1996;57:120–126.

Dow C, Michel KE, Love M, Brown DC. Evaluation of optimal sampling interval for activity monitoring in companion dogs. Am J Vet Res 2009;70:444–448.

Dupuis J, Harari J, Papageorges M, et al. Evaluation of fibular head transposition for repair of experimental cranial cruciate ligament injury in dogs. Vet Surg 1994;23:1–12.

Evans RB, Gordon W, Conzemius M. The effect of velocity on ground reaction forces in dogs with lameness attributable to tearing of the cranial cruciate ligament. Am J Vet Res 2003;64:1479–1481.

Evans R, Horstman C, Conzemius M. Accuracy and optimization of force platform gait analysis in Labradors with cranial cruciate disease evaluated at the walking gait. Vet Surg 2005;34:445–449.

Gordon WJ, Conzemius MG, Riedesel E, et al. The relationship between limb function and radiographic osteoarthrosis in dogs with stifle osteoarthrosis. Vet Surg 2003;32:451–454.

Hill CM, Conzemius MG, Smith GK, et al. Bacterial culture of the canine stifle joint following surgical repair of ruptured cranial cruciate ligament. Vet Comp Orthop Traumatol 1999;12:1–5.

Hoffmann DE, Miller JM, Ober CP, et al. Tibial tuberosity advancement in 65 canine stifles. Vet Comp Orthop Traumatol 2006;19:219–227.

Horstman CL, Conzemius MG, Evans R, Gordon WJ. Assessing the efficacy of perioperative oral carprofen after cranial cruciate surgery using noninvasive, objective pressure platform gait analysis. Vet Surg 2004;33:286–289.

Jevens DJ, DeCamp CE, Hauptman J, et al. Use of force-plate analysis of gait to compare two surgical techniques for treatment of cranial cruciate ligament rupture in dogs. Am J Vet Res 1996;57:389–393.

Luther JK, Cook CR, Cook JL. Meniscal release in cruciate ligament intact stifles causes lameness and medial compartment cartilage pathology in dogs 12 weeks postoperatively. Vet Surg 2009;38:520–529.

Marsolais GS, McLean S, Derrick T, Conzemius MG. Kinematic analysis of the hind limb during swimming and walking in healthy dogs and dogs with surgically corrected cranial cruciate ligament rupture. J Am Vet Med Assoc 2003;222:739–743.

Stein S, Schmoekel H. Short-term and eight to 12 months results of a tibial tuberosity advancement as treatment of canine cranial cruciate ligament damage. J Small Anim Pract 2008;49:398–404.

Voss K, Damur DM, Guerrero T, et al. Force plate gait analysis to assess limb function after tibial tuberosity advancement in dogs with cranial cruciate ligament disease. Vet Comp Orthop Traumatol 2008;21:243–249.

Waxman AW, Robinson DA, Evans R, et al. Relationship between objective and subjective assessment of limb function in normal dogs with an experimentally induced lameness. Vet Surg 2008;37:241–246.

Welsch GH, Mamisch TC, Marlovits S, et al. Quantitative T2 mapping during follow-up after matrix-associated autologous chondrocyte transplantation (MCAT): Full-thickness and zonal evaluation to visualize the maturation of cartilage repair tissue. J Orthop Res 2009;27:957–963.

Section V

Medical Management of Cruciate Rupture

Introduction

Although several new nonsteroidal anti-inflammatory drugs have entered the veterinary market over the last several years, a limited number of different types of drug are available for treatment of stifle arthritis. In contrast a plethora of nutritional supplements are available, although evidence of clinical efficacy for many nutritional supplements is limited. Until recently, the role of rehabilitation for dogs affected with the cruciate rupture arthropathy has been underappreciated.

This section provides a detailed discussion of current medical therapies commonly used for treatment of dogs affected with the cruciate rupture arthropathy.

35 Medical Therapy for Stifle Arthritis

Gayle H. Jaeger and Steven C. Budsberg

Introduction

Osteoarthritis (OA) of the stifle joint is a progressive degenerative disease that can have a profound impact on quality of life (Vasseur & Berry 1992; Lazar et al. 2005). The clinical signs of stifle OA include discomfort, limited joint range of motion, loss of muscle mass and muscle tone, and decreased overall limb use. Additionally, chronic discomfort and nociceptive input can lead to modulation of the central nervous system, referred to as "spinal windup," amplifying the primary disease and systemic effect while impairing the response to therapy (Johnston 1997). Although OA is considered a chronic progressive disease, the clinical picture may be quite dynamic with intermittent periods of acute signs or "flare ups" and periods of clinical quiescence. In addition, there also appears to be variation in the clinical impact between individual dogs.

The goals of medical management are to minimize the clinical signs of OA, maintain or improve limb use, and, if possible, slow the progression of the disease. Multimodal therapy can yield a better

Advances in the Canine Cranial Cruciate Ligament,
Edited by Peter Muir, © 2010 ACVS Foundation, This Work is a co-publication between the American College of Veterinary Surgeons Foundation and Wiley-Blackwell.

response in the treatment of OA through the synergism of various therapies acting in noncompeting modes of action. This allows for the administration of collectively lower doses of medication, decreasing the potential side effects of any one treatment prescribed (Altman et al. 2000). In addition to nonsteroidal anti-inflammatory drugs (NSAIDs), multimodal therapy for the treatment of OA also incorporates weight loss, exercise modification, rehabilitation, and dietary changes (Argoff 2002; Budsberg & Bartges 2006; Johnston et al. 2008). Additionally, adjunctive analgesics, chondromodulating agents, nutraceuticals, and other dietary supplements may be used.

Weight management

The importance of weight management in the prevention and treatment of OA cannot be overestimated. A substantial portion of our patient population is obese. Obesity, defined as 15–20% over the ideal body weight, places excessive forces on the joint and articular cartilage and is exacerbated by inactivity, propagating a vicious cycle of muscle atrophy and a decline in overall fitness (Impellizeri et al. 2000; Kealy et al. 2000). There is not a clear cause and effect relationship between obesity and OA; however, fat is considered a metabolically active tissue promoting inflammation

(Greenberg & Obin 2006). There is speculation that obesity, while predisposing patients to OA, may also be directly related to cranial cruciate ligament (CrCL) tears. Leptin, a fat derived hormone elevated in the synovial fluid of obese patients, has been proposed to play a role in the development of CrCL tears in dogs by the alteration of ligamentocytes and collagenase activity. However, more research is needed to substantiate this claim (Comerford et al. 2005; Otero et al. 2006). Weight reduction has been shown to ameliorate the clinical signs associated with OA and can have preventive effects. Burkholder et al. (2000) demonstrated in a population of overweight dogs with clinical signs of hip dysplasia that appropriate weight loss markedly improved ground reaction forces and joint mobility. There are a series of studies that assess the protective benefits of a calorically restricted diet for the development of OA (Impellizeri et al. 2000; Kealy et al. 2000, 2002; Mlacnik et al. 2006; Smith et al. 2006).

Nonsteroidal anti-inflammatory drugs

NSAIDs are the most commonly prescribed class of medications to alleviate the clinical signs of OA. NSAIDs reduce the formation of inflammatory prostaglandins and thromboxane production by inhibiting cyclo-oxygenase (COX) enzymes in the arachadonic acid pathway, thereby decreasing synovitis and limiting cartilage matrix degradation associated with OA.

With the inhibition of COX isoenzymes, NSAIDs have a local effect at the site of injury as well as a central effect minimizing spinal nociception and central sensitization. NSAIDs may also sensitize μ receptors to the effects of opioids, explaining the synergism between these two medications. The benefit exerted by NSAIDs in the treatment of OA is indisputable. However, there are adverse effects, including gastrointestinal ulceration, impeded healing of the gastric mucosa, renal dysfunction, and transient hepatotoxicosis, when the constitutive forms of COX (both COX-1 and COX-2) are inhibited (Cullison 1984).

The primary selection of an NSAID is based on individual response (analgesic and adverse). Despite similar efficacies between different NSAIDs, there can be significant differences in individual responses. It is common to sequence different NSAIDs until acceptable analgesia is obtained or the patient experiences an adverse response. With chronic administration, an individual may become refractory to an NSAID at which point another should be selected. Currently, there is extensive debate concerning the length of washout between the administration of sequential NSAIDs. There is a unique occurrence with aspirin which emphasizes the importance of a washout period after this class of medication. Lipoxins are anti-inflammatory lipid mediators that have protective effects on the stomach lining, in which a specific form is induced by aspirin, Aspirin Triggered Lipoxin (ATL). ATLs diminish gastric mucosal injury from the nitric oxide produced by traumatized vascular endothelium (Souza et al. 2003). Concurrent or immediate administration of other NSAIDs, particularly COX-2 selective or COX-1 sparing, will completely block these lipoxins and their protective effects, increasing the risk of gastric ulceration. It is also of concern since COX-2 selective medications have been shown to impede gastric healing once present.

Additional analgesics

Although NSAIDs are traditionally the first line of pharmaceuticals used to treat OA, they incompletely suppress the inflammatory process through a limited mechanism of action and, therefore, are not completely effective at obviating the clinical signs of OA. A multimodal approach incorporating additional analgesics with differing mechanisms and sites of action is often indicated for improved pain control while lowering the therapeutically effective dose and thereby minimizing the adverse effects of NSAIDs (Lascelles et al. 2008).

Tramadol

Tramadol is an opioid analgesic acting at the μ receptor while inhibiting serotonin uptake and norepinephrine reuptake (Raffa et al. 1992). Tramadol also inhibits central pro-inflammatory cytokines and NFκβ, and influences various neuronal cation channels while locally decreasing IL-6 and substance P (Marincsak et al. 2008). Although tramadol is often paired clinically with NSAIDs for the management of OA, there is only one referenced study, in abstract form, available evaluating the benefits of this therapeutic combination (Lambert et al. 2004).

Amantadine

First recognized as an antiviral agent, amantadine has gained popularity for the treatment of chronic pain disorders via inhibition of NMDA receptors. NMDA receptor activation, secondary to chronic stimulation of alpha D and C fibers, is believed to be the primary component leading to "spinal windup." A recent study by Lascelles et al. (2008) compared the effects of adjunctive amantadine with meloxicam in a population of dogs with chronic OA refractory to NSAID therapy alone. Dogs treated with meloxicam in conjunction with amantadine had improved client-specific outcome measure scores and overall activity compared with dogs treated with meloxicam alone.

Gabapentin

Gabapentin is structurally similar to the central inhibitory neurotransmitter gamma-aminobutyric acid (GABA). GABA is synthesized from glutamate, an excitatory neurotransmitter. During periods of chronic pain there is up-regulation of glutamate and subsequent NMDA receptor activation with a relative decrease in GABA concentration. This results in loss of an endogenous feedback mechanism and an uninhibited nociceptive pathway. Although gabapentin's mechanism of action was initially assumed to be through GABAergic transmission, the therapeutic effects are believed to be moderated through the alpha2 subunit of voltage-gated calcium channels resulting in central analgesia (Davies et al. 2007). To the authors' knowledge, there are no clinical or experimental studies available evaluating the role of gabapentin in the treatment of OA in dogs.

Chondromodulating agents

There has recently been an increased interest in the alternative management of OA, not only to alleviate clinical signs associated with the disease, but also to slow the process of cartilage degradation and promote cartilage synthesis.

Polysulfated glycosaminoglycan

Polysulfated glycosaminoglycan (PSGAG) is a synthetic mixture of highly sulfated GAGs, principally chondroitin sulfate, extracted from bovine lung and tracheal cartilage (Todhunter & Lust 1994). PSGAGs are beneficial in the treatment of OA as they inhibit cartilage-degradative enzymes such as IL-1, matrix metalloproteinases (MMPs), lysosomal elastase, cathepsin g, as will as inhibiting prostaglandin E2 (PGE2), the formation of oxygen radicals, and components of the complement cascade such as C3a, and C5a (Todhunter & Lust 1994; Sevalla et al. 2000; Mertens et al. 2003; Fujiki et al. 2007). PSGAGs stimulate cartilage repair processes by promoting protein synthesis and collagen formation and by increasing GAG and hyaluronan concentration (Glade 1990). PSGAGs also maintain chondrocyte viability and stimulate chondrocyte division, thereby slowing the process of extracellular matrix degradation (Glade 1990; Sevalla et al. 2000). Since PSGAGs are a heparin analog, their use in dogs with coagulopathies or concurrent with administration of NSAIDs, particularly those with strong COX-1 (anti-thromboxane) activity, is contraindicated. There is some limited clinical data that support the use of PSGAG in dogs with OA (Lust et al. 1992; McNamara et al. 2007; Fujiki et al. 2007).

Hyaluronic acid

Hyaluronic acid (HA) is a linear non-sulfated GAG that is the primary constituent of synovial fluid. HA interacts with the aggrecan monomer through noncovalent association via link proteins to produce the large aggregating polyglycosaminoglycans of articular cartilage (McNamara et al. 1997). Administered HA is speculated to increase synovial viscosity by viscosupplementation. A variety of clinical and experimental trials are available evaluating the efficacy of HA for the treatment of CrCL rupture. However, these studies yield conflicting data on HA's ability to ameliorate the progression of stifle OA (Schiavinato et al. 1989; Marshall et al. 2000; Smith et al. 2001, 2005; Hellström et al. 2003; Canapp et al. 2005).

Nutritional supplements

Glucosamine and chondroitin sulfate

The majority of nutritional supplements available on the market for the management of OA are glucosamine and chondroitin sulfate formulations. Glucosamine is an amino-monosaccharide used in the synthesis of the disaccharide units of glycosaminoglycan (Neil et al. 2005; McNamara et al. 1997). Glucosamine can then be incorporated into the large-aggregating and small-non-aggregating proteoglycans of articular cartilage or as part of the disaccharide units of hyaluronan. Chondroitin sulfate is a long-chain polymer of repeating disaccharide units of galactosamine sulfate and glucuronic acid that constitutes the majority of glucosaminoglycans within articular cartilage (Neil et al. 2005; McNamara et al. 1997).

The mechanisms of action of chondroitin sulfate are synergistic with that of glucosamine and can stimulate the synthesis of endogenous glycosaminoglycans and inhibit the synthesis of degradative enzymes including MMPs. Additionally, chondroitin sulfate inhibits both IL-1-induced type II collagen degeneration and histamine-induced inflammation, and has the unique ability to improve synovial fluid viscosity by increasing hyaluronan concentration (McNamara et al. 1997; Kelly 1998; Canapp et al. 1999; Lippiello et al. 2000; Neil et al. 2005).

Notably, two studies evaluating the use of glucosamine and chondroitin sulfate to improve clinical signs associated with OA yield conflicting results. McCarthy et al. (2007) demonstrated a positive effect on pain score, weight-bearing, and severity of clinical condition in dogs with hip and elbow OA, while another study (Moreau et al. 2003) showed no effect.

Avocado and soybean oil unsaponifiables

Avocado and soybean oil unsaponifiables (ASUs) are biologically active lipids believed to have anti-inflammatory and anti-osteoarthritic properties. ASUs decrease the expression of inflammatory mediators and cartilage degradation (TNFa, IL-1b, COX-2, iNOS, and MMPs) and stimulate matrix synthesis by up-regulating TGF-β expression by chondroblasts and osteoblasts (Altinel et al. 2007; Au et al. 2007). A recent experimental study reported the protective effects of ASU in dogs with CrCL transection (Boileau et al. 2009). Compared with the placebo group, dogs treated with ASU had smaller macroscopic lesions on the tibial plateau. Histologically, these dogs had decreased severity of tibial and femoral cartilage lesions, synovitis, and a decreased loss of subchondral bone as well as a decreased loss of calcified cartilage thickness compared with the placebo group.

Omega-3 fatty acids

Nutritional supplementation with Omega-3 (n-3) fatty acids has been proposed as an adjunctive therapy for the management of OA. The most prevalent polyunsaturated fatty acids (PUFAs) comprising the cell membrane is the Omega-6 (n-6) fatty acid, arachidonic acid (AA). When the cell membrane, and therefore AA, is metabolized by the COX enzyme, proinflammatory and vasoactive mediators of 2- and 4-series prostaglandins, thromboxanes, and leukotrienes are produced. During the process of OA, there is an increase in serum, cartilage, and synovial fluid concentrations of n-6 PUFAs that propagate an inflammatory reaction. Incorporation of n-3 PUFAs, eicosapentaenoic acid (EPA), into the cell membrane will compete with AA for cyclo-oxygenase metabolism, which results in the production of 3- and 5-series prostaglandins, thromboxanes, and leukotrienes that are significantly less inflammatory and vasoactive, curtailing the inflammatory response (Bauer 2007). Several n-3 fatty acids are available, including EPA, docosahexaenoic acid (DHA), and alpha-linolenic acid (ALA), although EPA is the only n-3 PUFA with selectivity for the chondrocyte cell membrane. Several studies clinically support diet supplementation with n-3 fatty acids in the management of OA (Miller et al. 1992; Bartges et al. 2001; Roush et al. 2005). Current interest in n-3 dietary supplementation has spurred the advent of several commercial diets including Hill's J/D diet (Hill's Pet Nutrition Inc., Topeka, KS), CNM Joint Mobility JM diet (Nestlé Purina PetCare, St. Louis, MO), and the Royal Canin JS diet (Royal Canine USA Inc., St. Charles, MO).

Conclusion

The goals of multimodal medical therapy are to simultaneously maximize analgesia while minimizing the incidence and severity of adverse effects, and, if possible, to slow disease progression. This can be achieved by targeting multiple sites along the nociceptive pathway with the inclusion of medications with varying mechanisms of action. It is important when creating, maintaining, and adjusting multimodal treatment regimens to remember that no individual responds the same and no individual disease progresses the same. It is imperative to continually reassess the patient's response and adapt treatment as indicated.

References

Altinel L, Saritas ZK, Kose KC et al. Treatment with unsaponifiable extracts of avocado soybean increases TGFB1 and TGFB2 levels in canine joint fluid. Tohoku J Exp Med 2007;211:181–186.

Altman RD, Hochberg MC, Moskowitz RW et al. Recommendations for the medical management of osteoarthritis of the hip and knee. Arthritis Rheum 2000;43:1905–1915.

Argoff CE. Pharmacologic management of chronic pain. J Am Osteopath Assoc 2002;102:S21–27.

Au RY, Al-Talib TK, Au AY, et al. Avocado soybean unsaponifiables (ASU) suppress TNFA, IL1b COX 2 iNOS gene expression, and prostaglandin E2 and nitric oxide production in articular condrocytes and monocytes/macrophages. Osteoarthritis Cartilage 2007;15:1249–1255.

Bartges JW, Budsberg SC, Pazak HE, et al. Effects of different n6:n3 fatty acid ratio diets on canine stifle osteoarthritis. *Proceedings of the Orthopedic Research Society Annual Meeting.* San Francisco, CA, 2001; 47:462.

Bauer JE. Responses of dogs to dietary omega-3 fatty acids. J Am Vet Med Assoc 2007;231:1657–1661.

Boileau C, Martel-Pelletier J, Caron J, et al. Protective effects of total fraction of avocado/soybean unsaponifiables on the structural changes in experimental dog osteoarthritis: Inhibition of nitric oxide synthase and matrix metalloproteinase-13. Arthritis Res Ther 2009;11:R41.

Budsberg SC, Bartges JW. Nutrition and osteoarthritis in dogs: Does it help? Vet Clin North Am Small Anim Pract 2006;36:1307–1323.

Burkholder WJ, Taylor L, Hulse DA. Weight loss to optimal body condition increases ground reactive force in dogs with osteoarthritis. Compen Contin Educ Pract Vet 2000;23:74.

Canapp SO, McLaughlin RM, Hoskinson JJ, et al. Scintigraphic evaluation of dogs with acute synovitis after treatment with glucosamine hydrochloride and chondroitin sulfate. Am J Vet Res 1999;60:1552–1557.

Canapp SO, Cross AR, Brown MP, et al. Examination of synovial fluid and serum following intravenous injections of hyaluronan for the treatment of osteoarthritis in dogs. Vet Comp Orthop Traumatol 2005;18:169–174.

Comerford EJ, Tarlton JF, Innes JF, et al. Metabolism and composition of the canine anterior cruciate ligament relate to difference in knee joint mechanics and predisposition to ligament rupture. J Orthop Res 2005;23:61–66.

Cullison RF. Acetaminophen toxicosis in small animals: Clinical signs, mode of action, and treatment. Compend Cont Ed Pract Vet 1984;4:173–178.

Davies A, Hendrich J, Van Minh AT, et al. Functional biology of the alpha(2)delta subunits of voltage-gated calcium channels. Trends Pharmacol Sci 2007;28:220–228.

Fujiki M, Shineha J, Yamanokucki K, et al. Effects of treatment of polysulfated glycosaminoglycan on serum cartilage olgomeric matrix protein and C-reactive protein concentrations, serum matrix metalloproteinase-2 and -9 activities, and lameness in dogs with osteoarthritis. Am J Vet Res 2007;68:827–833.

Glade MJ. Polysulfated glycosaminoglycan accelerates net synthesis of collagen and glycosaminoglycans by arthritic equine cartilage tissues and chondrocytes. Am J Vet Res 1990;51:779–785.

Greenberg AS, Obin MS. Obesity and the role of adipose tissue in inflammation and metabolism. Am J Clin Nutr 2006;83:S461–S465.

Hellström LE, Carlsson C, Boucher JF, Michanek P. Intra-articular injections with high molecular weight sodium hyaluronate as a therapy for canine arthritis. Vet Rec 2003;153:89–90.

Impellizeri JA, Tetrick MA, Muir P. Effect of weight reduction on clinical signs of lameness in dogs with hip osteoarthritis. J Am Vet Med Assoc 2000;216:1089–1091.

Johnston SA. Osteoarthritis. Joint anatomy, physiology, and pathobiology. Vet Clin North Am Small Anim Pract 1997;27:699–723.

Johnston SA, McLaughlin RM, Budsberg SC. Nonsurgical management of osteoarthritis in dogs. Vet Clin N Amer Sm Anim Pract 2008;38:1449–1470.

Kelly GS. The role of glucosamine sulfate and chondroitin sulfates in the treatment of degenerative joint disease. Altern Med Rev 1998;3:27–39.

Kealy RD, Lawler DF, Ballam JM, et al. Evaluation of the effect of limited food consumption on radiographic evidence of osteoarthritis in dogs. J Am Vet Med Assoc 2000;217:1678–1680.

Kealy RD, Lawler DF, Ballam JM, et al. Effects of diet restriction on life span and age-related changes in dogs. J Am Vet Med Assoc 2002;220:1315–1320.

Lambert C, Bianchi E, Keroack S, et al. Reduced dosage of ketoprofen alone or with tramadol for long-term treatment of osteoarthritis in dogs (abstract). Vet Anaesth Analg 2004;31:23.

Lascelles BDX, Gaynor JS, Smith ES, et al. Amantidine in a multimodal analgesic regimen for alleviation of refractory osteoarthritis pain in dogs. J Vet Intern Med 2008;22:53–59.

Lazar TP, Berry CR, deHaan JJ, et al. Long-term radiographic comparison of tibial plateau leveling osteotomy versus extracapsular stabilization for cranial cruciate ligament rupture in the dog. Vet Surg 2005;34:133–141.

Lippiello L, Woodward J, Karpman R, et al. In vivo chondroprotection and metabolic synergy of glucosamine and chondroitin sulfate. Clin Orthop Relat Res 2000;381:229–240.

Lust G, Williams AJ, Burton-Wurster N, et al. Effects of intramuscular administration of glycosaminoglycan polysulfates on signs of incipient hip dysplasia in growing pups. Am J Vet Res 1992;53:1836–1843.

McCarthy G, O'Donovan J, Jones B, et al. Randomized double-blind, positive-controlled trial to assess the efficacy of glucosamine/chondroitin sulfate for the treatment of dogs with osteoarthritis. Vet J 2007;174:54–61.

Marincsak R, Toth BI, Czifra G, et al. The analgesic drug, tramadol, acts as an agonist of the transient receptor potential vanilloid-1. Anesth Analg 2008;106:1890–1896.

Marshall KW, Manolopoulos V, Mancer K, et al. Amelioration of disease severity by intraarticular hylan therapy in bilateral canine osteoarthritis. J Orthop Res 2000;18:416–425.

McNamara PS, Johnston SA, Todhunter RJ. Slow-acting disease-modifying osteoarthritis agents. Vet Clin North Am Small Anim Pract 1997;27:863–881.

Mertens WD, MacLead JN, Fubini L, et al. Polysulphated glycosaminoglycans modulate transcription of interleukin-1B treated chondrocytes in monolayer culture. Vet Comp Orthop Traumatol 2003;2:93–98.

Miller WH, Scott DW, Wellington JR. Treatment of dogs with hip arthritis with a fatty acid supplement. Canine Pract 1992;17:6–8.

Mlacnik E, Bockstahler BA, Muller M, et al. Effects of caloric restriction and a moderate or intense physiotherapy program for treatment of lameness in overweight dogs with osteoarthritis. J Am Vet Med Assoc 2006;229:1756–1760.

Moreau M, Dupuis J, Bonneau NH, et al. Clinical evaluation of a nutraceutical, carprofen and meloxicam for the treatment of dogs with osteoarthritis. Vet Rec 2003;152:323–329.

Neil KM, Caron JP, Orth MW. The role of glucosamine and chondroitin sulfate in treatment for and prevention of osteoarthritis in animals. J Am Vet Med Assoc 2005;226:1079–1088.

Otero M, Lago R, Gomez R, et al. Leptin: A metabolic hormone that functions like a proinflammatory adipokine. Drug News Perspect 2006;19:21–26.

Raffa RB, Friderichs E, Reimann W, et al. Opioid and nonopioid components independently contribute to the mechanism of action of tramadol, an "atypical" opioid analgesic. J Pharmacol Exp Ther 1992;260:275–285.

Roush JK, Cross AR, Renberg WC, et al. Effects of feeding a high omega-3 fatty acid diet on serum fatty acid profiles and force plate analysis in dogs with osteoarthritis. Vet Surg 2005;34:E21.

Schiavinato A, Lini E, Guidolin D, et al. Intraarticular sodium hyaluronate injections in the Pond-Nuki experimental model of osteoarthritis in dogs. II. Morphological findings. Clin Orthop Relat Res 1989;241:286–299.

Sevalla K, Todhunter RJ, Verneir-Singer M, et al. Effect of polysulfated glycosaminoglycan on DNA content and proteoglycan metabolism in normal and osteoarthritic canine articular cartilage explants. Vet Surg 2000;29:407–414.

Smith GN, Jr., Mickler EA, Myers SL, Brandt KD. Effect of intraarticular hyaluronan injection on synovial fluid hyaluronan in the early stage of canine post-traumatic osteoarthritis. J Rheumatol 2001;28:1341–1346.

Smith G Jr, Myers SL, Brandt KD, et al. Effect of intraarticular hyaluronan injection on vertical ground reaction force and progression of osteoarthritis after anterior cruciate ligament transection. J Rheumatol 2005;32:325–334.

Smith GK, Paster ER, Powers MY, et al. Lifelong diet restriction and radiographic evidence of osteoarthritis of the hip joint in dogs. J Am Vet Med Assoc 2006;229:690–693.

Souza MH, de Lima OM, Jr., Zamuner SR, et al. Gastritis increases resistance to aspirin-induced mucosal injury via COX-2-mediated lipoxin synthesis, Am J Physiol Gastrointest Liver Physiol 2003;285:54–61.

Todhunter RJ, Lust G. Polysulfated glycosaminoglycan in the treatment of osteoarthritis. J Am Vet Med Assoc 1994;8:1245–1251.

Vasseur PB, Berry CR. Progression of stifle osteoarthrosis following reconstruction of the cranial cruciate ligament in 21 dogs. J Am Anim Hosp Assoc 1992;28:129–136.

36 Rehabilitation for Dogs with Cranial Cruciate Ligament Rupture

Courtney J. Arnoldy

Introduction

The aim of physical rehabilitation for patients with cranial cruciate ligament (CrCL) rupture is to improve functional stability for a safe return to higher activity levels. Scientific evidence confirms rehabilitation programs facilitate functional recovery in humans after anterior cruciate ligament (ACL) reconstruction (Kvist 2004; Gerber et al. 2007; Risberg et al. 2007; Grodski & Marks 2008; Palmieri-Smith et al. 2008). Similarly, early rehabilitation programs contribute to successful functional outcomes in dogs after stifle stabilization (Millis & Levine 1997; Marsolais et al. 2002; Monk et al. 2006; Jandi & Schulman 2007). Rehabilitation programs must be individualized, follow tissue healing time frames, and modified and progressed based on reassessments during the recovery process. The type and timing of therapeutic intervention is important as inappropriate therapeutic techniques can have a deleterious effect leading to poor functional outcomes. This chapter concentrates on current scientific evidence and general principles to assist in the clinical reasoning process for treatment of patients with CrCL rupture.

Advances in the Canine Cranial Cruciate Ligament,
Edited by Peter Muir, © 2010 ACVS Foundation, This Work is a co-publication between the American College of Veterinary Surgeons Foundation and Wiley-Blackwell.

Literature review and considerations

Research in human literature may be used as a foundation for principles utilized during the rehabilitative process. However, one must use caution when extrapolating evidenced-based practice and specific techniques to the canine patient. Common rehabilitation goals for patients with ACL-deficiency and after reconstruction include restoration of passive and active range-of-motion, minimizing quadriceps inhibition, improvement of lower extremity muscle strength, and neuromuscular control. Various rehabilitative strategies have been suggested, but it is not known which are most efficacious. Additional research is needed to identify optimal therapeutic activities to normalize lower extremity strength and dynamic joint stability.

Lower extremity strength and neuromuscular control have been shown to play a role in restoring dynamic joint stability (Risberg et al. 2007). Initiation of strengthening exercises emphasizing the hamstring and quadriceps muscles is essential. Quadriceps muscle weakness is often a persistent deficit in humans after ACL reconstruction. Weakness of this muscle group has been related to poor functional outcomes and may contribute to early onset of osteoarthritis (Palmieri-Smith et al. 2008). Rehabilitation programs including eccentric training in the early postoperative phase have been

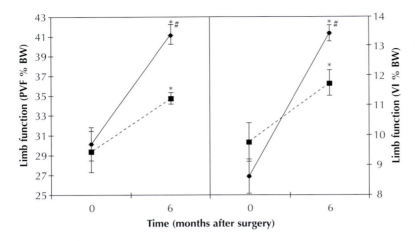

Figure 36.1 Vertical forces (peak vertical force [PVF], vertical impulse [VI]) before surgery (time 0) and 6 months after surgical treatment of cranial cruciate ligament rupture for dogs with rehabilitation (solid line) and exercise-restricted (dashed line) groups. *Significant ($p < 0.05$) difference between time 0 and 6. #Significant ($p < 0.05$) difference between groups. % BW: percentage of the dog's body weight. Reproduced from Marsolais et al. (2002), with permission from the American Veterinary Medical Association.

shown to produce a twofold greater increase in quadriceps peak cross-sectional area and volume (Gerber et al. 2007). Gains in muscle strength can promote joint stability and improved limb function. Together, these data suggest that if muscle weakness and reduced neuromuscular control are present in dogs with CrCL rupture, it is reasonable to introduce progressive strength (including eccentric exercise) and neuromuscular training into a comprehensive rehabilitation program to improve functional outcomes.

Research is limited on the effects of rehabilitation in dogs with CrCL rupture. Patients with CrCL rupture have stifle instability, joint inflammation, and lameness. If untreated, the dog will develop progressive osteoarthritis causing pain and decreased function. Conservative management for the patient with CrCL rupture has been reported and is most suitable for dogs weighing less than 15 kg (Edge-Hughes & Nicholson 2007; Vasseur 2003). Nonsurgical management may include low-impact exercises, controlled activity, isometric strengthening, and proprioceptive training for 2–3 months.

Rehabilitation programs after surgical stabilization have been shown to facilitate gains in thigh circumference, passive mobility, and improved limb use. A review of the literature analyzing rehabilitation in dogs after extracapsular stabilization reveals benefits in limb function demonstrated by a significant increase in peak vertical force (PVF) and vertical impulse (VI) values as measured by gait analysis (Marsolais et al. 2002; Figure 36.1). Rehabilitation programs initiated immediately in the postoperative period after a tibial plateau leveling osteotomy (TPLO) procedure may also hasten the return of limb function and decrease pain by preventing muscle atrophy and increasing muscle strength. In one study, thigh circumference was larger six weeks after a TPLO procedure in a group receiving rehabilitation compared with a home exercise-only group (Monk et al. 2006; Figure 36.2). Thigh circumference has also been found to decrease in the first 5 weeks after transection of the CrCL (Millis et al. 1999). Based on this evidence, rehabilitation for at least the first 5–6 weeks is recommended to prevent atrophy and increase muscle mass.

Normalizing passive stifle mobility is crucial in the early postoperative period, as mobility may be more difficult to achieve if improvements are not appreciated in the first 2 weeks (Millis et al. 1997). Passive flexion and extension of the stifle joint was significantly greater at 6 weeks after rehabilitation in patients that underwent a TPLO (Monk et al. 2006) (Figure 36.3 and 36.4). A loss of passive stifle joint extension or flexion ≥10° has also been shown to be responsible for higher clinical lameness scores in dogs after a TPLO procedure (Jandi & Schulman 2007).

Scientific evidence, although limited in dogs, has demonstrated the benefits of rehabilitation programs to improve function. Based on this knowledge, it is reasonable to initiate rehabilita-

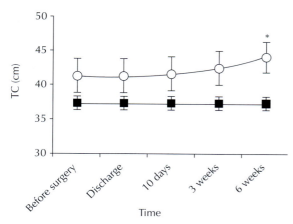

Figure 36.2 Mean ± SEM thigh circumference (TC) for affected limbs of dogs in the rehabilitation (open circles) and home exercise (solid squares) groups over time. Measurements were obtained before surgery, on the day the dogs were discharged to the owners (1 day after surgery), and 10 days and 3 and 6 weeks after surgery. *Within a time point, values differ significantly ($p < 0.05$) between groups. Reproduced with from (Monk et al. 2006), with permission from the American Veterinary Medical Association.

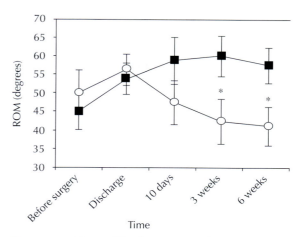

Figure 36.4 Mean ± SEM flexion range-of-motion (ROM) of the stifle joint for the rehabilitation (open circles) and home exercise (solid squares) groups over time. Improvement is indicated by a decrease in the ROM measurement. See Figure 36.2 for the remainder of the key. Reproduced with from Monk et al. (2006), with permission from the American Veterinary Medical Association.

tion immediately in the postoperative period. The use of evidence-based medicine should guide interventions chosen to achieve optimal results.

Rehabilitation principles and guidelines

Management of the patient with CrCL rupture is multifaceted. Before establishing a rehabilitation program, an understanding of the biomechanical behavior of the cruciate ligament, pelvic limb kinematics, neuromuscular control patterns, and tissue healing time frames is required. It is important for the rehabilitative practitioner to be cognizant of how osteoarthritis may impact treatment and long-term outcome. Awareness of possible postoperative complications is also essential in order to identify potential problems during the recovery process.

Therapy must be tailored, modified, and progressed based on the patient's response to treatment and tissue healing time frames. If surgically managed, each procedure has unique challenges. During each phase of tissue healing, appropriate stresses should be applied to the healing tissue. Phases will overlap; therefore, it is important for the practitioner to progress the rehabilitation program systematically. General rehabilitation

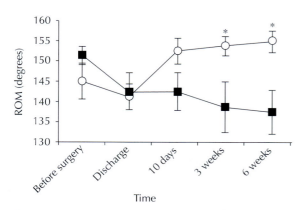

Figure 36.3 Mean ± SEM extension range-of-motion (ROM) of the stifle joint for the rehabilitation (open circles) and home exercise (solid squares) groups over time. Improvement is indicated by an increase in the ROM measurement. See Figure 36.2 for the remainder of the key. Reproduced with from Monk et al. (2006), with permission from the American Veterinary Medical Association.

goals for the postoperative patient in the inflammatory stage of tissue healing through the reparative phase include decreasing pain and edema, restoring range-of-motion, and improving stifle arthrokinematics, muscle mass, and functional limb strength. As healing progresses into the remodeling and maturation phases of healing, general goals consist of normalizing range-of-motion (active and passive), strength, proprioception, and neuromuscular control, and addressing dysfunctional movement patterns. A gradual increase in therapeutic exercise designed to simulate functional activities or demands of a sport that the patient will return to are advanced in order to achieve patient-specific goals in the later phases of tissue healing.

Evaluation and plan of care

A rehabilitation program begins with a thorough patient evaluation. This information guides all elements of management including goal setting, intervention selection, and outcome measures. Factors that require consideration include the patient's size, personality, comorbidities, surgical technique (if applicable), and the owner's goals. Information gained from the initial evaluation may include degree of lameness, presence of inflammation, active and passive mobility, presence of soft tissue tension, thigh muscle mass, and quality of movement during functional activities. The synthesis of objective findings gained during the evaluation and predicted prognosis determine functional goals. This information allows the practitioner to develop and implement appropriate therapeutic interventions. Decisions about interventions are contingent on the patient's response to treatment and progress toward expected outcomes (Rothstein et al. 2003). It is important that clinical reasoning skills and professional judgment based on scientific evidence guide the rehabilitative process. The TPLO Activity Guideline used at the University of Wisconsin Veterinary Medical Teaching Hospital is located at the following Web site: http://uwveterinarycare.wisc.edu/hosp_services/rehab/tplo.html. The guideline should be adjusted and modified based on the individual patient.

Future research

Numerous studies have documented the benefits of early intensive rehabilitation in human medicine for return to function. There is a lack of prospective randomized clinical research in veterinary medicine to substantiate the effectiveness of rehabilitation for a dog with CrCL rupture. Further studies are warranted to add scientific evidence to establish more effective and efficient therapeutic strategies to facilitate a safe return to function. An interesting focus for future research may include the benefits of neuromuscular training and effects on functional stability.

References

Edge-Hughes L, Nicholson H. Canine treatment and rehabilitation. In: *Animal Physiotherapy Assessment, Treatment and Rehabilitation of Animals*, McGowan C, Goff L, Stubbs N (eds). Oxford: Blackwell Publishing, 2007, p. 211.

Gerber JP, Marcus RL, Dibble LE, et al. Effects of early progressive eccentric exercise on muscle structure after anterior cruciate ligament reconstruction. J Bone Joint Surg Am 2007;89:559–570.

Grodski M, Marks R. Exercises following anterior cruciate ligament reconstructive surgery: biomechanical considerations and efficacy of current approaches. Res Sports Med 2008;16:75–96.

Jandi A, Schulman A. Incidence of motion loss of the stifle joint in dogs with naturally occurring cranial cruciate ligament rupture surgically treated with tibial plateau leveling osteotomy: Longitudinal clinical study of 412 cases. Vet Surg 2007;36:114–121.

Kvist J. Rehabilitation following anterior cruciate ligament injury: current recommendations for sports participation. Sports Med 2004;34:269–280.

Marsolais G, Dvorak G, Conzemius M. Effects of postoperative rehabilitation on limb function after cranial cruciate ligament repair in dogs. J Am Vet Med Assoc 2002;220:1325–1330.

Millis DL, Levine D. The role of exercise and physical modalities in the treatment of osteoarthritis. Vet Clin North Am Small Anim Pract. 1997;27:913–930.

Millis DL, Levine D, Taylor RA, et al. A preliminary study of early physical therapy following surgery for cranial cruciate ligament rupture in dogs. Vet Surg 1997;26:434.

Millis DL, Levine D, Mynatt T. Changes in muscle mass following transaction of the cranial cruciate ligament and immediate stifle stabilization. *Proceedings of the 1st International Symposium on Rehabilitation and Physical*

Therapy in Veterinary Medicine. Corvalis, OR, 1999, p. 155.

Monk ML, Preston CA, McGowen CM. Effects of early intensive physiotherapy on limb function after tibial plateau leveling osteotomy in dogs with deficiency of the cranial cruciate ligament. Am J Vet Res 2006;67:529–536.

Palmieri-Smith R, Thomas A, Wojtys E. Maximizing quadriceps strength after ACL reconstruction. Clin Sports Med 2008;27:405–424.

Risberg MA, Holm I, Myklebust G, Engebretsen L. Neuromuscular training versus strength training during first 6 months after anterior cruciate ligament reconstruction: A randomized clinical trial. Phys Ther 2007;87:737–750.

Rothstein J, Echternach J, Riddle D. The hypothesis-oriented algorithm for clinicians II (HOAC II): A guide for patient management. Phys Ther 2003;83: 455–470.

Vasseur PB. Stifle joint. In: *Textbook of Small Animal Surgery*, Slatter D (ed.), third edition. Philadelphia: WB Saunders, 2003, pp. 2090–2133.

Section VI

Future Directions

Introduction

Recent advances in knowledge regarding the cruciate rupture arthropathy have begun to challenge past dogma regarding this condition. This work will undoubtedly lead to new innovations in treatment in the future. These advances are likely to include innovations in both surgical and medical management. Given the emerging role of joint inflammation in the pathogenesis of cranial cruciate ligament (CrCL) rupture, a combination of both medical and surgical treatment will likely be required for improved outcomes. Genetic susceptibility, particularly involving the major histocompatibility complex, is an important risk factor for the development of persistent joint inflammation in human beings. Whether similar susceptibilities predispose dogs to development of stifle arthritis and CrCL rupture is an important question that remains to be answered in the future.

A major controversy in this field has been how to evaluate clinical outcomes in dogs that receive surgical treatment for stifle arthritis. Although computational gait analysis remains the gold-standard method for objective quantification of lameness using either a force platform or a pressure mat, use of client-specific outcome measures and accelerometers has now been validated as alternative measures of outcome. In future work, further careful validation and evaluation of such instruments used in combination with objective analysis of gait are likely to generate higher levels of evidence (Innes 2007) from clinical trials.

This section discusses several emerging areas of investigation relevant to the management of dogs affected with the cruciate rupture arthropathy.

Reference

Innes JF. Outcomes-based medicine in veterinary surgery: Levels of evidence. Vet Surg 2007;36: 610–612.

37 Client-Specific Outcome Measures

John F. Innes

Introduction

To improve the efficacy of treatments for dogs with cranial cruciate ligament (CrCL) rupture, it is imperative that the efficacy of treatments can be measured. Objective measures of outcomes are desirable because of their lack of bias and potential for greater reliability; such measures are likely, at the current time, to produce clinical evidence of a higher level (Innes 2007; Sanderson et al. 2009). However, such objective measures may be limited in their availability at the current time because of the cost and time involved in administering them. In addition, such measures may only capture certain dimensions of the condition. For example, the force platform is a robust outcome measure but it is generally used to measure certain force parameters in the affected limb on a runway. Thus, there are aspects of stifle joint function (and dysfunction) that the force platform cannot measure, such as "inactivity stiffness" and "ability to climb stairs." Therefore, in a chronic situation such as the postsurgical stifle, it

Advances in the Canine Cranial Cruciate Ligament, Edited by Peter Muir, © 2010 ACVS Foundation, This Work is a co-publication between the American College of Veterinary Surgeons Foundation and Wiley-Blackwell.

is likely to be useful to use client-specific outcome measures. In fact, veterinarians have done this for a long time in a relatively informal way; feedback from clients is part of a clinician's follow-up consultations, and veterinarians in the clinic typically translate and interpret a client's informal feedback into clinical notes. In past decades in published clinical studies, clinicians may have used a variety of client-administered questionnaires to standardize and formalize this feedback. These questionnaires have generally been paper- or telephone-based and have varied widely in the literature. Importantly, very few of these questionnaires have been validated. In the last 10–15 years, there has been an interest in developing validated questionnaires, or "clinical metrology instruments" for use in canine orthopaedic outcomes assessment, including stifle arthritis. The advantages of using such instruments are that it should result in more robust and reliable data, one can understand the limitations of the instrument, and one can start to compare between published reports. This chapter will discuss the process of designing such an instrument, the issues around validation of the instrument, the use of such instruments in clinical studies, and how such instruments relate to other disease outcome measures.

Designing a client-specific outcomes measure

Designing a clinical metrology instrument can involve several steps. An important aspect of any evaluative index is a strategy for the measurement of all clinically important treatment effects. Item generation is followed by testing *validity*, *reliability*, and *responsiveness* of the instrument (Bellamy et al. 1985).

Item generation

Initially, instrument development involves the generation of items (questions) that represent theoretic constructs (i.e., disease variables). Considering that the instrument will be completed by dog owners, it seems logical to involve dog owners in generation of the measures, and this approach has been taken in one instrument, the Canine Brief Pain Inventory, which is designed to measure chronic pain in dogs (Brown et al. 2008). Alternatively, items may be generated by veterinarians with expert knowledge of the condition in question, and this approach has also been reported for the Liverpool Osteoarthritis in Dogs (LOAD) instrument in a canine elbow osteoarthritis cohort (Hercock et al. 2009).

Item scaling

Item scaling refers to the various options for types of scale that are available for owners in answering each question. The most simple scale is a dichotomous one, for example, is the dog lame or not? This type of scale is preferred by some of the regulatory authorities and has been used in clinical trials of nonsteroidal anti-inflammatory drugs (NSAIDs) for licensing purposes (Pollmeier et al. 2006). However, such a scale is inherently poorly responsive (see below; Kirschner & Guyatt 1985). When an investigator requires grading of response or disease activity, there is a need for a discontinuous ordinal scales (Hercock et al. 2009) or visual analog scales (VASs; Hielm-Bjorkman et al. 2003; Burton et al. 2009). Five, seven, or nine-point rating scales are popular, with five-point

scales perhaps representing the best compromise between responsiveness and reliability. Such scales are often presented as "none, mild, moderate, severe, extreme," numerical rating scales. In human rheumatology, after much debate, the discontinuous ordinal scales appear to be preferred (Bolognese et al. 2003).

Validity

Once all items have been generated, one must consider the validity of the instrument. Validity refers to the extent to which the instrument is able to measure what is intended. There are various aspects to validity. *Face validity* is present if it "looks like" the instrument is going to measure what it is supposed to measure, and in this situation, this would be assessed by veterinarians (Hercock et al. 2009). *Content validity* is also judgmental and is said to be satisfied when the measure, or a combination of measures, comprehensively captures the important areas of the domain which it is attempting to represent (Frost et al. 2007). *Construct validity* is concerned with the extent to which a particular measure relates to other measures in a manner that is consistent with theoretically derived hypotheses concerning the constructs (or concepts) that are being measured. For instance, if other measures of the disease (e.g., veterinarian's assessment) produce a similar signal (i.e., good correlation) to the new index, construct validity may be supported. Similar, but not synonymous, *criterion validity* refers to the extent to which an instrument produces the same results as a "gold standard." This is a difficult issue in dogs with CrCL rupture because there is no current consensus on a gold standard. One might consider the force platform a gold standard, but, as already stated, it measures particular disease dimensions and the metrology instrument may be designed to capture more widely. Nevertheless, in one study, investigators were unable to find a significant correlation between items on an instrument relating to "lameness" and peak vertical force in a cohort of dogs with elbow osteoarthritis (Hercock et al. 2009). In addition, another study addressing a cohort of dogs with elbow dysplasia again found no significant relationship between owner assessment of lameness on a VAS and a total moment support ratio derived from inverse dynamics estimates of total joint moments (Burton et al. 2009). Further work is required to assess the construct and criterion validity of client-specific outcome measures in dogs with CrCL rupture.

Reliability

Reliability is the extent to which an instrument records the same numerical values on repeated occasions, assuming no underlying change in the index condition between assessment intervals (Bellamy & Buchanan 1990). This is evaluated in a "test–retest" scenario when the disease has become stable (Deyo et al. 1991; Hudson et al. 2004; Hercock et al. 2009). Reliability should be measured using a statistic that reflects *agreement* between the two assessments, such as the intraclass correlation coefficient (ICC; Fleiss & Cohen 1973). The ICC ranges from 0 to 1, with 1 representing perfect agreement. It should be noted that agreement is not the same as correlation in that there may be a good correlation with poor agreement due to systematic bias. In dogs with CrCL rupture, one study demonstrated overall good reliability of an owner-administered questionnaire with concordance correlation coefficients between 0.549 and 0.916 (Innes & Barr 1998). That study also suggested that owners are more reliable for more generic items and that very specific items showed poorer reliability. In canine osteoarthritis, Hudson and colleagues demonstrated that as an additional step internal consistency of the instrument may be assessed by investigating the correlation between items that assess the same disease dimension (Hudson et al. 2004; Brown et al. 2008; Hercock et al. 2009).

Responsiveness

Responsiveness is a measure of the extent to which an instrument can detect clinically important, statistically significant changes in health status (Bellamy & Buchanan 1990); it is particularly relevant to clinical outcomes measures tools.

Responsiveness should be tested using standard treatments, relevant types of patients, and conventional sample sizes. There are a variety of approaches to assess responsiveness. *Sensitivity* is the ability to detect change statistically, whereas *relevant change* is the change that is clinically meaningful. Therefore, responsiveness statistics are divided in to sensitivity measures on the one hand, and methods designed to assess the ability of an instrument to separate clinically relevant change from irrelevant change. Examples of sensitivity statistics are the standardized response mean (SRM) and the effect size. These indicate the magnitude of the change in comparison with the standard deviation of change, or the standard deviation at baseline, respectively. The larger the SRM or effect size, the greater the sensitivity to change. Although there are no absolute standards for effect size, it has been suggested that in comparative studies, examples of small, medium and large effect sizes might have values of 0.2, 0.5 and 0.8, respectively (Cohen 1977).

Responsiveness of clinical outcomes measures has received a limited amount of attention in veterinary orthopaedics. One previous study looked at the responsiveness of an instrument (Bristol osteoarthritis in Dogs [BrOAD]) using surgical intervention for dogs with CrCL rupture as the test treatment (Innes & Barr 1998). In that study, the authors reported effect sizes of 0.68 to 2.75 for various items, but the design of that study was less than optimal in that clients had to recall the pretreatment evaluation and there was no objective outcome measure. Thus, the BrOAD instrument had sensitivity; however, without criterion and construct validity, one cannot be certain that this was a relevant change. In another study, responsiveness of the LOAD instrument was considered low, as tested in a cohort of dogs with chronic elbow osteoarthritis using a licensed NSAID as the test treatment (Hercock et al. 2009). However, concomitant force platform data confirmed that the response to the treatment in this population was small and did not reach statistical significance with any measure. Thus, further testing of LOAD is required in alternative patient groups to assess responsiveness. At the current time, no client-specific outcome measure can be said to have proven responsiveness.

260 Future Directions

Table 37.1 Canine client-specific outcome measures in orthopaedic diseases in the peer-reviewed literature

Instrument	Supporting literature (see reference list for full citation)	Download or contact details	Validation status
Bristol Osteoarthritis in Dogs (BrOAD)	Innes and Barr 1998	NA	Partial
Canine Brief Pain Inventory (CBPI)	Brown et al. 2008	http://research.vet.upenn.edu/PennChart/AvailableTools/CBPI/tabid/1970/Default.aspx	Partial
Helsinki Chronic Pain Index	Hielm-Bjorkman et al. 2003	anna.hielm-bjorkman@helsinki.fi	Partial
Liverpool Osteoarthritis in Dogs (LOAD)	Hercock et al. 2009	http://www.liv.ac.uk/sath/services/LOAD.pdf http://www.liv.ac.uk/sath/services/NOTES.pdf	Partial
Texas A&M instrument	Hudson et al. 2004	Dr M.R. Slater, Department of Veterinary Anatomy and Public Health, College of Veterinary Medicine, Texas A&M University, College Station, TX 77843, USA	Partial

Note: Summary as of June 2009.
NA: not available.

Refinement and internal consistency of clinical metrology instruments

The instruments design process may generate multiple items, and it may then be possible to apply statistical techniques to reduce the number of items without losing information. In this way, one can reduce respondent burden. There are various approaches to this including principal components analysis (Hudson et al. 2004) and internal consistency testing (Brown et al. 2008). However, for an evaluative index, it is particularly important that nonresponsive items are deleted as they only contribute to random error (Kirschner & Guyatt 1985).

Summary

It is encouraging to see increasing interest in client-specific outcomes measures in veterinary orthopaedics (Table 37.1). However, as a community, we must strive to ensure that such instruments are carefully validated and evaluated before they are generally accepted into clinical practice. Most instruments have only limited publications on their validity and the data thus far are insufficient to consider any instrument validated for clinical use.

References

Bellamy N, Buchanan W. Assessment of antirheumatic activity in man. Ballieres Clin Rheumatol 1990;4:433–465.

Bellamy N, Buchanan W, Goldsmith C, et al. Validation of WOMAC: A health status instrument for measuring clinically important patient relevant outcomes to antirheumatic drug therapy in patients with osteoarthritis of the hip or knee. J Rheumatol 1985;15:1833–1840.

Bolognese JA, Schnitzer TJ, Ehrich EW. Response relationship of VAS and Likert scales in osteoarthritis efficacy measurement. Osteoarthritis Cartilage 2003;11:499–507.

Brown DC, Boston RC, Coyne JC, et al. Ability of the Canine Brief Pain Inventory to detect response to treatment in dogs with osteoarthritis. J Am Vet Med Assoc 2008;233:1278–1283.

Burton N, Owen M, Colborne G, et al. Can owners and clinicians assess outcome in dogs with fragmented medial coronoid process? Vet Comp Orthop Traumatol 2009;22:183–189.

Cohen J. *Statistical Power Analysis for the Behavioural Sciences*. New York: Academic Press, 1977.

Deyo R, Diehr P, Patrick D. Reproducibility and responsiveness of health status measures. Control Clin Trial 1991;12:142–158.

Fleiss JL, Cohen J. Equivalence of weighted kappa and intraclass correlation coefficient as measures of reliability. Educ Psychol Meas 1973;33:613–619.

Frost MH, Reeve BB, Liepa AM, et al. What is sufficient evidence for the reliability and validity of patient-reported outcome measures? Value Health 2007;10:S94–S105.

Hercock C, Pinchbeck G, Giejda A, et al. Validation of a client-based clinical metrology instrument for the evaluation of canine elbow osteoarthritis. J Small Anim Pract 2009;50:266–271.

Hielm-Bjorkman AK, Kuusela E, Liman A, et al. Evaluation of methods for assessment of pain associated with chronic osteoarthritis in dogs. J Am Vet Med Assoc 2003;222:1552–1558.

Hudson JT, Slater MR, Taylor L, et al. Assessing repeatability and validity of a visual analogue scale questionnaire for use in assessing pain and lameness in dogs. Am J Vet Res 2004;65:1634–1643.

Innes JF. Outcomes-based medicine in veterinary surgery: Levels of evidence. Vet Surg 2007;36:610–612.

Innes JF, Barr AR. Can owners assess outcome following surgical treatment of canine cranial cruciate ligament deficiency? J Small Anim Pract 1998;39:373–378.

Kirschner B, Guyatt G. A methodological framework for assessing health indices. J Chronic Dis 1985;38:27–36.

Pollmeier M, Toulemonde C, Fleishman C, et al. Clinical evaluation of firocoxib and carprofen for the treatment of dogs with osteoarthritis. Vet Rec 2006;159:547–551.

Sanderson RC, Beata C, Flipo RM, et al. Systematic review of management of canine osteoarthritis. Vet Rec 2009;164:418–424.

38 Total Knee Replacement in the Dog

Matthew J. Allen, William D. Liska, and Katy L. Townsend

History of total knee replacement in the dog

In humans, total knee replacement (TKR) has become a routine and highly successful procedure for patients with pain or disability associated with arthritic disorders of the knee joint. The long-term survival of TKR prostheses is comparable to that of total hip replacement prostheses, with approximately 10% of patients requiring revision surgery within the first 10 postoperative years (Robertsson et al. 2001). The most common cause of implant failure is aseptic loosening of the implant.

In the late 1980s, Dr. Tom Turner described the development of a condylar-style TKR prosthesis for the dog (Turner et al. 1989). Although initially used as a preclinical model for studying the effects of different fixation methods on bone apposition and bone ingrowth in cementless tibial components (Berzins et al. 1994; Sumner et al. 1994), the research implants were subsequently used

Advances in the Canine Cranial Cruciate Ligament,
Edited by Peter Muir, © 2010 ACVS Foundation, This Work is a co-publication between the American College of Veterinary Surgeons Foundation and Wiley-Blackwell.

in selected clinical cases with subjectively acceptable initial results (Dr. T. Turner, personal communication).

Allen et al. recently reported 1-year follow-up data on a series of 24 skeletally mature purpose-bred dogs that underwent cemented TKR with a research implant system consisting of a cobalt–chromium (Co–Cr) alloy femoral component and an ultra-high molecular weight polyethylene (UHMWPE) tibial insert enclosed in a Co–Cr tibial tray (Allen et al. 2009). Follow-up examinations were performed at 6, 12, 26, and 52 weeks postoperatively. The results were encouraging in all animals. However, the design of the femorotibial articulation was deemed less than optimal, and a commercial implant was not subsequently developed.

Liska et al. described the use of a custom-designed cemented canine TKR implant to reconstruct a stifle joint with femoral bone loss secondary to traumatic injury (Liska et al. 2007). Subsequent to this initial report, a modular implant system and associated instrumentation have been developed and released for clinical use. This implant system (Canine Total Knee System, BioMedtrix LLC, Boonton, NJ) is in trial use in a number of veterinary referral centers in North America and overseas.

264 Future Directions

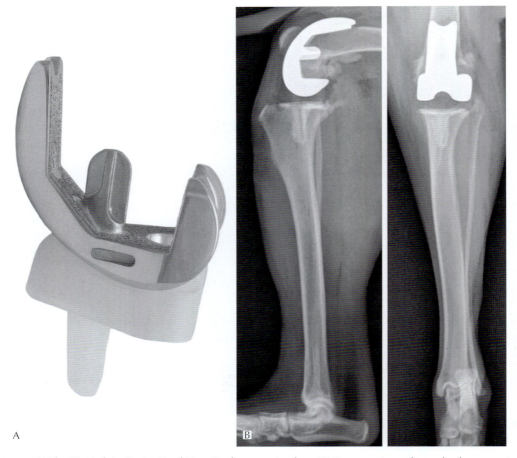

Figure 38.1 (A) The BioMedtrix Canine Total Knee Replacement implant. (B) Postoperative radiographs demonstrating successful implantation of the BioMedtrix TKR in a clinical case.

Design rationale for the BioMedtrix TKR implant

The BioMedtrix TKR implant consists of two elements: a femoral component manufactured from Co–Cr alloy, and a monobloc tibial component that is machined from UHMWPE (Figure 38.1). The fixation surface of the femoral component is covered with Co–Cr beads and is intended for cementless (biological) fixation. The UHMPWE tibial component is designed for polymethylmethacrylate (PMMA) bone cement fixation.

Case selection—indications and contraindications for surgery

The primary indication for canine TKR is degenerative joint disease, most commonly secondary to cranial cruciate ligament (CrCL) rupture. The majority of dogs present with a history of at least one previous surgical procedure. Conversion of a failed extracapsular repair is relatively straightforward and can be performed as a one-stage procedure. Conversion from a tibial plateau leveling osteotomy (TPLO) is best performed as a two-

Total Knee Replacement in the Dog   265

Surgical technique

Details of the surgical technique can be found in the literature (Allen et al. 2009; Liska & Doyle 2009). TKR can be performed through either a medial or lateral stifle arthrotomy. The patella is luxated to improve exposure of the distal femur and proximal tibia. The infrapatellar fat pad, cruciate ligaments, and menisci are excised. Custom-designed instruments and cutting blocks are used to guide the tibial osteotomy (Figure 38.3A) and the four femoral osteotomies (Figure 38.3B,C).

The osteotomized bone surfaces are prepared to accommodate the keel of the tibial implant and the post of the femoral implant. Rearticulated trial components are used to confirm proper implant size and position. The trials also facilitate evaluation of joint stability, collateral ligament tension, and range-of-motion. Upon completion of bone preparation, the bone surfaces are cleaned of debris with pulsatile lavage and suction. The tibial component is implanted first using PMMA (Figure 38.3D) and the femoral component is implanted in cementless press-fit or cemented fashion (Figure 38.3E). Range-of-motion is evaluated with the joint reduced. The joint space is lavaged copiously to remove all debris. The joint capsule, subcutaneous tissue, and skin are closed in routine fashion while assuring proper patella tracking. A sterile dressing is applied over the incision. There is no need for a bandage or splint unless complications (e.g., collateral ligament injury) are encountered during surgery.

Postoperative management

Postoperative pain management following TKR includes the use of a combination of opiate analgesics and nonsteroidal anti-inflammatory agents. Cold packs are applied immediately after surgery and at regular intervals thereafter to reduce pain and swelling. The dog's activity is restricted for the first 2 weeks, after which a controlled program of physical rehabilitation and leash exercise can begin. Recommendations for physical rehabilitation following TKR have been published (Liska & Doyle 2009). The goal of rehabilitation is to achieve a pain-free normal passive range-of-motion (PROM) in the operated joint.

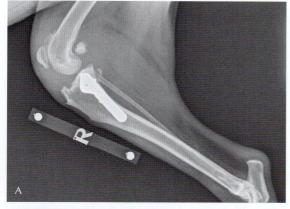

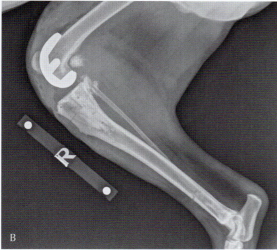

Figure 38.2 Conversion from TPLO (A) to TKR (B) in the dog. This is performed as a two-step procedure, with removal of the TPLO implants, followed 6–8 weeks later by implantation of the TKR. Images courtesy of Dr. Noel Fitzpatrick.

stage procedure with plate/screw removal as stage 1 several weeks before TKR (Figure 38.2). Since infection is an absolute contraindication for total joint replacement, it is recommended that synovial fluid analysis and tissue culture are undertaken if previous surgery has been performed or if infection is suspected.

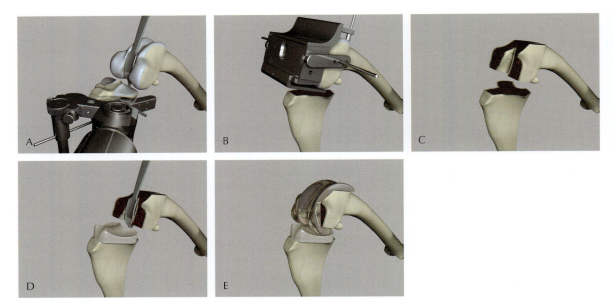

Figure 38.3 Key steps in the surgical procedure for canine total knee replacement. (A) Tibial osteotomy using an extramedullary tibial alignment guide. (B) Femoral cutting block used for the four femoral osteotomies. (C) Completed femoral and tibial osteotomies. (D) Implantation of tibial component. (E) Implantation of femoral component and rearticulation of the stifle joint. Images courtesy of Tim Vojt, The Ohio State University.

Clinical results with cemented canine TKR

Liska and Doyle recently published clinical follow-up on a series of six client-owned dogs that underwent TKR for end-stage osteoarthritis (Liska & Doyle 2009). Outcome measures included radiographic assessment, physical examination (including measurements of stifle joint range-of-motion and thigh circumference), and force-plate gait analysis. Data were recorded preoperatively and at 6 weeks, 3 months, 6 months, and 1 year after surgery. Rehabilitation was provided for each dog.

Joint extension, excursion, peak vertical force, and impulse parameters showed statistically significant improvement ($p \leq 0.01$) starting at 3 months. At the end of the study, joint extension (152°) and excursion (115°) were only 9° and 6° less than normal (Jaegger et al. 2002), respectively. Peak vertical force and impulse were 82% and 103% of the normal contralateral limb, respectively. Video during ambulation at the same intervals confirmed the owner's subjective evaluation that minimal or no gait abnormalities remained after rehabilitation in spite of the severity of the preoperative status.

Potential complications and their management

Infection

Infection is a devastating complication of total joint replacement (Figure 38.4). There are currently no published data on the incidence of infection in canine TKR. Management of an infected TKR would ideally be similar to that for an infected THR—a combination of systemic antibiotics combined with device removal. In contrast to the hip, however, removal of an infected TKR is problematic because it is not feasible to leave the joint to form a pseudarthrosis. Until improved revision strategies are developed, current solutions include arthrodesis or amputation of the affected limb.

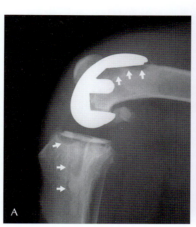 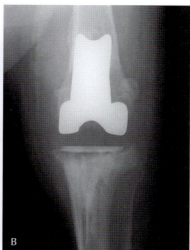

Figure 38.4 Radiographs from an infected canine total knee replacement. (A) There is an extensive zone of radiolucency below the tibial component and along the tibial keel (arrows). There is also lucency around the femoral component (B). The presence of lucencies on both sides of the joint suggests septic rather than aseptic loosening. Options for managing this case include arthrodesis or amputation.

Joint and/or implant instability

Instability following TKR may be due to deficiencies in implant design but is most commonly the result of surgeon error.

At surgery, tibial and femoral osteotomies are made to balance the joint space in flexion and extension while at the same time preserving the axial alignment of the joint. Excessive laxity will lead to instability and an increased risk of device subluxation and concomitant implant wear. Excessive tension on the soft tissues will restrict range-of-motion and may lead to an increased risk of collateral ligament failure.

Another cause of instability is ligament injury, either intraoperatively or in the early postoperative period. The medial collateral ligament is susceptible to iatrogenic injury during the tibial osteotomy. Care should be taken to ensure that the ligament is located and protected during the osteotomy. If a collateral ligament is inadvertently damaged, primary repair should be performed immediately. The repair should be protected with a Robert Jones bandage, a brace, or a splint.

Neurovascular injury

The popliteal artery is a major structure caudal and medial to the joint. It is at risk of injury during the tibial osteotomy as the saw blade exits the caudal-tibial cortex. The risk of vascular injury is reduced by flexing the joint during the osteotomy. This reduces the tension on the artery and allows it, along with the adjacent neurovascular bundles, to move caudally away from the exit point of the blade. Direct protection is achieved by placing a blunt-ended retractor tip immediately caudal to the tibial plateau between the tibia and the joint capsule/popliteal artery.

Wear

Wear of the metallic, and more commonly UHMWPE, components of a TKR implant is an important cause of long-term implant failure in humans (Reay et al. 2009). Any articulating implant material will undergo a variable amount of mechanical wear. *In vivo* material wear rates are influenced by both iatrogenic (e.g., implant malalignment) and environmental (e.g., activity level, body weight) factors. In preclinical research studies with canine TKR implants, wear was found to be relatively mild at time points out to 12 months after surgery (Allen et al. 2009; Figure 38.5). However, the long-term performance of TKR implants has not been assessed and will likely only be determined through biomechanical testing and a systematic analysis of implants that

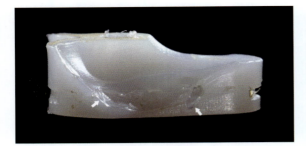

Figure 38.5 Wear of the UHMWPE component of a canine TKR. A large area of the UHMWPE (arrows) has delaminated from the lateral margin of this implant. The biological response to this fragmented UHMWPE can lead to osteolysis, fixation failure, and aseptic loosening. The wear seen with this research implant was at least in part a result of suboptimal implant design. Wear rates with the new clinical TKR implant system has not been determined to date.

are retrieved either at the time of revision surgery or through retrieval studies.

Aseptic loosening

A presumptive diagnosis of aseptic loosening is made on the basis of radiographic evidence of periprosthetic osteolysis in the face of negative bacterial cultures. As with aseptic loosening after total hip replacement, there is insufficient data to determine the incidence of aseptic loosening in canine TKR. One case of femoral component loosening was reported in a recent preclinical study (Allen et al. 2009; Figure 38.6), but the clinical experience with the BioMedtrix implant has been encouraging, with good implant stability in the short term and a low incidence of loosening in the early clinical cases (Liska & Doyle 2009).

Summary and conclusion

TKR improves joint function in dogs with end-stage osteoarthritis. As in humans (Noble et al. 2005), some subclinical degree of functional limitation may be present even in normal dogs that have undergone TKR surgery. The clinical impli-

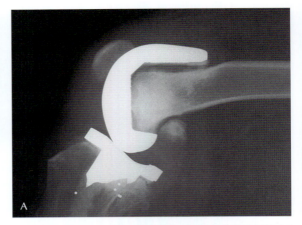
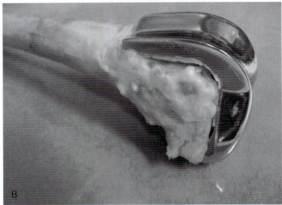

Figure 38.6 Aseptic loosening of a cemented canine TKR. (A) Radiograph demonstrating a wide, radiolucent line at the implant–cement interface of a cemented femoral component. On retrieval, the femoral component was found to be grossly loose with soft tissue between the implant and the cement mantle (B).

cations of this potential mild dysfunction do not appear to be significant considering the severity of pain and dysfunction present in TKR candidates. The subjective and objective data collected to date from clinical patients indicate that TKR is effective in the short term. The long-term success of the procedure can only be determined through additional controlled clinical trials by collecting objective data with long-term implant survival over the entire life of the patient.

References

Allen MJ, Leone KA, Lamonte K, et al. Cemented total knee replacement in 24 dogs: Surgical technique, clinical results, and complications. Vet Surg 2009;38:555–567.

Berzins A, Sumner DR, Turner TM, Natarajan R. Effects of fixation technique on displacement incompatibilities at the bone-implant interface in cementless total knee replacement in a canine model. J Appl Biomater 1994;5:349–352.

Jaegger G, Marcellin-Little DJ, Levine D. Reliability of goniometry in Labrador Retrievers. Am J Vet Res 2002;63:979–986.

Liska W, Doyle N. Canine total knee replacement: Surgical technique and 1-year outcome. Vet Surg 2009;38:568–582.

Liska W, Marcellin-Little D, Eskelinen E, et al. Custom total knee replacement in a dog with femoral condyle bone loss. Vet Surg 2007;36:293–301.

Noble PC, Gordon MJ, Weiss JM, et al. Does total knee replacement restore normal knee function? Clin Orthop Relat Res 2005;431:157–165.

Reay E, Wu J, Holland J, Deehan D. Premature failure of Kinemax Plus total knee replacements. J Bone Joint Surg Br 2009;91:604–611.

Robertsson O, Knutson K, Lewold S, Lidgren L. The Swedish Knee Arthroplasty Register 1975–1997. An update with special emphasis on 41,223 knees operated on in 1988–1997. Acta Orthop Scand 2001;72:503–513.

Sumner DR, Berzins A, Turner TM, et al. Initial *in vitro* stability of the tibial component in a canine model of cementless total knee replacement. J Biomech 1994;27:929–939.

Turner TM, Urban RM, Sumner DR, et al. Bone ingrowth into the tibial component of a canine total condylar knee replacement prosthesis. J Orthop Res 1989;7:893–901.

39 Regenerative Medicine and Cranial Cruciate Ligament Repair

Martha M. Murray and Patrick Vavken

Introduction

Given the fact that cranial cruciate (CrCL) insufficiency is the most common cause of lameness in dogs, it is not surprising that in recent years there has been considerable development in treatment options. Earlier chapters have outlined the spectrum of these procedures in much detail, and while new methods are gaining in popularity, tibial plateau leveling osteotomy (TPLO) is generally considered the most effective option in medium and large breed dogs and, thus, has become widely accepted as standard of care. TPLO consistently produces convincing clinical outcomes, but there are a number of potential shortcomings that should be addressed. Peri- and postoperative complications can arise that are implant-related or relate to the complicated nature of the procedure, such as nonunion or poor tibial plateau angle (TPA) adjustment. These complications can be minimized with meticulous technique. Other shortcomings result from the fact

that TPLO does not address the insufficient CrCL per se and, consequently, the passive stability of the stifle joint. Rather, TPLO creates a situation of dynamic stability during the gait cycle by reducing cranial tibial subluxation during weight-bearing. In point of fact, Ballagas and colleagues showed that peak vertical force and vertical impulse measured by force-plate analysis did not change between the preoperative and 18 weeks postoperative measurements after TPLO in dogs with experimentally induced CrCL insufficiency (Ballagas et al. 2004). The high risk of meniscal injury after TPLO further suggests the existence of inadequate, unbalanced biomechanical stressors (Slocum & Slocum 1993). These published findings also align well with a significantly increased risk of stifle osteoarthritis (OA) despite TPLO (Rayward et al. 2004). The role of the postulated increase in caudal tibial thrust, and the subsequent effects on the caudal cruciate ligament, is still unclear to date.

Parallel to TPLO, other surgical techniques are available for treatment of CrCL rupture (as has been detailed in prior chapters). Tibial tuberosity advancement (TTA) is another osteotomy that aims at the normalization of vertical force by aligning the patellar ligament perpendicular to the tibial plateau. Potential shortcomings and complications in TTA include nonunion, iatrogenic patella (sub)luxation, and the need for specialized

---

Advances in the Canine Cranial Cruciate Ligament,
Edited by Peter Muir, © 2010 ACVS Foundation, This Work is a co-publication between the American College of Veterinary Surgeons Foundation and Wiley-Blackwell.

Table 39.1 Results from the comparison of cruciate ligaments, which do not heal at all, and medial collateral ligaments (MCL), which heal spontaneously, in humans and a number of animal species

	Cell proliferation	Extracellular matrix production	Cell migration	Clot bridges defect
CrCL	Yes	Yes	Yes	No
MCL	Yes	Yes	Yes	Yes

Note: The crucial difference between these ligaments is that factors associated with the intra-articular location of the cranial cruciate ligament (CrCL) inhibits clot formation from bridging the defect, thus prohibiting healing.

implants. As a relatively new technique, there is still little published evidence for the effectiveness and safety of TTA. Another, technically less complicated method is extracapsular stabilization (ECS), using circumfabellar sutures to stabilize the joint. ECS, however, has been shown to result in residual craniocaudal instability, which, in turn, leads to premature OA. One recent study reports an approximately sixfold increase of radiographic signs of OA in dogs at 12 months after ECS compared with TPLO (Lazar et al. 2005). Recent advances in ECS include the TightRope® (Arthrex Vet Systems, Naples, FL) procedure, which employs a strong type of suture and fixation to bone, rather than a transosseous loop, leading to better outcomes in strength and stiffness and less displacement during cyclic loading (Cook et al. 2010).

In summary, these findings suggest that TPLO, ECS such as TightRope, and TTA provide consistently good clinical results regarding gross, dynamic stability in the CrCL-insufficient stifle, but insufficient protection against micromotion and passive instability, resulting in undue biomechanical stress on the meniscus and articular cartilage, thus leading to premature OA and progression of arthritis. This observation begs the question of whether the CrCL could be repaired or regenerated. A repaired ligament could potentially provide both dynamic and passive stability while preserving proprioception and much of the original tissue architecture at the same time. However, any endeavor to stimulate CrCL healing starts with the question of why it fails to heal after the initial trauma.

Why cruciate ligaments do not heal

The fact that cruciate ligaments do not heal has been baffling veterinarians as well as human physicians. This incapacity to heal is even more surprising in the light of the fact that collateral ligaments heal spontaneously with only minimal treatment, as has been extensively studied in humans (Murray & Spector 1999; Murray et al. 2000a,b, 2002, 2007b). This discrepancy offers a unique opportunity to study the reasons for the failure of cruciate healing. Early investigators theorized that the main reason for the lack of cruciate healing was the constant disruption of the ligament stumps during joint motion, and thus simple suture repair techniques were devised and tested. However, these techniques showed excessive failure rates. Subsequent studies returned to the original observation of differences in cruciate ligament and collateral ligament healing and compared these tissues at the cellular and tissue level. While no such studies were carried out for canine cells, studies on human, lapine, and caprine cells showed consistently that cells from cruciate and collateral ligaments have equal capabilities in proliferation, migration, and biosynthesis, ruling out these factors as reasons for differences in healing (Frank et al. 1983a,b; Hannafin et al. 1999). One important difference that was revealed by such comparative analysis was that cruciate injuries, as opposed to collateral ligament injuries, did not form a clot between the ruptured tissue ends; consequently, there was no scaffold for cell migration and tissue repair (Table 39.1; Murray et al. 2000a). High intra-articular levels of plasminogen after

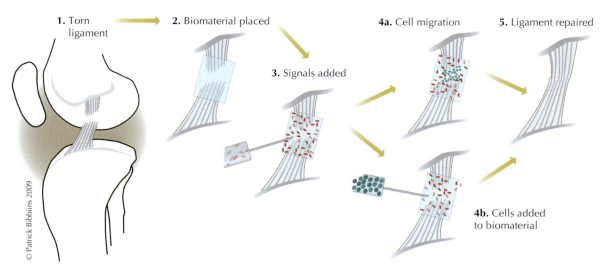

Figure 39.1 Principle of tissue engineering. The triad of cells, biomaterials, and signals are used to stimulate healing or to create a biological substitute to restore or replace lost tissue or organ function.

cruciate injuries are one possible reason for this deficiency in clot formation (Brommer et al. 1992, Rosc et al. 2002). The observation that the provisional scaffold is deficient for the anterior cruciate ligament (ACL) has led to new lines of inquiry into substitute provisional scaffolds designed for intra-articular use.

Tissue engineering to enhance ligament healing

Tissue engineering is currently the most promising method in regenerative medicine. By definition, tissue engineering is "an interdisciplinary field that applies the principles of engineering and life sciences toward the development of biological substitutes that restore, maintain, or improve tissue function or a whole organ" (Langer & Vacanti 1993). In other words, tissue engineering is the orchestrated application of cells, biomaterials, and signals aiming at the stimulation of healing processes (Figure 39.1). For the situation of the cruciate ligament, this means that an appropriate biomaterial, together with appropriate signaling, can be used to stimulate cruciate repair.

The biomaterial

The first question is what biomaterial to use. Among potential biomaterials, collagen has a long-standing record as a biocompatible, biodegradable, and safe material for orthopaedic applications and is the main constituent of the cruciate ligament (Lynn et al. 2004). Furthermore, collagen can be applied as a hydrogel in and on the defect, thus filling the defect easily and completely or as a sponge, allowing better handling intraoperatively and suture fixation. Studies of human and bovine *in vitro* models have demonstrated that fibroblasts are capable of migrating from the stump of the torn cruciate ligament into such a collagenous biomaterial; hence, it is not required to add exogenous cultured cells to the repair site (Murray et al. 2000b, 2002; Murray & Spector 2001).

Signaling

It is crucial to the success of any tissue-engineered repair procedure to consider that the fibrin clot that typically serves as a scaffold for cellular migration is also an important source of growth

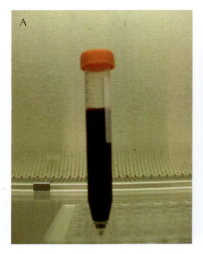 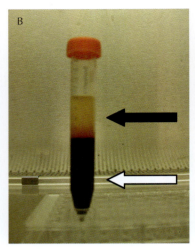 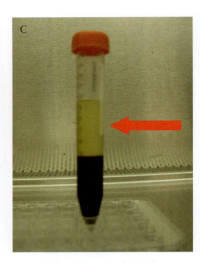

Figure 39.2   To produce a platelet concentrate, whole blood (A) is drawn and carefully centrifuged. This results in the separation of plasma-rich in platelets (black arrow in B) from the remaining blood constituents (white arrow in B). If centrifugation is too vigorous (C), the resulting plasma is poor in platelets; thus, clear (red arrow) and a buffy coat containing platelets and white blood cells is seen at the interface.

factors, extracellular matrix proteins, and other cytokines that stimulate and regulate the inflammatory process that leads to tissue remodeling and finally defect healing. Yet the exact mechanisms at work in physiological wound healing are too complicated to be replicated with currently available biological methods. An elegant way to obviate this problem is to supplement the biomaterial with a platelet concentrate. Autologous platelets at sufficient concentrations can easily be obtained by venipuncture and processed pre- or intra-operatively by simple centrifugation (Figure 39.2). The platelets are activated on contact with collagen and act as a natural growth factor delivery system that also suppresses inflammation (El-Sharkawy et al. 2007; Fufa et al. 2008).

Potential future applications for CrCL repair

Methods such as those described above may someday be used to expand the options in the treatment of CrCL rupture. First, collagenous biomaterials, in association with a platelet concentrate, can be used to enhance classical cruciate replacement techniques. One study applying such a technique in experimental cruciate-deficient goats found reduced craniocaudal laxity with the use of the platelet collagen–platelet composite 6 weeks after the procedure (Spindler et al. 2009). However, while tissue engineering methods can be used to further improve the outcome of cruciate reconstruction, they do not mitigate the problems associated with such procedures, such as the almost unabatedly high rate of osteoarthritis despite treatment, the loss of proprioceptive innervation, and important histological differences between an original ligament and a graft (Abe et al. 1993; Cho et al. 2004; Lanzetta et al. 2004; Gomez-Barrena et al. 2008).

A body of work has been presented describing progress toward developing a successful method of primary cruciate repair, supported by a collagenous biomaterial and platelet concentrate (Murray et al. 2006, 2007a,b; Spindler et al. 2009). While such research builds on studies in porcine and caprine models, it should be regarded as a scientific proof-of-principle and may eventually be applicable in the canine stifle too. Initial *in vitro* studies have shown, as mentioned earlier, that

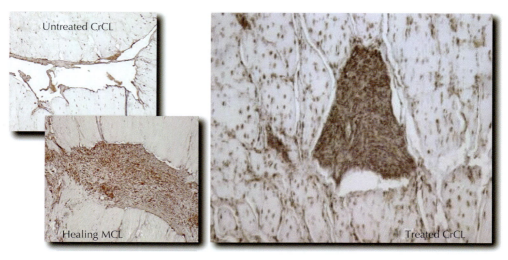

Figure 39.3 The untreated cranial cruciate ligament (CrCL) shows no bridging of the defect; thus, no healing occurs, in contrast to the medical collateral ligament (MCL), which forms a clot that spans the defect and serves as scaffold for cell migration and remodeling and consequently heals. Treatment of the ACL with a collagen–platelet composite produced results similar to what is seen in the MCL.

cells migrate from the stumps of an injured cruciate into a collagen-based biomaterial. The addition of a platelet concentrate stimulates cell migration, proliferation, and biosynthesis further. These findings were subsequently translated into a canine model of a central cruciate defect. In this model it was demonstrated that the use of a collagen platelet concentrate results in superior defect fill and biomechanical properties in dogs (Figure 39.3; Murray et al. 2006). The histological characteristics of the repair tissue were similar to those of successfully healing tissues such as the medial collateral ligament or the patellar tendon (Murray et al. 2007b).

While such models confirm the effectiveness of the procedure, they do not focus on the usual clinical problem, which is a complete cruciate rupture, and not a central defect. Hence, further studies were carried out using a porcine complete cruciate transection model. This model clearly demonstrated that the combination of both collagen as biomaterial and a platelet concentrate is needed to obtain optimal results (Murray et al. 2007a,b, 2009). The beneficial effect of a collagen platelet concentrate on cruciate biomechanics could be seen to persist for as long as 14 weeks (Joshi et al. 2009).

Summary

While TPLO, a procedure that consistently produces satisfactory results, is currently accepted as the standard of care for treatment of CrCL insufficiency in medium and large breeds, there remains interest in developing and validating improved methods of care of CrCL ruptures in the dog. Methods from regenerative medicine, in particular tissue engineering applications, have been shown to be a viable and effective next step in cruciate ligament treatment by offering a potential solution in enhanced primary repair. Such a technique holds much promise, not only for better outcomes in immediate stability, but also, and maybe even more importantly, for less invasive but still effective procedures. While most of the pertinent evidence for safety and efficacy originates from porcine and caprine models, there is no reason to believe that this evidence will not translate to some degree to the canine patient. However, these findings, techniques, and implants need to be optimized for dogs. Future studies will be needed to accurately define the differences in outcomes between TPLO, tissue engineering-enhanced primary repair, and other future methods of cruciate treatment.

References

Abe S, Kurosaka M, Iguchi T. Light and electron microscopic study of remodeling and maturation process in autogenous graft for anterior cruciate ligament reconstruction. Arthroscopy 1993;9:394–405.

Ballagas AJ, Montgomery RD, Henderson RA, Gillette R. Pre- and postoperative force plate analysis of dogs with experimentally transected cranial cruciate ligaments treated using tibial plateau leveling osteotomy. Vet Surg 2004;33:187–190.

Brommer EJ, Dooijewaard G, Dijkmans BA, Breedveld FC. Depression of tissue-type plasminogen activator and enhancement of urokinase-type plasminogen activator as an expression of local inflammation. Thromb Haemost 1992;68:180–184.

Cho S, Muneta T, Ito S. Electron microscopic evaluation of two-bundle anatomically reconstructed anterior cruciate ligament graft. J Orthop Sci 2004;9:296–301.

Cook JL, Luther JK, Beetem J, et al. Clinical comparison of a novel extracapsular stabilization procedure and tibial plateau leveling osteotomy for treatment of cranial cruciate ligament deficiency in dogs. Vet Surg 2010;39:315–323.

El-Sharkawy H, Kantarci A, Deady J, et al. Platelet-rich plasma: Growth factors and pro- and anti-inflammatory properties. J Periodontol 2007;78:661–669.

Frank C, Amiel D, Akeson W. Healing of the medial collateral ligament of the knee. A morphological and biochemical assessment in rabbits. Acta Orthop Scand 1983a;54:917–923.

Frank C, Woo SL, Amiel D, et al. Medial collateral ligament healing. A multidisciplinary assessment in rabbits. Am J Sports Med 1983b;11:379–389.

Fufa D, Shealy B, Jacobson M, et al. Activation of platelet-rich plasma using soluble type I collagen. J Oral Maxillofac Surg 2008;66:684–690.

Gomez-Barrena E, Bonsfills N, Martin JG, et al. Insufficient recovery of neuromuscular activity around the knee after experimental anterior cruciate ligament reconstruction. Acta Orthop 2008;79:39–47.

Hannafin JA, Attia ET, Warren RF, Bhargava M. Characterization of chemotactic migration and growth kinetics of canine knee ligament fibroblasts. J Orthop Res 1999;17:398–404.

Joshi S, Mastrangelo A, Murray M. Collagen-platelet composite enhances histologic healing of the ACL. Am J Sports Med 2009;37:2401–2410.

Langer R, Vacanti JP. Tissue engineering. Science 1993;260:920–926.

Lanzetta A, Corradini C, Verdoia C, et al. The nervous structures of anterior cruciate ligament of human knee, healthy and lesioned, studied with confocal scanning laser microscopy. Ital J Anat Embryol 2004;109:167–176.

Lazar TP, Berry CR, deHaan JJ, et al. Long-term radiographic comparison of tibial plateau leveling osteotomy versus extracapsular stabilization for cranial cruciate ligament rupture in the dog. Vet Surg 2005;34:133–141.

Lynn AK, Yannas IV, Bonfield W. Antigenicity and immunogenicity of collagen. J Biomed Mater Res B Appl Biomater 2004;71:343–354.

Murray MM, Spector M. Fibroblast distribution in the anteromedial bundle of the human anterior cruciate ligament: The presence of alpha-smooth muscle actin-positive cells. J Orthop Res 1999;17:18–27.

Murray MM, Spector M. The migration of cells from the ruptured human anterior cruciate ligament into collagen-glycosaminoglycan regeneration templates in vitro. Biomaterials 2001;22:2393–2402.

Murray MM, Martin SD, Martin TL, Spector M. Histological changes in the human anterior cruciate ligament after rupture. J Bone Joint Surg Am 2000a;82:1387–1397.

Murray MM, Martin SD, Spector M. Migration of cells from human anterior cruciate ligament explants into collagen-glycosaminoglycan scaffolds. J Orthop Res 2000b;18:557–564.

Murray MM, Bennett R, Zhang X, Spector M. Cell outgrowth from the human ACL in vitro: Regional variation and response to TGF-beta1. J Orthop Res 2002;20:875–880.

Murray MM, Forsythe B, Chen F, et al. The effect of thrombin on ACL fibroblast interactions with collagen hydrogels. J Orthop Res 2006;24:508–515.

Murray MM, Spindler KP, Abreu E, et al. Collagen-platelet rich plasma hydrogel enhances primary repair of the porcine anterior cruciate ligament. J Orthop Res 2007a;25:81–91.

Murray MM, Spindler KP, Ballard P, et al. Enhanced histologic repair in a central wound in the anterior cruciate ligament with a collagen-platelet-rich plasma scaffold. J Orthop Res 2007b;25:1007–1017.

Murray MM, Palmer M, Abreu E, et al. Platelet-rich plasma alone is not sufficient to enhance suture repair of the ACL in skeletally immature animals: An in vivo study. J Orthop Res 2009;27:639–645.

Rayward RM, Thomson DG, Davies JV, Innes JF, et al. Progression of osteoarthritis following TPLO surgery: A prospective radiographic study of 40 dogs. J Small Anim Pract 2004;45:92–97.

Rosc D, Powierza W, Zastawna E, et al. Post-traumatic plasminogenesis in intraarticular exudate in the knee joint. Med Sci Monit 2002;8:CR371–C378.

Slocum B, Slocum TD. Tibial plateau leveling osteotomy for repair of cranial cruciate ligament rupture in the canine. Vet Clin North Am Small Anim Pract 1993;23:777–795.

Spindler KP, Murray MM, Carey JL, et al. The use of platelets to affect functional healing of an anterior cruciate ligament (ACL) autograft in a caprine ACL reconstruction model. J Orthop Res 2009;27:631–638.

40 Disease-Modifying Medical Therapy

Sara A. Colopy

Introduction

Osteoarthritis (OA) is the most common form of joint disease in both human beings and companion animals (Boileau et al. 2009; Connor et al. 2009). Medications used to treat OA can be categorized as either symptom-modifying (analgesics, nonsteroidal anti-inflammatory drugs [NSAIDs], corticosteroids, and viscosupplementation) or structure-modifying (Fajardo & Di Cesare 2005). Current treatment options for OA are primarily symptomatic, focused on reducing pain and inflammation, and improving or maintaining joint mobility. These drugs do not delay, stabilize, or reverse the degenerative processes of OA. In addition, adverse effects of these drugs may be serious. Although NSAIDs are very effective in controlling clinical signs of OA, they can be associated with gastrointestinal hemorrhage and renal dysfunction (Fajardo & Di Cesare 2005). The initial response rate to glucocorticoids may be as high as 81% in dogs with inflammatory arthritis (Clements et al. 2004). However, in addition to polyuria, polydypsia, and polyphagia, adverse effects may

Advances in the Canine Cranial Cruciate Ligament,
Edited by Peter Muir, © 2010 ACVS Foundation, This Work is a co-publication between the American College of Veterinary Surgeons Foundation and Wiley-Blackwell.

include spontaneous tendon and ligament rupture, making glucocorticoids a poor choice for dogs with stifle synovitis. Apoptosis, inhibition of cellular proliferation, and reduction in collagen synthesis are likely important mechanisms here (Hossain et al. 2008). There is great need to develop disease-modifying osteoarthritis drugs (DMOADs) that target specific processes in the pathogenesis of OA and prevent irreversible destruction of articular cartilage. At present, there are no DMOADs approved for treatment of OA in human beings or animals (Qvist et al. 2008).

Cranial cruciate ligament (CrCL) rupture is the leading cause of OA in dogs (Hegemann et al. 2005). Although the underlying disease mechanism has yet to be elucidated, there is increasing evidence that cruciate rupture is associated with synovitis, which is similar histologically and pathophysiologically to rheumatoid arthritis and other immune-mediated arthropathies (Hegemann et al. 2005; Muir et al. 2007; refer to Section 2 of this book for further detail). Given the high prevalence of bilateral arthritis and CrCL rupture (Doverspike et al. 1993), the presence of osteophytosis at the time of diagnosis (Muir et al. 2005), the similarities to immune-mediated arthritis (Hegemann et al. 2005; Muir et al. 2007), and evidence that inflammation may actually precede cruciate rupture (Bleedorn et al. 2009), there is increasing support for the hypothesis that cruciate ligament

277

rupture is a pathologic process secondary to chronic joint inflammation. Thus, disease-modifying therapy may not only prove to be helpful in preventing progression of OA, but may also be beneficial in preventing further degradation of cruciate ligament.

MMP inhibitors

Up-regulation of degradative enzymes, such as the matrix metalloproteinases (MMPs) and aggrecanase, by pro-inflammatory cytokines is a characteristic feature of OA (Fernandes et al. 2002). Much effort has been focused on finding small molecule inhibitors of MMPs that act downstream in the pathophysiologic cascade of OA. Many of these agents have failed in clinical trials due to painful musculoskeletal side effects, which are likely related to broad-spectrum MMP inhibition (Hutchinson et al. 1998; Fajardo & Di Cesare 2005; Pelletier & Martel-Pelletier 2007; Qvist et al. 2008). Development of specific MMP inhibitors and inhibitors of aggrecanase family members involved in OA pathophysiology are currently being investigated. Clinical data regarding these compounds are still lacking (Pelletier & Martel-Pelletier 2007; Qvist et al. 2008).

Antibacterials of the tetracycline class (including doxycycline and minocycline) have also been found to inhibit MMP activity and thus have been studied as potential DMOADs. *In vitro* studies show that doxycycline inhibits degradation of type XI collagen in articular cartilage, results in lower levels of active collagenase and gelatinase, and can inhibit mRNA for inducible nitric oxide synthase (an enzyme responsible for secretion of MMPs by chondrocytes) (Yu et al. 1991; Amin et al. 1996; Smith et al. 1996; Lotz 1999; Fajardo & Di Cesare 2005). *In vivo*, doxycycline reduces cartilage gelatinase and collagenase in human beings and dogs with OA, and reduces the incidence and progression of joint pathology in a canine model of OA (Yu et al. 1992; Smith et al. 1998; Brandt et al. 2005). In a randomized double-blind placebo-controlled study, doxycycline administration slowed joint space narrowing in obese women with OA of the medial tibiofemoral compartment. The frequency of follow-up visits at which patients reported a ≥20% increase in pain relative to the previous visit was less in patients receiving doxycycline (Brandt et al. 2005). Doxycycline has not yet been approved by the Food and Drug Administration as a chondroprotective agent (Qvist et al. 2008).

Bisphosphonates

Evidence documenting changes in subchondral bone integrity and bone metabolic activity in patients with OA has prompted investigation of bisphosphonates as potential DMOADs (Agnello et al. 2005; Qvist et al. 2008). Bisphosphonates interfere with osteoclast activity and thus have the ability to inhibit bone resorption. In a study involving experimental CrCL transection in dogs, zoledronate inhibited an increase in osteocalcin and prevented loss of subchondral bone mineral density. Lameness and markers of cartilage metabolism were not evaluated in this study (Agnello et al. 2005). However, in several large placebo-controlled studies in people with OA, bisphosphonates (primarily risedronate) failed to prevent structural deterioration of the cartilage, despite beneficial effects seen in the subchondral bone (Qvist et al. 2008). Thus, at this time, there is a lack of evidence supporting the use of bisphosphonates for disease-modifying therapy in OA.

T cell inhibitors

Given the similarities between inflammatory arthritis associated with CrCL rupture and rheumatoid arthritis, there are several disease-modifying drugs used successfully for rheumatoid arthritis that may be of benefit in dogs with stifle synovitis. We are currently investigating leflunomide, a newer immunomodulating drug, as a potential disease-modifying therapy in dogs with inflammatory arthritis. The active metabolite of leflunomide, A77-1726, is a malononitriloamide analog that inhibits T and B cell proliferation, suppresses immunoglobulin production, and interferes with leukocyte adhesion and diapedesis. Many targets of A77-1726 have been described, with inhibition of tyrosine kinases being the primary mechanism of immunomodulation (Silva & Morris 1997; Gregory et al. 1998a,b; Chong et al.

1999; Kirsch et al. 2005; Ranganath & Furst 2007). Tyrosine kinase signaling is important for activation of the T cell receptor and several cytokine receptors, including the IL-2 receptor (Mattar et al. 1993; Williams et al. 1994). A77-1726 also inhibits the mitochondrial enzyme dihydroorotate dehydrogenase (DHODH), an enzyme necessary for *de novo* pyrimidine synthesis. Subsequent depletion of nucleotides inhibits lymphocyte proliferation (Silva & Morris 1997; Kirsch et al. 2005).

Leflunomide is an effective disease-modifying drug for rheumatoid arthritis in people, and decreases symptoms and radiographic progression, and systemic levels of MMPs and pro-inflammatory cytokines (Litinsky et al. 2006; Marder & McCune 2007). We have recently documented successful treatment of dogs with immune-mediated polyarthritis using leflunomide. Of the 14 dogs in this study, eight dogs demonstrated complete initial resolution of clinical signs; five dogs demonstrated partial response to therapy; and one dog demonstrated no response to therapy (Colopy et al. 2010). Leflunomide is well tolerated in dogs; significant toxicity has not been reported thus far when used clinically at a dosage of 3–4 mg/kg/day (Gregory et al. 1998b; Colopy et al. 2010). We are currently exploring the use of this drug for treatment of dogs with evidence of primarily mononuclear synovitis and a stable stifle with partial CrCL rupture. However, until trial data are available, the value of this therapeutic approach is unclear.

Other DMOADs

Other drugs that have been studied as potential DMOADs include diacerein, cathepsin k, and cathepsin S inhibitors, a cyclo-oxygenase/5-lipoxygenase (COX/5-LOX) inhibitor, inducible nitric oxide synthase inhibitors, and inhibitors of pro-inflammatory cytokines (Bendele et al. 1996; Dougados et al. 2001; Fernandes et al. 2002; Gerwin et al. 2006; Pelletier & Martel-Pelletier 2007; Qvist et al. 2008; Connor et al. 2009; Williams & Spector 2009). Many of these compounds have shown benefit in experimental or *in vitro* analysis and may prove to be effective DMOADs in the future. However, data regarding significant clinical efficacy are currently lacking.

Difficulties in developing reliable DMOADs arise from several issues. These include a lack of specific, sensitive, and quantitative biomarkers to detect and monitor changes in OA progression, and a lack of reliable animal models that mimic naturally occurring disease. Measurement of joint space narrowing on weight-bearing radiographs is most commonly used to assess OA progression and efficacy of DMOADs in human beings. However, this method does not readily detect subtle changes in a slowly progressing disease. Magnetic resonance imaging is more sensitive than computed radiography for detection of osteophytosis, changes in the subchondral bone, and changes in the articular cartilage, and could better discriminate between joint effusion and synovial thickening (D'Anjou et al. 2008; Qvist et al. 2008). Further analysis and validation of both diagnostic imaging and reliable biomarkers is critical to the development and approval of new DMOADs in human and veterinary medicine.

Conclusion

In summary, there is a clear need for new disease-modifying therapies in both human beings and animals with OA. It is likely that future directions in research and treatment of OA will be based on the pathophysiologic events that modulate the initiation and progression of this disease. Given evidence that synovitis occurs concurrently with and may *precede* CrCL rupture in dogs, it is possible that new disease-modifying drugs for OA could prevent degradation of the CrCL over time.

References

Agnello KA, Trumble, TN, Chambers JN, et al. Effects of zoledronate on markers of bone metabolism and subchondral bone mineral density in dogs with experimentally induced cruciate-deficient osteoarthritis. Am J Vet Res 2005;66:1487–1495.

Amin AR, Attur MG, Thakker GD, et al. A novel mechanism of action of tetracyclines: Effects on nitric oxide synthases. Proc Natl Acad Sci U S A 1996;93: 14014–14019.

Bendele AM, Bendele RA, Hulman JF, Swann BP. Beneficial effects of treatment with diacerhein in guinea pigs with osteoarthritis. Rev Prat 1996;46:S35–S39.

Bleedorn JA, Greuel E, Manley PA, et al. Synovitis precedes development of joint instability in dogs with degenerative cranial cruciate ligament rupture. Vet Surg 2009;38:E26.

Boileau C, Martel-Pelletier J, Caron J, et al. Protective effects of total fraction of avocado/soybean unsaponifiables on the structural changes in experimental dog osteoarthritis: Inhibition of nitric oxide synthase and matrix metalloproteinase-13. Arthritis Res Ther 2009;11:R41.

Brandt KD, Mazzuca SA, Katz BP, et al. Effects of doxycycline on progression of osteoarthritis: Results of a randomized, placebo-controlled, double-blind trial. Arthritis Rheum 2005;52:2015–2025.

Chong AS-F, Huang W, Liu W, et al. *In vivo* activity of leflunomide: Pharmacokinetic analyses and mechanism of immunosuppression. Transplantation 1999;68:100–109.

Clements DN, Gear RN, Tattersall J, et al. Type I immune-mediated polyarthritis in dogs: 39 cases (1997–2002). J Am Vet Med Assoc 2004;224:1323–1327.

Colopy SA, Baker TA, Muir P. Therapeutic efficacy of leflunomide for treatment of immune-mediated polyarthritis in dogs: 14 cases (2006–2008). J Am Vet Med Assoc 2010;236:312–318.

Connor JR, LePage C, Swift BA, et al. Protective effects of a cathepsin K inhibitor, SB-553484, in the canine partial medial meniscectomy model of osteoarthritis. Osteoarthritis Cartilage 2009;17:1236–1243..

D'Anjou MA, Moreau M, Troncy E, et al. Osteophytosis, subchondral bone sclerosis, joint effusion and soft tissue thickening in canine experimental stifle osteoarthritis: comparison between 1.5T magnetic resonance imaging and computed radiography. Vet Surg 2008;37:166–177.

Dougados M, Nguyen M, Berdah L, et al. Evaluation of the structure-modifying effects of diacerein in hip osteoarthritis: ECHODIAH, a three-year, placebo-controlled trial. Evaluation of the chondromodulating effect of diacerein in OA of the hip. Arthritis Rheum 2001;44:2539–2547.

Doverspike M, Vasseur PB, Harb MF, Walls CM. Contralateral cranial cruciate ligament rupture: Incidence in 114 dogs. J Am Anim Hosp Assoc 1993;29:167–170.

Fajardo M, Di Cesare PE. Disease-modifying therapies for osteoarthritis. Drugs Aging 2005;22:141–161.

Fernandes JC, Martel-Pelletier J, Pelletier JP. The role of cytokines in osteoarthritis pathophysiology. Biorheology 2002;39:237–246.

Gerwin N, Hops C, Lucke A. Intraarticular drug delivery in osteoarthritis. Adv Drug Deliv Rev 2006;58:226–242.

Gregory CR, Silva HT, Patz JD, Morris RE. Comparative effects of malononitriloamide analogs of leflunomide on whole blood lymphocyte stimulation in humans, rhesus macaques, cats, dogs, and rats. Transplant Proc 1998a;30:1047–1048.

Gregory CR, Stewart A, Sturges B, et al. Leflunomide effectively treats naturally occurring immune-mediated and inflammatory diseases of dogs that are unresponsive to conventional therapy. Transplant Proc 1998b;30:4143–4148.

Hegemann N, Wondimu A, Kohn B, et al. Cytokine profile in canine immune-mediated polyarthritis and osteoarthritis. Vet Comp Orthop Traumatol 2005;18:67–72.

Hossain MA, Park J, Choi SH, Kim G. Dexamethasone induces apoptosis in proliferative canine tendon cells and chondrocytes. Vet Comp Orthop Traumatol 2008;21:337–342.

Hutchinson JW, Tierney GM, Parsons SL, Davis TR. Dupuytren's disease and frozen shoulder induced by treatment with a matrix metalloproteinase inhibitor. J Bone Joint Surg Br 1998;80:907–908.

Kirsch BM, Zeyda M, Stuhlmeier K, et al. The active metabolite of leflunomide, A77 1726, interferes with dendritic cell function. Arthritis Res Ther 2005;7;R694–R703.

Litinsky I, Paran D, Levartovsky D, et al. The effects of leflunomide on clinical parameters and serum levels of IL-6, IL-10, MMP-1 and MMP-3 in patients with resistant rheumatoid arthritis. Cytokine 2006;33:106–1110.

Lotz M. The role of nitric oxide in articular cartilage damage. Rheum Dis Clin North Am 1999;25:269–82.

Marder W, McCune WJ. Advances in immunosuppressive therapy. Semin Respir Crit Care Med 2007;28:398–417.

Mattar T, Kochhar K, Bartlett R, et al. Inhibition of the epidermal growth factor receptor tyrosine kinase activity by leflunomide. Fed Euro Biochem Soc 1993;334:161–164.

Muir P, Schamberger BM, Manley PA, Hao Z. Localization of cathepsin K and tartrate-resistant acid phosphatase in synovium and cranial cruciate ligament in dogs with cruciate disease. Vet Surg 2005;34:239–246.

Muir P, Oldenhoff WE, Hudson AP, et al. Detection of DNA from a range of bacterial species in the knee joints of dogs with inflammatory knee arthritis and associated degenerative anterior cruciate ligament rupture. Microb Pathog 2007;42:47–55.

Pelletier JP, Martel-Pelletier J. DMOAD developments: present and future. Bull NYU Hosp Jt Dis 2007;65:242–248.

Qvist P, Bay-Jensen AC, Christiansen C, et al. The disease modifying osteoarthritis drug (DMOAD): Is it in the horizon? Pharmacol Res 2008;58:1–7.

Ranganath VK, Furst MD. Disease-modifying antirheumatic drug use in the elderly rheumatoid arthritis patient. Rheum Dis Clin North Am 2007;33:197–217.

Silva HT, Morris RE. Leflunomide and malonitriloamides. Exp Opin Invest Drugs 1997;6:51–64.

Smith GN, Jr., Brandt KD, Hasty KA. Activation of recombinant human neutrophil procollagenase in the presence of doxycycline results in fragmentation of the enzyme and loss of enzyme activity. Arthritis Rheum 1996;39:235–244.

Smith GN, Jr., Yu L, Jr., Brandt K, Capello W. Oral administration of doxycycline reduces collagenase and gelatinase activities in extracts of human osteoarthritic cartilage. J Rheumatol 1998;25:532–535.

Williams JW, Xiao F, Foster P, et al. Leflunomide in experimental transplantation. Control of rejection and alloantibody production, reversal of acute rejection, and interaction with cyclosporine. Transplantation 1994;57:1223–1231.

Williams FMK, Spector TD. A new 5-lipoxygenase inhibitor seems to be safe and effective for the treatment of osteoarthritis. Nat Clin Pract Rheumatol 2009;5:132–133.

Yu LP, Smith GN, Hasty KA, Brandt KD. Doxycycline inhibits type XI collagenolytic activity of extracts from human osteoarthritic cartilage and of gelatinase. J Rheumatol 1991;18:1450–1452.

Yu LP, Smith GN, Brandt KD, et al. Reduction of the severity of canine osteoarthritis by prophylactic treatment with oral doxycycline. Arthritis Rheum 1992;35:1150–1159.

Index

Note: Page numbers in *italics* refer to figures, those in **bold** to tables. The abbreviation CrCL is used throughout for cranial cruciate ligament.

abnormal stifle, 119–121, *119, 120, 121*

accelerometers, use in assessing limb function after stifle stabilization surgery, 234–235

ACL injury in humans. *See* anterior cruciate ligament injury in humans

activity level, as risk factor for CrCL rupture, 97

age

    and CrCL rupture, 54, 95, **96**

    effect on ligament biomechanical properties, 17

allografts

    and healing potential of reconstructed CrCL, 24

    in intra-articular stabilization, 192

amantadine, use in stifle arthritis, 243

analgesics, use in stifle arthritis, 242–243

anatomy of cruciate ligaments, 3

    functional, 10–11

    innervation, 9–10

    macroanatomy, 5–6, *6, 7*

    microanatomy, 6, *8*

    synovium, 6–7, 189–190

    vascular supply, 7–9, *9, 10*

anatomy of stifle, as risk factor for CrCL rupture, **96,** 96–97

anterior cruciate ligament injury in humans, 55, 57, 59–60, 65–66, 68, 69, 105, 213, 249–250

antibacterials, use in arthritis, 278

antibodies to type I and II collagen, 77–79, *78*

antigen-specific immune responses in joint tissues, 88

apoptosis in joint tissues, 72, 75

arthritis, stifle, *40, 41, 43,* 135

    biochemical markers, and disease mechanisms, 231–232

clinical signs, 241

and CrCL-deficient stifle, 229–232, *230, 231*

joint lavage, as treatment for, 159, *160,* **160,** 161

and lameness, 236–237

medical therapy for, 234, 241–245, 277–279

nitric oxide, role of, 75

and obesity, 241–242

pathomechanics theory of, *40*

progression of after stifle stabilization, 229–232, *230,* 236–237

and weight management, 241–242

arthrography, computed tomographic, 123, *124*

arthroscopic evaluation of synovial membrane, 82–83

arthroscopic follow-up after stifle stabilization, 201–208, *202, 203, 204, 205, 206, 207, 208, 209,* 210–212, *210, 211*

arthroscopic-assisted arthrotomy, 152–154, *153, 154, 155, 156–158*

arthroscopy, 145, 147, 149, *149, 150, 151,* 151–152, *152. See also* arthroscopic-assisted arthrotomy

arthrotomy, 145–147, *146, 148, 149, 150. See also* arthroscopic-assisted arthrotomy

articular cartilage, identification of pathological change, 152, *152*

aseptic loosening, as complication in total knee replacement, 268, *268*

Aspirin Triggered Lipoxins, 242

ASUs (avocado and soybean oil unsaponifiables), use in stifle arthritis, 244

ATLs (Aspirin Triggered Lipoxins), 242

autografts, in intra-articular stabilization, 190–192, *191, 192*

284 Index

avocado and soybean oil unsaponifiables, use in stifle
    arthritis, 244
avulsion fracture, 110, 111, 126, *127–130*, 133

bilateral disease, and CrCL rupture, 96, **97**
bilateral lameness, 102, *102*
biochemical markers, and arthritis disease
    mechanisms, 231–232
biologic factors affecting ligament biomechanical
    properties, 17–19
    age, 17
    breed, 17
    grafts, biomechanics of, *18*, 18–19
    isometric points, 18
    ligament rupture, sites of, 17
    reproductive status, 17
    synovitis, 17–18
    use/disuse, 17
    weight, 17
biological stabilization methods in extracapsular
    stabilization, 164–165, **165**
biomechanics of cruciate ligaments, 13–19
    biomechanical properties, 14–16
    CrCL-deficient stifle treated by tibial osteotomies,
        195–199, *196, 198*
    ligament composition, 13–14, *14*, 59
    viscoelasticity, 16–17
biomechanics of grafts, *18*, 18–19
biomechanics of joint, effect of meniscal release,
    224–225, *224, 225, 226*
biomechanics of stifle, 37–41, 177–179, *179, 180, 181,*
    195–199, *196, 198*
BioMedtrix Canine Total Knee Replacement implant,
    263, 264, *264*, 268
bisphosphonates, use in arthritis, 278
blood supply. *See* vascular supply
body condition, as risk factor for CrCL rupture, 96, **96.**
    See also weight
bone
    magnetic resonance imaging of, 138, *141*
    screws, in tibial plateau leveling osteotomy,
        171–172
breed
    effect on ligament biomechanical properties, 17
    as risk factor for CrCL rupture, 53, 95–96, **96**
Bristol Osteoarthritis in Dogs outcome measure, 259,
    260
BrOAD (Bristol Osteoarthritis in Dogs) outcome
    measure, 259, **260**

CaCL. *See* caudal cruciate ligament
CaCL rupture. *See* rupture, CaCL
candidate gene analyses, 54–55, **56**
Canine Brief Pain Inventory, 233–234, 258, **260**
caudal articular nerve, 9–10

caudal cruciate ligament, 5–6
    rupture of, 103–104, 109–111, *110*
    and tibial plateau leveling osteotomy, 111
    ultrasonography of, 118–119
caudal hemimeniscectomy, 218, **219**
caudal lateral bundle of CrCL. *See* caudolateral
    subdivision
caudolateral subdivision (caudal lateral bundle) of
    CrCL, 5, *6*, 10–11, 14, 105, 115, 190
CBPI (Canine Brief Pain Inventory), 233–234, 258, **260**
chondroitin sulfate, use in stifle arthritis, 244
chondromodulating agents, use in stifle arthritis,
    243–244
CL (caudal lateral bundle) of CrCL. *See* caudolateral
    subdivision
clinical signs of CrCL rupture, 102–104, *102, 103*
CM (cranial medial bundle) of CrCL. *See* craniomedial
    subdivision
collagen
    antibodies to type I and II, 77–79, *78*
    antigenicity, 77
    in cruciate ligaments, 6, *8*, 46, 59, 77
    in ligaments, 13
    in menisci, 30, 32, 33
    in tissue engineering, 273
completely ruptured CrCL
    debridement, 214, *215*
    healing potential of, 22–23, **23**
computational gait analysis, use in assessing limb
    function after stifle stabilization surgery, 235–236,
    236
computed tomographic arthrography, 123, *124*
computed tomography of stifle, 123–126, *124, 125, 126,*
    127, 128, 129, 130, 131, 132, 133
concurrent meniscal injury, 217–221, *218, 219, 220, 221,*
    221, 223
conformation, as risk factor for CrCL rupture, **96,**
    96–97
cranial drawer motion, 105–106, **106**
cranial drawer test, 102–103, *103*
cranial medial bundle of CrCL. *See* craniomedial
    subdivision
cranial tibial closing wedge osteotomy, 196–197
cranial tibial subluxation, 197
cranial tibial thrust, 68, 172, *196*, 196, 197
cranial tibial thrust test, 102–103, *103*
cranial translation of tibia relative to femur, as clinical
    sign of CrCL rupture, 103
cranial-caudal instability, as clinical sign of CrCL
    rupture, 102–103
craniomedial subdivision (cranial medial bundle) of
    CrCL, 5, *6*, 10–11, 14, 105, 115, 190
CrCL rupture. *See* rupture, CrCL
CrCL-deficient stifle, *39*, 39–41, 195–199, *196, 198,*
    229–232, *230, 231*

creep, as characteristic of viscoelastic material, 16
crimp
    in CrCL, 46, *47*, 47–48, *49*
    in ligaments, 13, *14*, *15*
CT of stifle. *See* computed tomography of stifle
CTA (computed tomographic arthrography), 123, *124*
CTT. *See* cranial tibial thrust
CTWO (cranial tibial closing wedge osteotomy),
    196–197

debridement, 213–215, *215*
deformities of limb, angular/torsional, and tibial
    tuberosity advancement, 183
disease-modifying osteoarthritis drugs, 277–279
distal femur, morphology, 65–67, *66*, *67*, *68*
disuse, effect on ligament biomechanical properties,
    17
DMOADs (disease-modifying osteoarthritis drugs),
    277–279
doxycycline, use in arthritis, 278

ECM metabolism. *See* extracellular matrix metabolism
effusion, as clinical sign of CrCL rupture, 102
energy dissipation, as characteristic of viscoelastic
    material, 16–17
epidemiology of CrCL rupture, 95–97, **96, 97**
ES. *See* extracapsular stabilization
extracapsular ligament, healing potential of, 21–22,
    22
extracapsular stabilization, 18, 163–167, **165,** 272
    arthroscopic follow-up after, 210, *210*, *211*
    biological stabilization, 164–165, **165**
    conversion to total knee replacement, 264
    fixation points, isometric, 18, 164, *164*
    postoperative procedures, 167
    rehabilitation after, 250, *250*
    synthetic stabilization, 165–167, **165,** *166*
extracellular matrix metabolism, 59, 61, *61*, 62, *62*

fabella, mediodistal position of, 69
fascial/biceps tendon advancement/imbrication
    procedure, 164–165, **165**
femoropatellar joint space, 231
FHT (fibular head transposition), 164, 165, **165**
fibroblasts, in ligaments, 13, *14*, 59
fibrocartilagenous areas in CrCL, 49–51
fibular fractures, after tibial plateau leveling
    osteotomy, 172, *173*
fibular head transposition, 164, 165, **165**
force platform gait analysis, 235, *236*, 257
force-deformation curves, use in CrCL testing, *15*,
    15–16
FPJS (femoropatellar joint space), 231
fractures, as complication of tibial plateau leveling
    osteotomy, 172, *173*

function
    return to, 155, 158
    as risk factor for CrCL rupture, **96,** 97
functional anatomy of cruciate ligaments, 10–11

gabapentin, use in stifle arthritis, 243
gene analysis, 54–55, **56**
glucosamine, use in stifle arthritis, 244
grafts
    allografts, 24, 192
    autografts, 190–192, *191*, *192*
    biomechanics of, *18*, 18–19
    intra-articular, use in restoration of joint stability, *18*,
        18–19, 189–193
    patellar tendon, 190–191, *191*
    reconstructed CrCL graft, healing potential of,
        24–25, *25*
    reconstructed graft interface tissue, healing potential
        of, 25–26, *26*
GRF (ground reaction forces), as measure of gait,
    235–236
ground reaction forces, as measure of gait, 235–236

HA (hyaluronic acid), use in stifle arthritis, 243–244
healing potential
    of completely ruptured CrCL, 22–23, **23**
    of CrCL, 189–190, 272–273, **272**
    of extracapsular ligament, 21–22, *22*
    of partially ruptured CrCL, **23,** 23–24
    of reconstructed CrCL graft, 24–25, *25*
    of reconstructed graft interface tissue, 25–26,
        26
    of surgically repaired CrCL, **23,** 24
hemostasis, and inflammation phase of ligament
    healing, 21, *22*, 24
histology of CrCL rupture, 17, 45–51
histopathology of CrCL, 46–49, *47*, *48*, *49*, *50*
history provided for CrCL rupture, 101
hoop tension, 33, *34*, 224
hyaluronic acid, use in stifle arthritis, 243–244
hysteresis, as characteristic of viscoelastic material,
    16–17

ICN (intercondylar notch), 65–67, *66*, *67*
immune responses
    antigen-specific, within joint tissues, 88
    innate, within joint tissues, 88–90, *90*
    synovial, in stifle synovitis, 87–90, *88*, *89*, *90*
implant
    instability, as complication in total knee
        replacement, 267
    selection, in tibial plateau leveling osteotomy, *171*,
        171–172
    for tibial tuberosity advancement, 184
inducible nitric oxide synthase, 71, 72

286 Index

infection, as complication in total knee replacement, 266, *267*

inflammatory cell populations within stifle, 87–88, *88, 89*

innervation
of cruciate ligaments, 9–10
of menisci, 31–32
of stifle, 9–10, *11*

iNOS (inducible nitric oxide synthase), 71, 72

intended function, as risk factor for CrCL rupture, **96**, 97

intercondylar notch, 65–67, *66, 67*

intra-articular grafts, use in restoration of joint stability, *18*, 18–19, 189–193

intra-articular stabilization, 189–193
allografts, use in, 192
autografts, use in, 190–192, *191, 192*
intra-articular ligament replacement, 190–193, *191, 192*
intra-articular repair, 189–190
prosthetics, use in, 192

intracapsular stabilization, arthroscopic follow-up after, 210–212, *211*

isometric fixation points for joint stabilization/ ligament reconstruction, 18, 164, *164*

item generation, in client-specific outcome measures, 258

item scaling, in client-specific outcome measures, 234, 258

jig
use in tibial compression radiography, 114
use in tibial plateau leveling osteotomy, 170

joint/implant instability, as complication in total knee replacement, 267

joint lavage, 159, *160*, **160**, 161

kinematics, two-/three-dimensional, use in assessing limb function after stifle stabilization surgery, 236

knee replacement, total. *See* total knee replacement

lameness
bilateral, 102, *102*
and CaCL disruption, 109
as clinical sign of CrCL rupture, 101, 102, *102*
residual, after stifle stabilization surgery, 233–237, *236, 237*
unilateral, 102

lateral arthrotomy, 145, 146, *146*

lateral articular nerve, 10

lateral fabellotibial suture, 165–166, **165**, *166*

lateral meniscus, 29, *31*

lateral suture anchor technique, **165**, *166*, 166–167

lavage, 159, *160*, **160**, 161

laxity
and CrCL metabolism, 59–63, *61, 62, 63*
of knee, in human females, 59
tests, 195–196

leflunomide, use in arthritis, 278–279

LFTS (lateral fabellotibial suture), 165–166, **165**, *166*

ligamentous injuries to stifle, 110

ligaments
composition, 13–14, *14*, 59
fibroblasts in, 13, *14*, 59
injury of, as cause of joint/implant instability in total knee replacement, 267
magnetic resonance imaging of, 137–138, **138**, *139–141*
rupture of, sites, 17

limb deformities, angular/torsional, and tibial tuberosity advancement, 183

Liverpool Osteoarthritis in Dogs outcome measure, 258, 259, **260**

LOAD (Liverpool Osteoarthritis in Dogs) outcome measure, 258, 259, **260**

LSA (lateral suture anchor) technique, **165**, *166*, 166–167

macroanatomy of cruciate ligaments, 5–6, *6, 7*

magnetic resonance imaging of stifle, 135–142, *136, 137*, **138**, *139–141*

matrix metabolism of cruciate ligament, and development of laxity, 59–63, *61, 62, 63*

matrix metalloproteinases, 73–75
in CrCL, 61
influence on CrCL structure, 74
in stifle joint, *73*, 74

mechanoreceptors in CrCL, 213–214

medial arthrotomy, 145, 146

medial articular nerve, 9

medial meniscus, 29, *31*

medical therapy for stifle arthritis, 234, 241, 245, 277
analgesics, 242–243
antibacterials, 278
chondromodulating agents, 243–244
disease-modifying drugs, 277–279
nonsteroidal anti-inflammatory drugs, 242
nutritional supplements, 244–245
weight management, 241–242

meniscal injury, 137, *204, 206*, 207–208, 210, *211*, 215, 227, 237
concurrent, 217–221, *218, 219, 220, 221*, **221**, 223
magnetic resonance imaging, 137, *137*
postliminary, 223
subsequent, 223
ultrasonography, 120, *120*

meniscal release, 151, *151*, 154, *158*, 220, 220–221, **221**, 223–228, 237
clinical decision making, 227–228

effect on joint biomechanics, 224–225, *224*, *225*, *226*
surgical technique, 225–227, *227*
and tibial plateau leveling osteotomy, 170, 207–208, *209*, 210, 220
and tibial tuberosity advancement, 186
meniscal repair, 218
meniscal resection. *See* meniscectomy
meniscectomy, 151, 154, *157*, 207, 218–220, **219**, *220*
menisci
  arthroscopic-assisted arthrotomy, 154, *157–158*
  arthroscopy, 149, *150*, 151, *151*, 202
  arthrotomy, 147, *148*, *149*
  biomechanical/material properties, 32–33
  collagen in, 30, 32, 33
  composition, 30
  and computed tomography, 123, *124*
  function, 33–34
  hoop tension theory, 33, *34*, 224
  innervation, 31–32
  lateral, 29, *31*
  magnetic resonance imaging of, 137, *137*, *139*
  medial, 29, *31*
  and stifle stability, 33, 38
  structure, 30
  surgical anatomy, 29–30, *30*, *31*
  tie fibers in, 30
  ultrasonography of, 119, *119*
  vascular supply, 30–31, *32*
microanatomy of cruciate ligaments, 6, *8*
mid-substance tears, 109–110
minimally invasive arthrotomy, 147, *148*
MMP inhibitors, use in arthritis, 278
MMPs. *See* matrix metalloproteinases
modified retinacular imbrication technique, 165–166, **165**, *166*
morbidity, after stifle surgery, 154–155, 158
MRI of stifle. *See* magnetic resonance imaging of stifle
MRIT (modified retinacular imbrication technique), 165–166, **165**, *166*
muscles, magnetic resonance imaging of, 137–138, **138**, *139–141*

neurovascular injury, as complication in total knee replacement, 267
nitric oxide, 71, *72*
  arthritis, role of in, 75
  in articular tissues, 72
  influence on CrCL structure, 74–75
  in joint physiology, 72–73, *73*
nitric oxide synthase, 71, 75
NO. *See* nitric oxide
nonsteroidal anti-inflammatory drugs
  for postoperative pain, 155
  for stifle arthritis, 242
normal stifle, biomechanics of, 37–39

NOS (nitric oxide synthase), 71, 75
notch shape index, 66, *66*, 67
notch width, 66, *66*
notch width index, 66, *66*, 67
NRS (numeric rating scales), in assessing limb function after stifle stabilization surgery, 234
NSAIDs. *See* nonsteroidal anti-inflammatory drugs
NSI (notch shape index), 66, *66*, 67
numeric rating scales, in assessing limb function after stifle stabilization surgery, 234
nutritional supplements, use in stifle arthritis, 244–245
NW (notch width), 66, *66*
NWI (notch width index), 66, *66*, 67

obesity, and stifle arthritis, 241–242
Omega-3 fatty acids, use in stifle arthritis, 244–245
osteoarthritis. *See* arthritis, stifle
outcome measures, 233, 237, *237*, 257, 260, **260**
  accelerometers, 234–235
  computational gait analysis, 235–236, *236*
  design of, 258–259
  internal consistency of, **260**
  pedometers, 234–235
  questionnaires, 233–234, 257–260, **260**
  refinement of, **260**
  veterinary exam, 234
owner questionnaires, 233–234, 257–260, **260**

partial CrCL rupture, 105–106, *106*, **106**
  healing potential, **23**, 23–24
  ligament debridement, 214–215, *215*
partial meniscectomy, 218, **219**
patella/quadriceps mechanism, and Q angle, 68–69
patellar luxation, and tibial tuberosity advancement, *183*, 183–184
patellar tendon
  angle, 177, 178, *178*, 179, *179*, 197, 198
  enlargement, after tibial plateau leveling osteotomy, 172, *172*
  graft, 190–191, *191*
  insertion point, in tibial tuberosity advancement, 179, 181, *182*
  ultrasonography, 117, 120–121, *121*
patellofemoral joint, role in stifle biomechanics, 37–38
pathomechanics theory of stifle arthritis, *40*
patient size, and tibial tuberosity advancement, 184, *184*
pattern recognition receptors, 89
pedometers, use in assessing limb function after stifle stabilization surgery, 234–235
pelvic limb, *7*
periarticular fibrosis, as clinical sign of CrCL rupture, 102, *102*
peroxynitrite, 72–73, 75
pivot shift, 172

platelet concentrate, use in tissue engineering, 274, *274*

polysulfated glycosaminoglycan, use in stifle arthritis, 243

popliteal sesamoid, in interpretation of tibial compression radiographs, 114–115

population stratification, in genetic analyses, 54

postoperative pain
   after arthrotomy/arthroscopy, 154–155
   nonsteroidal anti-inflammatory drugs for, 155

postoperative procedures, in extracapsular stabilization, 167

pressure platform gait analysis, 235–236

proliferation phase of ligament healing, 21, *22*, 24–25

prosthetics, use in intra-articular stabilization, 192

proteoglycan in menisci, 30

PRR (pattern recognition receptors), 89

PSGAG (polysulfated glycosaminoglycan), use in stifle arthritis, 243

PTA. *See* patellar tendon angle

Q angle, and patella/quadriceps mechanism, 68–69

questionnaires, owner, 233–234, 257–260, **260**

radial transection. *See* meniscal release

radiography, stifle, 102, 113–115, *114, 115, 116*

reconstructed CrCL graft, healing potential of, 24–25, *25*

reconstructed graft interface tissue, healing potential of, 25–26, *26*

regenerative medicine, and CrCL repair, 271–275, **272,** *273, 274, 275*

rehabilitation
   for CrCL rupture, 249–252, *250, 251*
   after extracapsular stabilization, 250, *250*
   after tibial plateau leveling osteotomy, 250, *251*
   after total knee replacement, 265

relaxation, as characteristic of viscoelastic material, 16

reliability, in client-specific outcome measures, 259

remodeling phase of ligament healing, 21–22, *22*, 25

reproductive status
   effect on ligament biomechanical properties, 17
   as risk factor for CrCL rupture, 95, **96**

residual lameness, after stifle stabilization surgery, 233–237, *236, 237*

responsiveness, in client-specific outcome measures, 259

return to function, 155, 158

risk factors for CrCL rupture, 95–97, **96, 97**

rupture, CaCL, 103–104, 109–111, *110*
   presentation, 109–110
   treatment, 110–111

rupture, CrCL
   age of onset, 54
   and bilateral disease, 96, **97**
   causes, 54

   clinical signs, 102–104, *102, 103*
   ECM metabolism, 61, *61*, 62, *62*
   epidemiology, 95–97, **96, 97**
   genetics, 53–57, **56**
   healing potential of, 22–24, **23**
   histology, 17, 45–51
   history provided for, 101
   partial, **23**, 23–24, 105–106, *106*, **106**, 214–215, *215*
   pathology, 45–46
   rehabilitation, 249–252, *250, 251*
   risk factors for, 95–97, **96, 97**
   screening for, 53–54
   and tibial plateau angle, 68, 97

rupture, of ligaments, sites of, 17

screening for CrCL rupture, 53–54

segmental meniscectomy, 218, **219**

segregation analysis, 54

"sit test," 102

size of patient, and tibial tuberosity advancement, 184, *184*

Slocum TPLO plate, *171*, 171

stifle, *6*, 37, *38*
   abnormal, 119–121, *119, 120, 121*
   anatomy, as risk factor for CrCL rupture, **96**, 96–97
   biomechanics, 37–41, 177–179, *179, 180, 181*, 195–199, *196, 198*
   computed tomography of, 123–126, *124, 125, 126, 127, 128, 129, 130, 131, 132*, 133
   CrCL-deficient, *39*, 39–41, 195–199, *196, 198*
   inflammatory cell populations within, 87–88, *88, 89*
   innervation, 9–10, *11*
   instability, 83, *84*, 106, 237
   ligamentous injuries to, 110
   magnetic resonance imaging of, 135–142, *136, 137,* **138,** *139–141*
   matrix metalloproteinases, role of, *73*, 74
   mechanical integrity, role of CrCL, 60
   morphology, 65–69
   normal, 37–39
   radiography of, 102, 113–115, *114, 115, 116*
   stability, 33, 38–39, 195–196, 237
   ultrasonography, 117–121, *118, 119, 120, 121*
   vascular supply, 7, *9*
   "zone of homeostasis," 41

stress-strain curves, use in CrCL testing, *16*, 16–17

surgically repaired CrCL, healing potential of, **23**, 24

synovial immune responses, in stifle synovitis, 87–90, *88, 89, 90*

synovitis, 81–83, *82, 84*, 85
   and ligament biomechanics, 17–18
   in stable stifle, 83, *84*
   synovial immune responses, 87–90, *88, 89, 90*

synovium, 6–7, 74, 77, 81–82, 189–190
   arthroscopic evaluation, 82–83

and arthroscopic-assisted arthrotomy, 153, *154*
in CrCL rupture, 77, 78–79
magnetic resonance imaging of, *136*, 136–137
synthetic stabilization methods in extracapsular
stabilization, 165–167, **165,** *166*

T cell inhibitors, use in arthritis, 278–279
tendons, magnetic resonance imaging of, 137–138, **138,**
140
tibia
fractures of, after tibial plateau leveling osteotomy,
172
morphology, 68
tibial compression radiography, 113–115, *114, 115, 116,*
126, 133
tibial compression test, 113, *114*, 196
tibial osteotomies, biomechanics of CrCL-deficient
stifle treated by, 195–199, *196, 198*
tibial plateau angle, 169–170, *170*, 172, 173, 198
and cranial tibial closing wedge osteotomy, 196–197
and CrCL rupture, 68, 97
excessive, 172, 181, *182*, 183
tibial plateau leveling osteotomy, 169–174, *170*, 271,
272
and arthritis, progression of, 230–231
arthroscopic follow-up after, 202–208, *202, 203, 204,*
205, 206, 207, 208, 209, 210
and biomechanics of CrCL-deficient stifle, 197–198
bone screws, locking/conventional, 171–172
and CaCL damage, 111
complications after, 172–173, *172, 173*
conversion to total knee replacement, 264–265, *265*
implant selection, *171,* 171–172
and meniscal release, 170, 207–208, *209,* 210, 220
outcome after, 173–174
patient selection, 170–171
rehabilitation programs after, 250, *251*
tibial tuberosity, 69
fracture of, as complication of tibial plateau leveling
osteotomy, 172
in human knee joint, 177, *178*
tibial tuberosity advancement, 177–179, *178, 179, 180,*
181, *181, 182, 183,* 183–186, *184, 185,* 271–272
and biomechanics of CrCL-deficient stifle, 197–198
case selection, 179–185
complications, 184–186
implants used in, 184
and limb deformities, angular/torsional, 183
and meniscal release, 186
outcome, 184–186
and patellar luxation, *183,* 183–184
and patellar tendon insertion point, 179, 181,
182
and patient size, 184, *184*

and stifle biomechanics, 177–179, *179, 180, 181*
technical details, *185,* 186
and tibial plateau angle, excessive, 181, *182,* 183
tie fibers, in menisci, 30
TightRope CrCL procedure, **165,** *166,* 167, 272
TIMPs (tissue inhibitors of metalloproteinases), 73
tissue engineering, 273–275, *273, 274, 275*
tissue inhibitors of metalloproteinases, 73
TKR. *See* total knee replacement
total knee replacement, 263, 268
BioMedtrix Canine Total Knee Replacement implant,
263, 264, *264,* 268
case selection, 264–265, *265*
clinical results, 266
complications, 266–268, *267, 268*
conversion from extracapsular stabilization, 264
conversion from tibial plateau leveling osteotomy,
264–265, *265*
postoperative management, 265
rehabilitation after, 265
surgical technique, 265, *266*
total meniscectomy, 218, **219**
TPA. *See* tibial plateau angle
TPLO. *See* tibial plateau leveling osteotomy
TR (TightRope) CrCL procedure, **165,** *166,* 167, 272
tramadol, use in stifle arthritis, 242–243
TTA. *See* tibial tuberosity advancement

ultrasonography of stifle, 117–121, *118, 119, 120, 121*
unilateral lameness, 102
use/disuse, effect on ligament biomechanical
properties, 17

validity, in client-specific outcome measures, 258–259
VAS (visual analog scales), in assessing limb function
after stifle stabilization surgery, 234
vascular supply
cruciate ligaments, 7–9, *9, 10*
menisci, 30–31, *32*
stifle, 7, *9*
veterinary exam, in assessing limb function after stifle
stabilization surgery, 234
viscoelasticity, 16–17
visual analog scales, in assessing limb function after
stifle stabilization surgery, 234

wear, as complication in total knee replacement,
267–268, *268*
weight. *See also* body condition
effect on ligament biomechanical properties, 17
management of, in stifle arthritis, 241–242
as risk factor for CrCL rupture, 96, **96**

"zone of homeostasis," 41

Keep up with critical fields

Would you like to receive up-to-date information on our books, journals and databases in the areas that interest you, direct to your mailbox?

Join the **Wiley e-mail service** - a convenient way to receive updates and exclusive discount offers on products from us.

Simply visit www.wiley.com/email and register online

We won't bombard you with emails and we'll only email you with information that's relevant to you. We will ALWAYS respect your e-mail privacy and NEVER sell, rent, or exchange your e-mail address to any outside company. Full details on our privacy policy can be found online.

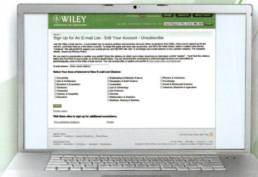

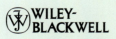

www.wiley.com/email

VETERINARY SURGICAL SPECIALISTS
E. 21 MISSION AVE.
SPOKANE, WA. 99202
(509) 324-0055   Fax (509) 328-7213